Mathematical Models for Communicable Diseases

CBMS-NSF REGIONAL CONFERENCE SERIES IN APPLIED MATHEMATICS

A series of lectures on topics of current research interest in applied mathematics under the direction of the Conference Board of the Mathematical Sciences, supported by the National Science Foundation and published by SIAM.

GARRETT BIRKHOFF, *The Numerical Solution of Elliptic Equations*
D. V. LINDLEY, *Bayesian Statistics, A Review*
R. S. VARGA, *Functional Analysis and Approximation Theory in Numerical Analysis*
R. R. BAHADUR, *Some Limit Theorems in Statistics*
PATRICK BILLINGSLEY, *Weak Convergence of Measures: Applications in Probability*
J. L. LIONS, *Some Aspects of the Optimal Control of Distributed Parameter Systems*
ROGER PENROSE, *Techniques of Differential Topology in Relativity*
HERMAN CHERNOFF, *Sequential Analysis and Optimal Design*
J. DURBIN, *Distribution Theory for Tests Based on the Sample Distribution Function*
SOL I. RUBINOW, *Mathematical Problems in the Biological Sciences*
P. D. LAX, *Hyperbolic Systems of Conservation Laws and the Mathematical Theory of Shock Waves*
I. J. SCHOENBERG, *Cardinal Spline Interpolation*
IVAN SINGER, *The Theory of Best Approximation and Functional Analysis*
WERNER C. RHEINBOLDT, *Methods of Solving Systems of Nonlinear Equations*
HANS F. WEINBERGER, *Variational Methods for Eigenvalue Approximation*
R. TYRRELL ROCKAFELLAR, *Conjugate Duality and Optimization*
SIR JAMES LIGHTHILL, *Mathematical Biofluiddynamics*
GERARD SALTON, *Theory of Indexing*
CATHLEEN S. MORAWETZ, *Notes on Time Decay and Scattering for Some Hyperbolic Problems*
F. HOPPENSTEADT, *Mathematical Theories of Populations: Demographics, Genetics and Epidemics*
RICHARD ASKEY, *Orthogonal Polynomials and Special Functions*
L. E. PAYNE, *Improperly Posed Problems in Partial Differential Equations*
S. ROSEN, *Lectures on the Measurement and Evaluation of the Performance of Computing Systems*
HERBERT B. KELLER, *Numerical Solution of Two Point Boundary Value Problems*
J. P. LASALLE, *The Stability of Dynamical Systems*
D. GOTTLIEB AND S. A. ORSZAG, *Numerical Analysis of Spectral Methods: Theory and Applications*
PETER J. HUBER, *Robust Statistical Procedures*
HERBERT SOLOMON, *Geometric Probability*
FRED S. ROBERTS, *Graph Theory and Its Applications to Problems of Society*
JURIS HARTMANIS, *Feasible Computations and Provable Complexity Properties*
ZOHAR MANNA, *Lectures on the Logic of Computer Programming*
ELLIS L. JOHNSON, *Integer Programming: Facets, Subadditivity, and Duality for Group and Semi-Group Problems*
SHMUEL WINOGRAD, *Arithmetic Complexity of Computations*
J. F. C. KINGMAN, *Mathematics of Genetic Diversity*
MORTON E. GURTIN, *Topics in Finite Elasticity*
THOMAS G. KURTZ, *Approximation of Population Processes*
JERROLD E. MARSDEN, *Lectures on Geometric Methods in Mathematical Physics*
BRADLEY EFRON, *The Jackknife, the Bootstrap, and Other Resampling Plans*
M. WOODROOFE, *Nonlinear Renewal Theory in Sequential Analysis*
D. H. SATTINGER, *Branching in the Presence of Symmetry*
R. TEMAM, *Navier–Stokes Equations and Nonlinear Functional Analysis*

Miklós Csörgo, *Quantile Processes with Statistical Applications*
J. D. Buckmaster and G. S. S. Ludford, *Lectures on Mathematical Combustion*
R. E. Tarjan, *Data Structures and Network Algorithms*
Paul Waltman, *Competition Models in Population Biology*
S. R. S. Varadhan, *Large Deviations and Applications*
Kiyosi Itô, *Foundations of Stochastic Differential Equations in Infinite Dimensional Spaces*
Alan C. Newell, *Solitons in Mathematics and Physics*
Pranab Kumar Sen, *Theory and Applications of Sequential Nonparametrics*
László Lovász, *An Algorithmic Theory of Numbers, Graphs and Convexity*
E. W. Cheney, *Multivariate Approximation Theory: Selected Topics*
Joel Spencer, *Ten Lectures on the Probabilistic Method*
Paul C. Fife, *Dynamics of Internal Layers and Diffusive Interfaces*
Charles K. Chui, *Multivariate Splines*
Herbert S. Wilf, *Combinatorial Algorithms: An Update*
Henry C. Tuckwell, *Stochastic Processes in the Neurosciences*
Frank H. Clarke, *Methods of Dynamic and Nonsmooth Optimization*
Robert B. Gardner, *The Method of Equivalence and Its Applications*
Grace Wahba, *Spline Models for Observational Data*
Richard S. Varga, *Scientific Computation on Mathematical Problems and Conjectures*
Ingrid Daubechies, *Ten Lectures on Wavelets*
Stephen F. McCormick, *Multilevel Projection Methods for Partial Differential Equations*
Harald Niederreiter, *Random Number Generation and Quasi-Monte Carlo Methods*
Joel Spencer, *Ten Lectures on the Probabilistic Method, Second Edition*
Charles A. Micchelli, *Mathematical Aspects of Geometric Modeling*
Roger Temam, *Navier–Stokes Equations and Nonlinear Functional Analysis, Second Edition*
Glenn Shafer, *Probabilistic Expert Systems*
Peter J. Huber, *Robust Statistical Procedures, Second Edition*
J. Michael Steele, *Probability Theory and Combinatorial Optimization*
Werner C. Rheinboldt, *Methods for Solving Systems of Nonlinear Equations, Second Edition*
J. M. Cushing, *An Introduction to Structured Population Dynamics*
Tai-Ping Liu, *Hyperbolic and Viscous Conservation Laws*
Michael Renardy, *Mathematical Analysis of Viscoelastic Flows*
Gérard Cornuéjols, *Combinatorial Optimization: Packing and Covering*
Irena Lasiecka, *Mathematical Control Theory of Coupled PDEs*
J. K. Shaw, *Mathematical Principles of Optical Fiber Communications*
Zhangxin Chen, *Reservoir Simulation: Mathematical Techniques in Oil Recovery*
Athanassios S. Fokas, *A Unified Approach to Boundary Value Problems*
Margaret Cheney and Brett Borden, *Fundamentals of Radar Imaging*
Fioralba Cakoni, David Colton, and Peter Monk, *The Linear Sampling Method in Inverse Electromagnetic Scattering*
Adrian Constantin, *Nonlinear Water Waves with Applications to Wave-Current Interactions and Tsunamis*
Wei-Ming Ni, *The Mathematics of Diffusion*
Arnulf Jentzen and Peter E. Kloeden, *Taylor Approximations for Stochastic Partial Differential Equations*
Fred Brauer and Carlos Castillo-Chavez, *Mathematical Models for Communicable Diseases*

FRED BRAUER
University of British Columbia
Vancouver, British Columbia
Canada

CARLOS CASTILLO-CHAVEZ
Arizona State University
Tempe, Arizona

Mathematical Models for Communicable Diseases

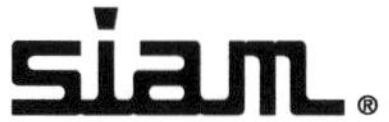
SOCIETY FOR INDUSTRIAL AND APPLIED MATHEMATICS
PHILADELPHIA

10 9 8 7 6 5 4 3 2 1

Library of Congress Cataloging-in-Publication Data

Brauer, Fred.
Mathematical models for communicable diseases / Fred Brauer, Carlos Castillo-Chavez.
p. ; cm. -- (CBMS-NSF regional conference series in applied mathematics ; 84)
Includes bibliographical references and index.
ISBN 978-1-611972-41-2
I. Castillo-Chavez, Carlos. II. Society for Industrial and Applied Mathematics. III. Title. IV. Series: CBMS-NSF regional conference series in applied mathematics ; 84.
[DNLM: 1. Communicable Diseases--epidemiology. 2. Models, Theoretical. 3. Communicable Disease Control. WC 16]

616.901'5118--dc23

2012030574

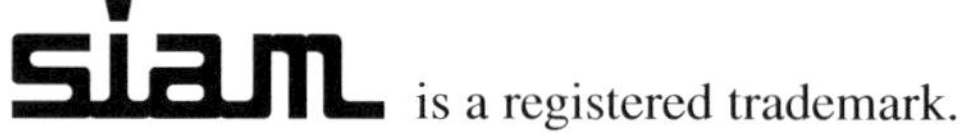

CCC would like to dedicate
his contribution to this effort
to his dad,
Carlos Castillo-Cruz,
who was unfortunately unable to see the final version.

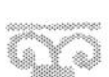

Contents

Preface

These lecture notes collect the material used for the talks delivered by Fred Brauer and Carlos Castillo-Chavez in the CBMS workshop *Mathematical Epidemiology with Applications* funded by the National Science Foundation and held at East Tennessee State University (ETSU) from July 25–29, 2011. The goal of the lectures was to reach *all participants*, a population that includes researchers with backgrounds in the biological, epidemiological, mathematical, and medical sciences as well as individuals involved in the development, implementation, and evaluation of public health policy. It was assumed that participants were cognizant of the value and utility of mathematical models in the study and control of infectious diseases because of their use to increase our understanding of disease dynamics, their value in the evaluation of possible prevention/intervention/control policies, their key role in the exploration of "what if" scenarios systematically, and their use in assessing and/or reducing the levels of uncertainty naturally associated with the unpredictability of disease outbreaks, disease severity, and disease evolution.

These notes describe a variety of topics, but are not meant to present a complete portrait of mathematical epidemiology. The interested reader may wish to consult other sources, such as the books [2, 5, 9], compilations of lectures [1, 4, 10], chapters in books on mathematical biology [3, 12], and the survey paper [8]. The notes were written using *primarily* the published research of both authors, classical articles, and research or expository articles that we have found useful.

Diseases have been important in shaping the course of history. The book [11] describes some of the influences of the impact of communicable diseases on history since ancient times. Disease dynamics biblical references include the description in the book of Exodus of the plagues that Moses brought down upon Egypt and the decision of Sennacherib, the king of Assyria, to abandon his attempt to capture Jerusalem about 700 BC because of the illness of his soldiers (Isaiah 37, 36–38).

The fall of empires has been attributed directly or indirectly to epidemic diseases. In the 2nd century AD the so-called Antonine plagues (possibly measles and smallpox) invaded the Roman Empire, causing drastic population reductions and economic hardships leading to disintegration of the empire which facilitated invasions. The Han empire in China collapsed in the 3rd century AD after a similar sequence of events. The defeat of a population of millions of Aztecs by Cortez and his 600 followers was facilitated by an outbreak of smallpox that devastated the Aztecs but had almost no impact on the invading Spaniards. Smallpox spread southward to the Incas in Peru and was an important factor in the success of Pizarro's invasion a few years later. Smallpox was followed by other diseases such as measles and diphtheria imported from Europe to North America. In some regions, the indigenous populations were reduced to one tenth of their previous levels by disease invasions. Between 1519 and 1530 the Indian population of Mexico was reduced from 30 million to 3 million.

The Black Death (probably bubonic plague) spread from Asia throughout Europe in several waves during the 14th century, beginning in 1346, and is estimated to have caused the death of as much as one-third of the population of Europe between 1346 and 1350. The disease recurred periodically in various regions of Europe for more than 300 years, notably as the Great Plague of London of 1665–1666. It gradually withdrew from Europe. As the plague struck some regions harshly while avoiding others, it had a profound effect on political and economic developments in medieval times. In the last bubonic plague epidemic in France (1720–1722), half the population of Marseilles, 60 percent of the population in nearby Toulon, 44 percent of the population of Arles, and 30 percent of the population of Aix and Avignon died, but the epidemic did not spread beyond Provence.

Many of the early developments in the mathematical modeling of communicable diseases are due to public health physicians. The first known result in mathematical epidemiology is a defense of the practice of inoculation against smallpox in 1760 by Daniel Bernoulli, a member of a famous family of mathematicians (eight spread over three generations) who had been trained as a physician. The first contributions to modern mathematical epidemiology are due to P.D. En'ko between 1873 and 1894 [6], and the foundations of the entire approach to epidemiology based on compartmental models were laid by public health physicians such as Sir R.A. Ross, W.H. Hamer, A.G. McKendrick, and W.O. Kermack between 1900 and 1935, along with important contributions from a statistical perspective by J. Brownlee.

The development of mathematical methods for the study of models for communicable diseases led to a divergence between the goals of mathematicians, who sought broad understanding, and public health professionals, who sought practical procedures for management of diseases. While mathematical modeling led to many fundamental ideas, such as the possibility of controlling smallpox by vaccination and the management of malaria by controlling the vector (mosquito) population, the practical implementation was always more difficult than the predictions of simple models. Fortunately, in recent years there have been determined efforts to encourage better communication between mathematicians, so that public health professionals can better understand the situations in which simple models may be useful and mathematicians can recognize that real-life public health questions are much more complicated than the worlds generated with simple models.

The philosophy behind the set of lectures by Fred Brauer may be partially characterized as one that focuses on the mathematical analyses of classical epidemic models from a perspective shaped not only by mathematical contributions to the field of epidemiology but also by the context of specific diseases such as influenza or SARS. Castillo-Chavez's lectures are driven by his desire to address *naturally* emerging epidemiological questions, that is, those that typically arise in the study of the dynamics of specific diseases. His lectures, complementary to those given by Fred Brauer, provide a personal overview on the way that Castillo-Chavez, as a member of a practitioner class of epidemiologists, broadly understood to include computational and theoretical biologists, public health experts, and evolutionary biologists, approaches the solution of the scientific challenges that emerge from the study of disease dynamics over multiple temporal and spatial scales, dynamics most often driven or shaped by evolving levels of heterogeneity, the kind *normally* found in co-evolving biological populations. Thus, in particular, there are two chapters on influenza, the first concerned with the basic structure of a single outbreak and the second viewing influenza in a broader context and including such questions as cross-immunity between different strains.

Communicable diseases such as measles, influenza, or tuberculosis are important in modern life. In this monograph, we will be concerned both with sudden disease outbreaks and endemic situations, in which a disease is always present. The AIDS epidemic, the recent SARS epidemic, recurring influenza, and the re-emergence of tuberculosis are events of concern and interest to many people. Every year millions of people die of measles, respiratory infections, diarrhea, and other diseases that are easily treated and not considered dangerous in the Western world. Diseases such as malaria, typhus, cholera, schistosomiasis, and sleeping sickness are endemic in many parts of the world. Further, the impact of sexually transmitted disease on the reproductive health of women, the devastating impact of sexually transmitted HIV on the young and very young all over the world, and the synergistic interactions between HIV and communicable diseases like tuberculosis or vector-transmitted diseases like malaria show that the effects of high disease mortality on mean life span and of disease debilitation and mortality on the economy in afflicted countries are considerable.

In the face of a disease outbreak it is not possible to do experiments comparing the effects of different management strategy, and predictions based on mathematical models may be essential when it comes down to addressing the impact of communicable diseases. Models must be based on some understanding of the etiology and epidemiology of the disease in question and in some instances on the social and behavioral dynamics of the populations affected. Generally, diseases transmitted by viral agents, such as influenza, measles, rubella (German measles), and chicken pox, confer immunity against reinfection. We will describe SIR (susceptible–infectious–recovered) models for such diseases. Diseases transmitted by bacteria, such as tuberculosis, meningitis, and gonorrhea, confer no immunity against reinfection, and we will describe SIS (susceptible–infectious–susceptible) models for such diseases.

Other diseases, such as malaria, are transmitted not directly from human to human but by vectors, agents (usually insects) who are infected by humans and who then transmit the disease to humans. Heterosexual transmission of HIV/AIDS is also a vector process in which transmission goes back and forth between males and females. Diseases with vector transmission require models for both host and vector populations and the interactions between them.

The distinction between epidemic and endemic situations will be highlighted in this book. An epidemic acts on a short time scale, a sudden outbreak of a disease that infects a substantial portion of the population in a region before it disappears, usually leaving many members untouched. In an endemic situation, a disease becomes established in a population and remains for a long time. In models for epidemics one usually ignores demographic effects (births and deaths not due to disease). The justification for ignoring demographic effects is that the demographic time scale is normally much longer than the disease time scale and may therefore be neglected. Endemic situations, on the other hand, may endure for years, and it is therefore necessary to include demographic effects in models that describe their dynamics.

There are many questions of interest to public health physicians confronted with a possible epidemic. For example, how severe will an epidemic be? This question may be interpreted in a variety of ways. For example, how many individuals will be affected and require treatment? What is the maximum number of people needing care at any particular time? How long will the epidemic last? How much good would quarantine of victims do in reducing the severity of the epidemic? Can treatment of infected individuals prevent the epidemic from spreading?

Scientific experiments are usually designed to obtain information and to test hypotheses. Experiments in epidemiology with controls are often difficult or impossible to design due to ethical questions. Sometimes data may be obtained after the fact from reports of epidemics or of endemic disease levels, but the data may be incomplete or inaccurate. In addition, data may contain enough irregularities to raise serious questions of interpretation, such as whether there is evidence of chaotic behavior [7]. Hence, parameter estimation and model fitting, a critical component of model validation, are difficult.

In the mathematical modeling of disease transmission, as in most other areas of mathematical modeling, there is always a trade-off between simple models, which omit most details and are designed only to highlight general qualitative behavior, and detailed models, usually designed for specific situations including short-term quantitative predictions. Detailed models are generally difficult or impossible to solve analytically, and hence their usefulness for theoretical purposes is limited although their strategic value may be high.

Simple models for epidemics predict that an epidemic will die out after some time, leaving a part of the population untouched by disease. This prediction holds true of models that include control measures. This qualitative principle is not by itself helpful in suggesting what control measures would be most effective in a given situation, but it implies that a detailed model describing the situation as accurately as possible might be indeed quite useful for public health professionals. Such a model might have many equations and in practice may be only solved approximately by numerical simulations. This has become feasible in recent years because of the developments in high-speed computing.

In these notes we concentrate mainly on simple models in order to establish broad principles. These simple models have value as they are the building blocks of models that include more detailed structure. One use is to compare the dynamics of simple and slightly more detailed models to see whether slightly different assumptions can lead to significant differences in qualitative behavior. In the first four lectures we describe general classes of models that should be viewed as templates to use in modeling specific diseases with the incorporation of properties of the disease.

However, it is important to recognize that mathematical models to be used for making policy recommendations tied in to management decisions must be quite different. Models needed for the exploration, development, and implementation of public health policy require the incorporation of a great deal of detail as they must often address scenarios accurately. For example, if the problem is to recommend what age group or groups should be the focus of attention in coping with a disease outbreak, it is essential to use a model that separates the population into a sufficient number of age groups and recognizes the interactions between different age groups. The increased availability of high-speed computing in the last few years has made use of such models possible. The intensive use of agent-based models has also brought to the forefront the use of computationally explicit models in the development of timely and reliable public policy.

Acknowledgments

The preparation of this notes expands and complements the lectures given for the CBMS workshop *Mathematical Epidemiology with Applications* funded by the National Science Foundation and held at East Tennessee State University (ETSU) from July 25–29, 2011

(NSF-CBMS Regional Research Conference in the Mathematical Sciences: Mathematical Epidemiology with Applications, National Science Foundation grant DMS-1040928; Ariel Cintron-Arias (PI); Anant Godbole (co-PI), Principal Lecturers: Carlos Castillo-Chavez and Fred Brauer). There are many individuals that we must thank. The 50+ participants that listened to us for a whole week certainly need to be thanked. Professors Ariel Cintron-Arias and Anant Godbole, who wrote the grant proposal that funded this workshop and carried out the administrative, organizational, intellectual, and social activities that are essential for a successful workshop, deserve a special note of appreciation. Kamal Barley did all schematic and graphic illustrations and helped with the graphic formatting, while Raquel Lopez and Emmanuel Morales provided invaluable assistance with LaTeX coding. The material presented in this monograph came from our own past research efforts, *some* classical articles, and published manuscripts that we have found useful, inspiring, or noteworthy. We have also made use of existing collections of articles that included one or both of us as editors. The American Mathematical Society (AMS), the American Institute of Mathematical Sciences (AIMS), the Mathematical Biosciences and Engineering (MBE), the Royal Netherlands Academy of Arts and Sciences (AIMS), Springer-Verlag of Heidelberg/Berlin are the journals or publishers that kindly gave us permission to use several of the figures and tables that appear in the text (or modifications). They came from earlier published articles as noted in the text. We thank them. The bulk of Castillo-Chavez's chapters were written while he spent two months in treatment for a (noncommunicable) disease and in residence at the Center for Communicable Disease Dynamics (CCDD) within the Harvard School of Public Health, a center supported by grant U54GM088558 from NIGMS to Marc Lipsitch. CCDD provided a wonderful intellectual environment that included the extraordinary support of Felisa Nobles and Mel Larsen. FB's research is supported in part by NSERC (National Sciences and Engineering Research Council of Canada). CCC's research is also partially supported by grant 1R01GM100471-01 from the National Institute of General Medical Sciences (NIGMS) at the National Institutes of Health. Finally, these were not the best of times but also not the worst of times for CCC. He thanks the support of David Harrington, Xiao-Li Meng, Marcello Pagano, and Marc Lipsitch at Harvard; The AstraZeneca Hope Lodge staff and residents; and Joanne Arruda, Kristen Bertone, Alicia Brodeur, Tom Eggleston, Aymen Elfiky, Sandra M. Kelly, and the incomparable Anthony D'Amico at the DFCI in Boston. Finally, the time provided to CCC for the completion of this work was substantially increased through the support of Deans Robert Page and Sander Van Der Leeuw, Provost Elizabeth Capaldi, and President Michael Crow. Finally, the time provided to CCC for the completion of this work was substantially increased through the support of Deans Robert Page and Sander Van Der Leeuw, Provost Elizabeth Capaldi, and President Michael Crow, and late revisions were supported by the Massachusetts Institute of Technology through the Dr. Martin Luther King, Jr., Visiting Professor Program.

Fred Brauer, Vancouver, BC, CA
Carlos Castillo-Chavez, Tempe, AZ, USA
June 25, 2012

Bibliography

[1] Anderson, R.M., ed. (1982) *Population Dynamics of Infectious Diseases: Theory and Applications,* Chapman and Hall, London, New York.

[2] Anderson, R.M. and R.M. May (1991) *Infectious Diseases of Humans,* Oxford Science Publications, Oxford.

[3] Brauer, F. and C. Castillo-Chavez (2012) *Mathematical Models in Population Biology and Epidemiology*, Springer-Verlag.

[4] Brauer, F., P. van den Driessche, and J. Wu, eds. (2008) *Mathematical Epidemiology*, Lecture Notes in Math. **1945**, Springer-Verlag, Berlin, Heidelberg, New York.

[5] Diekmann, O. and J.A.P. Heesterbeek (2000) *Mathematical Epidemiology of Infectious Diseases: Model Building, Analysis and Interpretation*, John Wiley.

[6] Dietz, K. (1988) *The first epidemic model: A historical note on P. D. En'ko*, Australian J. Stat. **30**: 56–65.

[7] Ellner, S., R. Gallant, and J. Theiler (1995) *Detecting nonlinearity and chaos in epidemic data*, in Epidemic Models: Their Structure and Relation to Data, D. Mollison, ed., Cambridge University Press, Cambridge: 229–247.

[8] Hethcote, H.W. (2000) *The mathematics of infectious diseases*, SIAM Rev. **42**: 599–653.

[9] Keeling, M.J. and P. Rohani (2008) *Modelling Infectious Diseases in Humans and Animals*, Princeton University Press, Princeton, NJ.

[10] Ma, Z., Y. Zhou, and J. Wu (2009) *Modelling and Dynamics of Infectious Diseases*, Higher Education Press, Beijing.

[11] McNeill, W.H. (1976) *Plagues and Peoples,* Doubleday, New York.

[12] Thieme, H.R. (2003) *Mathematics in Population Biology*, Princeton University Press, Princeton, NJ.

Lecture 1

Compartmental Epidemic Models

1.1 Introduction to Compartmental Models

We begin with a study of epidemic models, leaving the additional aspect of inclusion of demographic effects until the next lecture. We formulate our descriptions as *compartmental models*, with the population under study being divided into compartments and with assumptions about the nature and time rate of transfer from one compartment to another. Diseases that confer immunity have a different compartmental structure from diseases without immunity and from diseases transmitted by vectors. The rates of transfer between compartments are expressed mathematically as derivatives with respect to time of the sizes of the compartments, and as a result our models are formulated initially as *differential equations*. Models in which the rates of transfer depend on the sizes of compartments over the past as well as at the instant of transfer lead to more general types of functional equation, such as differential-difference equations or integral equations.

1.2 The Simple Kermack–McKendrick Model

One of the early triumphs of mathematical epidemiology was the formulation of a simple model by Kermack and McKendrick in [15] whose predictions are very similar to the behavior, observed in countless epidemics, of disease that invade a population suddenly, grow in intensity, and then disappear leaving part of the population untouched. The Kermack–McKendrick model is a compartmental model based on relatively simple assumptions on the rates of flow between different classes of members of the population. The SARS epidemic of 2002–2003 revived interest in epidemic models, which had been largely ignored since the time of Kermack and McKendrick in favor of models for endemic diseases. More recently, the threat of spread of avian flu raised in 2005 and the H1N1 influenza A pandemic of 2009 have provided a continuing source of important modeling questions.

In order to model such an epidemic we divide the population being studied into three classes labeled S, I, and R. We let $S(t)$ denote the number of individuals who are susceptible to the disease, that is, who are not (yet) infected at time t. $I(t)$ denotes the number of infected individuals, assumed infectious and able to spread the disease by contact with susceptibles. $R(t)$ denotes the number of individuals who have been infected and then removed from the possibility of being infected again or of spreading infection. Removal is carried out either through isolation from the rest of the population, immunization against infection, recovery from the disease with full immunity against reinfection, or death caused by the disease. These characterizations of removed members are different from an epidemiological perspective but are often equivalent from a modeling point of view which takes into account only the state of an individual with respect to the disease.

We will use the terminology SIR to describe a disease which confers immunity against reinfection, to indicate that the passage of individuals is from the susceptible class S to the infective class I to the removed class R. Epidemics are usually diseases of this type. We would use the terminology SIS to describe a disease with no immunity against reinfection, to indicate that the passage of individuals is from the susceptible class to the infective class and then back to the susceptible class. Usually diseases caused by a virus are of SIR type, while diseases caused by bacteria are of SIS type.

In addition to the basic distinction between diseases for which recovery confers immunity against reinfection and diseases for which recovered members are susceptible to reinfection, and the intermediate possibility of temporary immunity signified by a model of $SIRS$ type, more complicated compartmental structure is possible. For example, there are $SEIR$ and $SEIS$ models, with an exposed period between being infected and becoming infective. We shall describe such models in later sections, with the goal of formulating a general structure that includes all these models. The general model includes dependence of infectivity on the age of infection, that is, the time since becoming infected. What is often called the Kermack–McKendrick epidemic model is actually a special case of this general model introduced by Kermack and McKendrick in their 1927 paper.

We are assuming that the epidemic process is *deterministic*, that is, that the behavior of a population is determined completely by its history and by the rules which describe the model. In formulating models in terms of the derivatives of the sizes of each compartment we are also assuming that the number of members in a compartment is a differentiable function of time. This assumption is plausible once a disease outbreak has become established but is not valid at the beginning of a disease outbreak when there are only a few infectives. When there are only a few infected members the start of a disease outbreak depends on random contacts between small numbers of individuals. In the next section we will use this to describe an approach to the study of the beginning of a disease outbreak by means of branching processes, but we begin with a description of deterministic compartmental models.

The independent variable in our compartmental models is the time t, and the rates of transfer between compartments are expressed mathematically as derivatives with respect to time of the sizes of the compartments. As a result our models are formulated initially as differential equations.

The special case of the model proposed by Kermack and McKendrick in 1927, which is the starting point for our study of epidemic models, is

$$\begin{aligned} S' &= -a\frac{S}{N}I, \\ I' &= a\frac{S}{N}I - \alpha I, \\ R' &= \alpha I. \end{aligned} \tag{1.1}$$

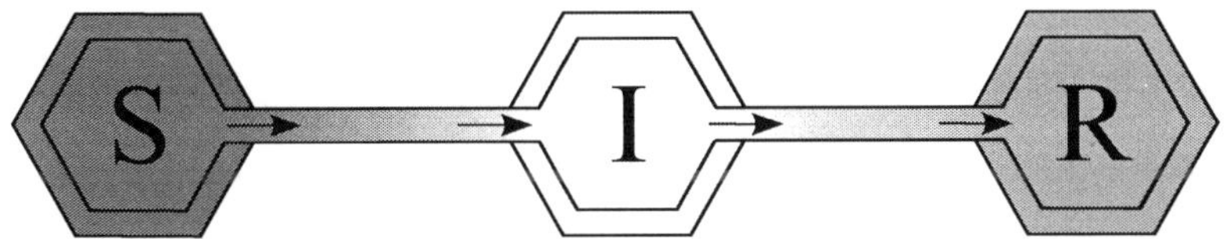

Figure 1.1. *Flow chart for the SIR model.*

A flow chart is shown in Figure 1.1. It is based on the following assumptions:

(i) An average member of the population makes contact sufficient to transmit infection with a others per unit time (mass-action incidence).

(ii) Infectives leave the infective class at rate αI per unit time.

(iii) There is no entry into or departure from the population, except possibly through death from the disease.

(iv) There are no disease deaths, and the total population size is a constant N.

According to (i), since the probability that a random contact by an infective is with a susceptible, who can then transmit infection, is S/N, the number of new infections in unit time per infective is $a\frac{S}{N}I$, giving a rate of new infections $a\frac{S}{N}I$. Alternately, we may argue that for a contact by a susceptible the probability that this contact is with an infective is I/N, and thus the rate of new infections per susceptible is $a(I/N)$, giving a rate of new infections $a(I/N)S = a\frac{S}{N}I$. Note that both approaches give the same rate of new infections; in models with more complicated compartmental structure one may be more appropriate than the other.

We need not give an algebraic expression for N since it cancels out of the final model, but we should note that for an SIR disease model $N = S + I + R$. Later, we will allow the possibility that some infectives recover, while others die of the disease. The hypothesis (iii) really says that the time scale of the disease is much faster than the time scale of births and deaths so that demographic effects on the population may be ignored. An alternative view is that we are only interested in studying the dynamics of a single epidemic outbreak.

The assumption (ii) requires a fuller mathematical explanation, since the assumption of a recovery rate proportional to the number of infectives has no clear epidemiological meaning. We consider the "cohort" of members who were all infected at one time and let $u(s)$ denote the number of these who are still infective s time units after having been infected. If a fraction α of these leave the infective class in unit time, then

$$u' = -\alpha u,$$

and the solution of this elementary differential equation is

$$u(s) = u(0)e^{-\alpha s}.$$

Thus, the fraction of infectives remaining infective s time units after having become infective is $e^{-\alpha s}$, so that the length of the infective period is distributed exponentially with mean $\int_0^\infty e^{-\alpha s}ds = 1/\alpha$, and this is what (ii) really assumes. If we assume, instead of (ii), that the fraction of infectives remaining infective at time τ after having become infective is $P(\tau)$, the second equation of (1.1) would be replaced by the integral equation

$$I(t) = I_0(t) + \int_0^\infty a\frac{S(t-\tau)}{N}I(t-\tau)P(\tau)d\tau,$$

where $I_0(t)$ represents the members of the population who were infective at time $t = 0$ and are still infective at time t.

The assumptions of a constant rate of contacts and of an exponentially distributed recovery rate are unrealistically simple. More general models can be constructed and analyzed, but our goal here is to show what may be deduced from extremely simple models. It will turn out that many more realistic models exhibit very similar qualitative behaviors.

In our model, R is determined once S and I are known, and we can drop the R equation from our model, leaving the system of two equations

$$\begin{aligned} S' &= -\frac{a}{N}SI, \\ I' &= \left(\frac{a}{N} - \alpha\right)I, \end{aligned} \tag{1.2}$$

together with initial conditions

$$S(0) = S_0, \quad I(0) = I_0, \quad S_0 + I_0 = N.$$

We think of introducing a small number of infectives into a population of susceptibles and ask whether there will be an epidemic. We remark that the model makes sense only as long as $S(t)$ and $I(t)$ remain nonnegative. Thus if either $S(t)$ or $I(t)$ reaches zero, we consider the system terminated. We observe that $S' < 0$ for all t and $I' > 0$ if and only if $S > \alpha N/a$. Thus I increases as long as $S > \alpha N/a$, but since S decreases for all t, I ultimately decreases and approaches zero. If $S_0 < \alpha N/a$, then I decreases to zero (no epidemic), while if $S_0 > \alpha N/a$, then I first increases to a maximum attained when $S = \alpha N/a$ and then decreases to zero (epidemic).

The quantity $aS_0/\alpha N$ is a threshold quantity, called the *basic reproduction number* [7, 12] and denoted by $\mathcal{R}_0$, which determines whether there is an epidemic or not. If $\mathcal{R}_0 < 1$, the infection dies out, while if $\mathcal{R}_0 > 1$, there is an epidemic. The basic reproduction number $\mathcal{R}_0$ is defined as the number of secondary infections caused by a single infective introduced into a wholly susceptible population of size $N \approx S_0$ over the course of the infection of this single infective. In this situation, an infective makes a contacts in unit time, all of which are with susceptibles and thus produce new infections, and the mean infective period is $1/\alpha$; thus the basic reproduction number is actually a/α rather than $aS_0/\alpha N$. Another way to view this apparent discrepancy is to consider two ways in which an epidemic may begin. One way would be an epidemic started by a member of the population being studied, for example, by returning from travel with an infection acquired away from home. In this case, we would have $I_0 > 0$, $S_0 + I_0 = N$. A second way would be for an epidemic to be started by a visitor from outside the population. In this case, we would have $S_0 = N$.

Since (1.2) is a two-dimensional autonomous system of differential equations, the natural approach would be to find equilibria and linearize about each equilibrium to determine its stability. However, since every point with $I = 0$ is an equilibrium, the system (1.2) has a line of equilibria and this approach is not applicable (the linearization matrix at each equilibrium has a zero eigenvalue).

Fortunately, there is an alternative approach that enables us to analyze the system (1.2). The sum of the two equations of (1.2) is

$$(S+I)' = -\alpha I.$$

Thus $S+I$ is a nonnegative smooth decreasing function and therefore tends to a limit as $t \to \infty$. Also, it is not difficult to prove that the derivative of a smooth decreasing function that tends to a limit must tend to zero, and this shows that

$$I_\infty = \lim_{t\to\infty} I(t) = 0.$$

Thus $S+I$ has limit S_∞.

Integration of the sum of the two equations of (1.2) from 0 to ∞ gives

$$\alpha \int_0^\infty I(t)dt = S_0 + I_0 - S_\infty = N - S_\infty.$$

Division of the first equation of (1.2) by S and integration from 0 to ∞ gives

$$\begin{aligned} \log\frac{S_0}{S_\infty} &= \frac{a}{N}\int_0^\infty I(t)dt \\ &= \frac{a}{\alpha N}[N - S_\infty] \\ &= \mathcal{R}_0\left[1 - \frac{S_\infty}{N}\right]. \end{aligned} \tag{1.3}$$

Equation (1.3) is called the *final size relation*. It gives a relation between the basic reproduction number and the size of the epidemic. Note that the final size of the epidemic, the number of members of the population who are infected over the course of the epidemic, is $N - S_\infty$. This is often described in terms of the *attack rate* $(1 - S_\infty/N)$. (Technically, the attack rate should be called an attack ratio, since it is dimensionless and is not a rate.)

The final size relation (1.3) can be generalized to epidemic models with more complicated compartmental structure than the simple SIR model (1.2), including models with exposed periods, treatment models, and models including quarantine of suspected individuals and isolation of diagnosed infectives. The original Kermack–McKendrick model [15] included dependence on the time since becoming infected (age of infection), and this includes such models.

Integration of the first equation and the sum of the two equations of (1.2) from 0 to t gives

$$\begin{aligned} \log\frac{S_0}{S(t)} &= \frac{a}{N}\int_0^t I(t)dt \\ &= \frac{a}{\alpha N}[N - S(t) - I(t)], \end{aligned}$$

and this leads to the form

$$I(t) + S(t) - \frac{\alpha N}{a}\log S(t) = N - \frac{\alpha N}{a}\log S_0. \tag{1.4}$$

This implicit relation between S and I describes the orbits of solutions of (1.2) in the (S,I) plane.

In addition, since the right side of (1.3) is finite, the left side is also finite, and this shows that $S_\infty > 0$. The final size relation (1.3) is valid for a large variety of epidemic models, as we shall see in later sections.

It is not difficult to prove that there is a unique solution of the final size relation (1.3). To see this, we define the function

$$g(x) = \log \frac{S_0}{x} - \mathcal{R}_0 \left[1 - \frac{x}{N}\right],$$

as in Figure 1.2.

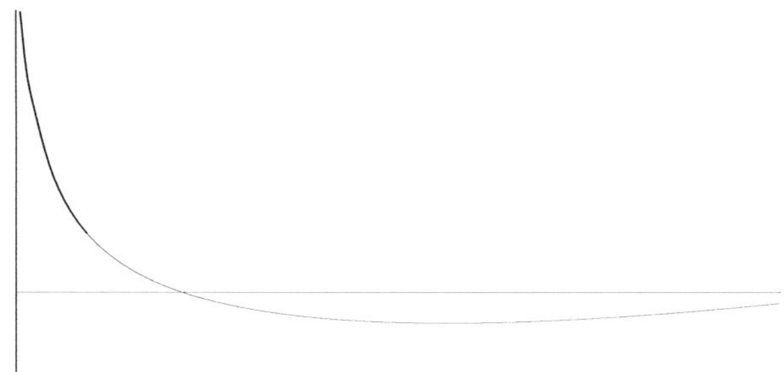

Figure 1.2. *The function g(x).*

Then

$$g(0+) > 0, \quad g(N) < 0,$$

and $g'(x) < 0$ if and only if

$$0 < x < \frac{N}{\mathcal{R}_0}.$$

If $\mathcal{R}_0 \leq 1, g(x)$ is monotone decreasing from a positive value at $x = 0+$ to a negative value at $x = N$. Thus there is a unique zero S_∞ of $g(x)$ with $S_\infty < N$.

If $\mathcal{R}_0 > 1, g(x)$ is monotone decreasing from a positive value at $x = 0+$ to a minimum at $x = N/\mathcal{R}_0$ and then increases to a negative value at $x = N_0$. Thus there is a unique zero S_∞ of $g(x)$ with

$$S_\infty < \frac{N}{\mathcal{R}_0}.$$

In fact,

$$\begin{aligned} g\left(\frac{S_0}{\mathcal{R}_0}\right) &= \log \mathcal{R}_0 - \mathcal{R}_0 + \frac{S_0}{N} \\ &\leq \log \mathcal{R}_0 - \mathcal{R}_0 + 1. \end{aligned}$$

Since $\log \mathcal{R}_0 < \mathcal{R}_0 - 1$ for $\mathcal{R}_0 > 0$, we actually have

$$g\left(\frac{S_0}{\mathcal{R}_0}\right) < 0$$

and

$$S_\infty < \frac{S_0}{\mathcal{R}_0}.$$

It is generally difficult to estimate the contact rate a, which depends on the particular disease being studied but may also depend on social and behavioral factors. The quantities S_0 and S_∞ may be estimated by serological studies (measurements of immune responses in blood samples) before and after an epidemic, and from these data the basic reproduction number $\mathcal{R}_0$ may be estimated by using (1.3). This estimate, however, is a retrospective one which can be derived only after the epidemic has run its course.

The maximum number of infectives at any time is the number of infectives when the derivative of I is zero, that is, when $S = \alpha N/a$. This maximum is given by

$$I_{max} = N - \frac{\alpha N}{a} \log \frac{\alpha N}{a} - \frac{\alpha N}{a}, \tag{1.5}$$

obtained by substituting $S = \alpha N/a$, $I = I_{max}$ into (1.4).

In order to prevent the occurrence of an epidemic if infectives are introduced into a population it is necessary to reduce the basic reproductive number $\mathcal{R}_0$ below one. This may sometimes be achieved by immunization, which has the effect of transferring members of the population from the susceptible class to the removed class and thus reducing $S(0)$. If a fraction p of the population is successfully immunized, the effect is to replace $S(0)$ by $S(0)(1-p)$, and thus to reduce the basic reproductive number to $aS(0)(1-p)/\alpha N$. The requirement $aS(0)(1-p)/\alpha N < 1$ gives $1-p < \alpha N/aS(0)$, or

$$p > 1 - \frac{\alpha N}{aS(0)} = 1 - \frac{1}{\mathcal{R}_0}.$$

Initially, the number of infectives grows exponentially because the equation for I may be approximated by

$$I' = (a-\alpha)I,$$

and the initial growth rate is

$$r = a - \alpha = \alpha(\mathcal{R}_0 - 1).$$

This initial growth rate r may be determined experimentally when an epidemic begins. Then since N and α may be measured a may be calculated as

$$a = \frac{r+\alpha}{N}.$$

However, because of incomplete data and underreporting of cases, this estimate may not be very accurate. This inaccuracy is even more pronounced for an outbreak of a previously unknown disease, where early cases are likely to be misdiagnosed. Because of the final size relation, estimation of a or $\mathcal{R}_0$ is an important question that has been studied by a variety of approaches. Estimation of the initial growth rate from data can provide an estimate of the contact rate a. However, this relation is valid only for the model (1.2) and does not hold for models with different compartmental structure, such as an exposed period.

There are serious shortcomings in the simple Kermack–McKendrick model as a description of the beginning of a disease outbreak, and a very different kind of model is required.

1.3 A Branching Process Disease Outbreak Model

The Kermack–McKendrick compartmental epidemic model assumes that the sizes of the compartments are large enough that the mixing of members is homogeneous, or at least that there is homogeneous mixing in each subgroup if the population is stratified by activity levels. However, at the beginning of a disease outbreak, there is a very small number of infective individuals and the transmission of infection is a stochastic event depending on the pattern of contacts between members of the population; a description should take this pattern into account.

Another approach would be to give a stochastic branching process description of the beginning of a disease outbreak to be applied as long as the number of infectives remains small, distinguishing a (minor) disease outbreak confined to this stage from a (major) epidemic, which occurs if the number of infectives begins to grow at an exponential rate. Once an epidemic has started we may switch to a deterministic compartmental model, arguing that in a major epidemic contacts would tend to be more homogeneously distributed. Implicitly, we are thinking of an infinite population, and by a major epidemic we mean a situation in which a nonzero fraction of the population is infected; by a minor outbreak we mean a situation in which the infected population may grow but remains a negligible fraction of the population.

We will not describe the branching process and network approach to epidemic models in detail here, referring the reader to such sources as [4, 6, 22, 23, 24, 26]. We confine ourselves to an outline and a description of the main results.

We assume that the infectives make contacts independently of one another and let p_k denote the probability that the number of contacts by a randomly chosen individual is exactly k, with $\sum_{k=0}^{\infty} p_k = 1$. In other words, $\{p_k\}$ is the degree distribution of the vertices of the graph describing the population network, where individuals correspond to vertices and contacts correspond to edges of the graph. For the moment, we assume that every contact leads to an infection, but we will relax this assumption later.

It is convenient to define the *generating function*

$$G_0(z) = \sum_{k=0}^{\infty} p_k z^k.$$

The mean degree, which we denote by $\langle k \rangle$ or z_1, is

$$\langle k \rangle = \sum_{k=1}^{\infty} k p_k = G_0'(1).$$

More generally, we define the moments

$$\langle k^j \rangle = \sum_{k=1}^{\infty} k^j p_k, \quad j = 1, 2, \ldots, \infty.$$

When a disease is introduced into a network, we think of it as starting at a vertex (patient zero) who transmits infection to every individual to whom this individual is connected, that is, along every edge of the graph from the vertex corresponding to this individual. We may think of this individual as being inside the population, as when a member of a population returns from travel after being infected, or as being outside the population, as when someone visits a population and brings an infection. For transmission of disease after this initial contact we need to use the *excess degree* of a vertex.

The probability that a vertex at the end of a random edge has excess degree $(k-1)$ is a constant multiple of kp_k with the constant chosen to make the sum over k of the probabilities equal to 1. Then the probability that a vertex has excess degree $(k-1)$ is

$$q_{k-1} = \frac{kp_k}{\langle k \rangle}.$$

This leads to a generating function $G_1(z)$ for the excess degree

$$G_1(z) = \sum_{k=1}^{\infty} q_{k-1} z^{k-1} = \sum_{k=1}^{\infty} \frac{kp_k}{\langle k \rangle} z^{k-1} = \frac{1}{\langle k \rangle} G_0'(z),$$

and the mean excess degree, which we denote by $\langle k_e \rangle$, is

$$\begin{aligned}
\langle k_e \rangle &= \frac{1}{\langle k \rangle} \sum_{k=1}^{\infty} k(k-1)p_k \\
&= \frac{1}{\langle k \rangle} \sum_{k=1}^{\infty} k^2 p_k - \frac{1}{\langle k \rangle} \sum_{k=1}^{\infty} kp_k \\
&= \frac{\langle k^2 \rangle}{\langle k \rangle} - 1 = G_1'(1).
\end{aligned}$$

We let $\mathcal{R}_0 = G_1'(1)$, the mean excess degree. This is the mean number of secondary cases infected by patient zero and is the basic reproduction number as usually defined; the threshold for an epidemic is determined by $\mathcal{R}_0$. The quantity $\langle k_e \rangle = G_1'(1)$ is sometimes written in the form

$$\langle k_e \rangle = G_1'(1) = \frac{z_2}{z_1},$$

where $z_2 = \sum_{k=1}^{\infty} k(k-1)p_k = \langle k^2 \rangle - \langle k \rangle$ is the mean number of second neighbors of a random vertex.

Our next goal is to calculate the probability that the infection will die out and will not develop into a major epidemic, proceeding in two steps. First we find the probability that a secondary infected vertex (a vertex which has been infected by another vertex in the population) will not spark a major epidemic.

The equation $G_1(z) = z$ has a root $z = 1$ since $G_1(1) = 1$. The equation $G_1(z) = z$ has at most two roots in $0 \le z \le 1$. If $\mathcal{R}_0 < 1$, the equation $G_1(z) = z$ has only one root, namely, $z = 1$. On the other hand, if $\mathcal{R}_0 > 1$, the equation $G_1(z) = z$ has a second root $z_\infty < 1$.

This root z_∞ is the probability that an infection transmitted along one of the edges at the initial secondary vertex will die out, and this probability is independent of the excess degree of the initial secondary vertex. It is also the probability that an infection originating outside the population, such as an infection brought into the population under study from outside, will die out.

Next, the probability that an infection originating at a primary infected vertex, such as an infection introduced by a visitor from outside the population under study, is the sum over k of the probabilities that the initial infection in a vertex of degree k will die out, weighted by the degree distribution $\{p_k\}$ of the original infection, and this is

$$\sum_{k=0}^{\infty} p_k z_\infty^k = G_0(z_\infty).$$

To summarize this analysis, we see that if $\mathcal{R}_0 < 1$, the probability that the infection will die out is 1. On the other hand, if $\mathcal{R}_0 > 1$, there is a solution $z_\infty < 1$ of

$$G_1(z) = z$$

and there is a probability $1 - G_0(z_\infty) > 0$ that the infection will persist and lead to an epidemic. However, there is a positive probability $G_0(z_\infty)$ that the infection will increase initially but produce only a minor outbreak and die out before triggering a major epidemic. This distinction between a minor outbreak and a major epidemic and the result that if $\mathcal{R}_0 > 1$, there may be only a minor outbreak and not a major epidemic are aspects of stochastic models not reflected in deterministic models.

1.3.1 Transmissibility

Contacts do not necessarily transmit infection. For each contact between an infected individual and a susceptible individual, there is a probability that infection will actually be transmitted. This probability depends on such factors as the closeness of the contact, the infectivity of the member who has been infected, and the susceptibility of the susceptible member. We assume that there is a mean probability T, called the *transmissibility*, of transmission of infection. The transmissibility depends on the rate of contacts, the probability that a contact will transmit infection, the duration time of the infection, and the susceptibility. Until now, we have been assuming that all contacts transmit infection, that is, that $T = 1$. Now, we will continue to assume that there is a network describing the contacts between members of the population whose degree distribution is given by the generating function $G_0(z)$, but we will assume in addition that there is a mean transmissibility T.

We define $\Gamma_0(z,T)$ be the generating function for the distribution of the number of occupied edges attached to a randomly chosen vertex, which is the same as the distribution of the infections transmitted by a randomly chosen individual for any (fixed) transmissibility T. Then

$$\Gamma_0(z,T) = G_0(1+(z-1)T). \tag{1.6}$$

For secondary infections we need the generating function $\Gamma_1(z,T)$ for the distribution of occupied edges leaving a vertex reached by following a randomly chosen edge. This is obtained from the excess degree distribution in the same way,

$$\Gamma_1(z,T) = G_1(1+(z-1)T).$$

The basic reproduction number is now

$$\mathcal{R}_0 = \Gamma_1'(1,T) = TG_1'(1).$$

The calculation of the probability that the infection will die out and not develop into a major epidemic follows the same lines as the argument for $T = 1$. The result is that if $\mathscr{R}_0 = TG_1'(1) < 1$, the probability that the infection will die out is 1. If $\mathscr{R}_0 > 1$, there is a solution $z_\infty(T) < 1$ of

$$\Gamma_1(z,T) = z,$$

and a probability $1 - \Gamma_0(z_\infty(T),T) > 0$ that the infection will persist and lead to an epidemic. However, there is a positive probability $\Gamma_1(z_\infty(T),T)$ that the infection will increase initially but will produce only a minor outbreak and die out before triggering a major epidemic.

Another interpretation of the basic reproduction number is that there is a *critical transmissibility* T_c defined by

$$T_c G_1'(1) = 1.$$

In other words, the critical transmissibility is the transmissibility that makes the basic reproduction number equal to 1. If the mean transmissibility can be decreased below the critical transmissibility, then an epidemic can be prevented.

The measures used to try to control an epidemic may include contact interventions, that is, measures affecting the network such as avoidance of public gatherings and rearrangement of the patterns of interaction between caregivers and patients in a hospital and transmission interventions such as careful hand washing or face masks to decrease the mean transmissibility.

As we have remarked, compartmental models for epidemics are not suitable for describing the beginning of a disease outbreak because they assume that all members of a population are equally likely to make contact with a very small number of infectives. Stochastic branching process models are better descriptions of the beginning of an epidemic. They allow the possibility that even if a disease outbreak has a reproduction number greater than 1, it may be only a minor outbreak and may not develop into a major epidemic. One possible approach to a more realistic description of an epidemic would be to use a branching process model initially and then make a transition to a compartmental model when the epidemic has become established and there are enough infectives that mass-action mixing in the population is a reasonable approximation. Another approach would be to continue to use a network model throughout the course of the epidemic [20, 21, 28]. It is possible to formulate this model dynamically, and the limiting case of this dynamic model as the population size becomes very large is the same as the compartmental model.

The network approach to disease modeling is a rapidly developing field of study, and there will undoubtedly be fundamental developments in our understanding of the modeling of disease transmission. Some useful references are [2, 18, 19, 22, 24, 26].

In the remainder of these notes, we assume that we are in an epidemic situation following a disease outbreak which has been modeled initially by a branching process. Thus we return to the study of compartmental models.

1.4 More Complicated Epidemic Models

We have established that the simple Kermack–McKendrick epidemic model (1.2) has the following basic properties:

1. There is a basic reproduction number $\mathscr{R}_0$ such that if $\mathscr{R}_0 < 1$, the disease dies out, while if $\mathscr{R}_0 > 1$, there is an epidemic.

2. The number of infectives always approaches zero and the number of susceptibles always approaches a positive limit as $t \to \infty$.

3. There is a relation between the reproduction number and the final size of the epidemic, which is an equality if there are no disease deaths.

In fact, these properties hold for epidemic models with more complicated compartmental structure. We will describe some common epidemic models as examples. These models may be considered as general templates which can be modified to fit the properties of specific diseases.

1.4.1 Exposed periods

In many infectious diseases there is an exposed period after the transmission of infection from susceptibles to potentially infective members but before these potential infectives develop symptoms and can transmit infection. To incorporate an exposed period with mean exposed period $1/\kappa$ we add an exposed class E and use compartments S, E, I, R and total population size $N = S + E + I + R$ to give a generalization of the epidemic model (1.2):

$$\begin{aligned} S' &= -a\frac{S}{N}I, \\ E' &= a\frac{S}{N}I - \kappa E, \\ I' &= \kappa E - \alpha I. \end{aligned} \tag{1.7}$$

A flow chart is shown in Figure 1.3.

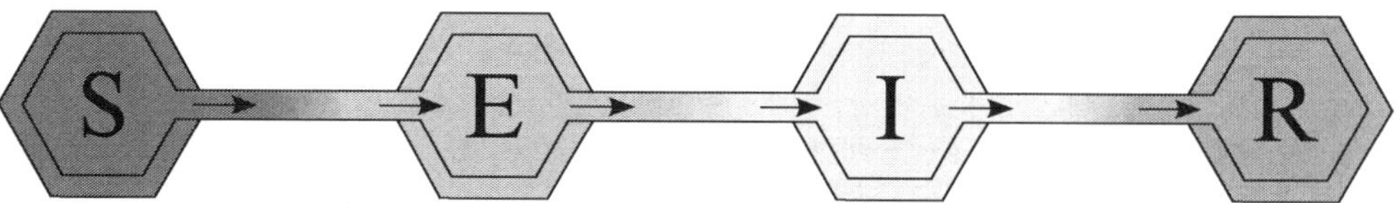

Figure 1.3. *Flow chart for the $SEIR$ model.*

The analysis of this model is the same as the analysis of (1.2), but with I replaced by $E + I$. That is, instead of using the number of infectives as one of the variables we use the total number of infected members, whether or not they are capable of transmitting infection.

For the model (1.7) it is no longer possible to distinguish whether there is an epidemic or not by determining whether the number of infectives grows or decreases initially. A more general characterization is given by whether the equilibrium with all members of the population susceptible is unstable (epidemic) or asymptotically stable (no epidemic). We will use a situation in which the disease-free equilibrium is unstable as our definition of an epidemic.

For the model (1.7), the matrix of the linearization at the equilibrium $S = N, E = 0, I = 0$ is

$$\begin{bmatrix} 0 & 0 & -a \\ 0 & -\kappa & a \\ 0 & \kappa & -\alpha \end{bmatrix}.$$

The eigenvalues of this matrix are zero and the eigenvalues of the 2×2 matrix

$$\begin{bmatrix} -\kappa & a \\ \kappa & -\alpha \end{bmatrix}.$$

These have negative real part, corresponding to stability of the equilibrium and failure of an epidemic to develop (since the trace of the matrix is negative) if and only if the determinant of the matrix is positive. The determinant is $\kappa(\alpha - a)$, and this is positive if and only if $\mathcal{R}_0 < 1$.

If there is an epidemic, the initial exponential growth rate is the largest eigenvalue of the matrix, and this is the largest root of the quadratic characteristic equation

$$\lambda^2 - (\alpha + \kappa)\lambda - \kappa(a + \alpha) = 0.$$

Since the constant term in this equation is negative if $\mathcal{R}_0 > 1$, there is one negative and one positive root, and the positive root is

$$\frac{-(\alpha+\kappa) + \sqrt{(\alpha-\kappa)^2 + 4\kappa a}}{2}.$$

This is the initial exponential growth rate. Note that it is not the same as the initial exponential growth rate for the SIR model (1.2). The effect of an exposed period is to decrease the initial exponential growth rate.

1.4.2 Infectivity in the exposed period

In some diseases there is some infectivity during the exposed period. This may be modeled by assuming infectivity reduced by a factor ε during the exposed period. A calculation of the rate of new infections per susceptible leads to the model

$$\begin{aligned} S' &= -\frac{a}{N} S(I + \varepsilon E), \\ E' &= \frac{a}{N} S(I + \varepsilon E) - \kappa E, \\ I' &= \kappa E - \alpha I. \end{aligned} \tag{1.8}$$

We take initial conditions

$$S(0) = S_0, \quad E(0) = E_0, \quad I(0) = I_0.$$

For this model

$$\mathcal{R}_0 = \frac{a}{\alpha} + \varepsilon \frac{a}{\kappa}.$$

This is seen most easily by recognizing that the first term in the expression for $\mathcal{R}_0$ is the number of secondary infections caused by an individual during the infective stage, and the second term is the number of secondary infections caused during the exposed stage.

For the model (1.8), the matrix of the linearization at the equilibrium $S = N, E = 0$, $I = 0$ is

$$\begin{bmatrix} 0 & -\varepsilon a & -a \\ 0 & \varepsilon a - \kappa & a \\ 0 & \kappa & -\alpha \end{bmatrix}.$$

The eigenvalues of this matrix are zero and the eigenvalues of the 2×2 matrix

$$\begin{bmatrix} \varepsilon a - \kappa & a \\ \kappa & -\alpha \end{bmatrix}.$$

These have negative real part, corresponding to stability of the equilibrium and failure of an epidemic to develop (since the trace of the matrix is negative) if and only if the determinant of the matrix is positive. The determinant is

$$-\alpha(\varepsilon a - \kappa) - \kappa a,$$

and this is positive if and only if $\mathcal{R}_0 < 1$. If $\mathcal{R}_0 < 1$, the trace of the matrix, which is

$$\varepsilon a - (\kappa + \alpha),$$

is negative, and this implies that the equilibrium is asymptotically stable if and only if $\mathcal{R}_0 < 1$, so that there is an epidemic if and only if $\mathcal{R}_0 > 1$.

If there is an epidemic, the initial exponential growth rate is the largest eigenvalue of the matrix, and this is the largest root of the quadratic characteristic equation

$$\lambda^2 + (\alpha + \kappa - \varepsilon a\lambda - \kappa a - \alpha(\varepsilon a - \kappa) = 0.$$

Since the constant term in this equation is negative if $\mathcal{R}_0 > 1$, there is one negative and one positive root, and the positive root, which is easy to calculate, is the initial exponential growth rate.

Integration of the sum of the equations of (1.7) from 0 to ∞ gives

$$N - S_\infty = \alpha \int_0^\infty I(s)ds.$$

Integration of the third equation of (1.8) gives

$$\kappa \int_0^\infty E(s)ds = \alpha \int_0^\infty I(s)ds - I_0,$$

and division of the first equation of (1.8) by S followed by integration from 0 to ∞ gives

$$\begin{aligned} \log \frac{S_0}{S_\infty} &= \int_0^\infty \frac{a}{N}[I(s) + \epsilon E(s)]ds \\ &= \frac{a}{N} \int_0^\infty [I(s) + \epsilon E(s)]ds \\ &= \frac{a}{N}\left[\epsilon + \frac{\kappa}{\alpha}\right] \int_0^\infty E(s)ds - \frac{\varepsilon \frac{a}{N} I_0}{\kappa} \\ &= \mathcal{R}_0 \left[1 - \frac{S_\infty}{N}\right] - \frac{\varepsilon \frac{a}{N} I_0}{\kappa}. \end{aligned}$$

In this final size relation there is an initial term $\frac{a}{N} I_0/\alpha$, caused by the assumption that there are individuals infected originally who are beyond the exposed stage in which they would have had some infectivity. In order to obtain a final size relation without such an initial term it is necessary to assume $I(0) = 0$, i.e., that initial infectives are in the first stage in which they can transmit infection. If $I(0) = 0$, the final size relation has the form (1.3).

1.4.3 Treatment models

One form of treatment that is possible for some diseases is vaccination to protect against infection before the beginning of an epidemic. For example, this approach is commonly used for protection against annual influenza outbreaks. A simple way to model this would be to reduce the total population size by the fraction of the population protected against infection.

In reality such inoculations are only partly effective, decreasing the rate of infection and also decreasing infectivity if a vaccinated person does become infected. This may be modeled by dividing the population into two groups with different model parameters, which would require some assumptions about the mixing between the two groups. This is not difficult, but we will not explore this direction here.

If there is a treatment once a person has been infected, this may be modeled by supposing that a fraction γ per unit time of infectives is selected for treatment, and that treatment reduces infectivity by a fraction δ. Suppose that the rate of removal from the treated class is η. This leads to the $SITR$ model, where T is the treatment class, given by

$$\begin{aligned} S' &= -\frac{a}{N}S[I+\delta T], \\ I' &= \frac{a}{N}S[I+\delta T]-(\alpha+\gamma)I, \\ T' &= \gamma I - \eta T. \end{aligned} \tag{1.9}$$

A flow chart is shown in Figure 1.4.

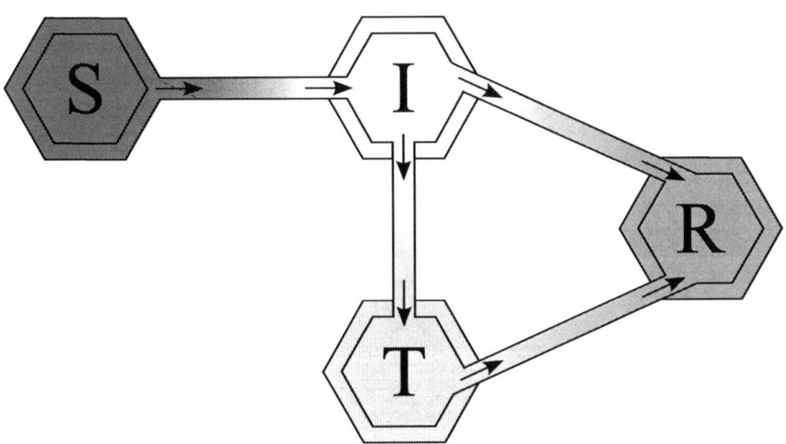

Figure 1.4. *Flow chart for the $SITR$ model.*

It is not difficult to prove, much as was done for the model (1.2), that

$$S_\infty = \lim_{t\to\infty} S(t) > 0, \quad \lim_{t\to\infty} I(t) = \lim_{t\to\infty} T(t) = 0.$$

In order to calculate the basic reproduction number, we may argue that an infective in a totally susceptible population causes a new infections in unit time, and the mean time spent in the infective compartment is $1/(\alpha+\gamma)$. In addition, a fraction $\gamma/(\alpha+\gamma)$ of infectives are treated. While in the treatment stage, the number of new infections caused in unit time is δa, and the mean time in the treatment class is $1/\eta$. Thus $\mathcal{R}_0$ is

$$\mathcal{R}_0 = \frac{a}{\alpha+\gamma} + \frac{\gamma}{\alpha+\gamma}\frac{\delta a}{\eta}. \tag{1.10}$$

It is also possible to establish the final size relation (1.3) by means very similar to those used for the simple model (1.2). We integrate the first equation of (1.9) to obtain

$$\begin{aligned}\log\frac{S_0}{S_\infty} &= \int_0^\infty \frac{a}{N}[I(t)+\delta T(t)]dt \\ &= \frac{a}{N}\int_0^\infty [I(t)+\delta T(t)]dt.\end{aligned}$$

Integration of the third equation of (1.9) gives

$$\gamma\int_0^\infty I(t)dt = \eta\int_0^\infty T(t)dt.$$

Integration of the sum of the first two equations of (1.9) gives

$$N - S_\infty = (\alpha+\gamma)\int_0^\infty I(t)dt.$$

Combination of these three equations and (1.10) gives (1.3).

For the model (1.9), the matrix of the linearization at the equilibrium $S=N, I=0$, $T=0$ is

$$\begin{bmatrix} 0 & -a & -\delta a \\ 0 & a-(\alpha+\gamma) & \delta a \\ 0 & \gamma & -\eta \end{bmatrix}.$$

The eigenvalues of this matrix are zero and the eigenvalues of the 2×2 matrix

$$\begin{bmatrix} a-(\alpha+\gamma) & \delta a \\ \gamma & -\eta \end{bmatrix}.$$

These have negative real part, corresponding to stability of the equilibrium and failure of an epidemic to develop if and only if the determinant of the matrix is positive and the trace is negative. The determinant is

$$-a(\eta+\delta\gamma)+\eta(\alpha+\gamma),$$

which is positive if and only if $\mathcal{R}_0 < 1$, and this condition implies that the trace is negative.

If there is an epidemic, the initial exponential growth rate is the largest eigenvalue of the matrix, and this is the largest root of the quadratic characteristic equation

$$\lambda^2 + [a-(\alpha+\gamma+\eta)]\lambda + a(\eta+\delta\gamma) - \eta(\alpha+\gamma) = 0.$$

Since the constant term in this equation is negative if $\mathcal{R}_0 > 1$, there is one negative and one positive root, and the positive root is the initial exponential growth rate. Notice that this rate depends on the treatment rate.

1.4.4 A quarantine-isolation model

For an outbreak of a new disease, where no vaccine is available, isolation of diagnosed infectives and quarantine of people who are suspected of having been infected (usually by tracing of contacts of diagnosed infectives) are the only control measures available. We formulate a model to describe the course of an epidemic, originally introduced for modeling the SARS epidemic of 2002–2003 [11], when control measures are begun under the following assumptions:

1. Exposed members may be infective with infectivity reduced by a factor $\varepsilon_E, 0 \le \varepsilon_E < 1$.
2. Exposed members who are not quarantined become infective at rate κ_E.
3. We introduce a class Q of quarantined members and a class J of isolated (hospitalized) members, and exposed members are quarantined at a proportional rate γ_Q in unit time (in practice, a quarantine will also be applied to many susceptibles, but we ignore this in the model). Quarantine is not perfect, but it reduces the contact rate by a factor ε_Q. The effect of this assumption is that some susceptibles make fewer contacts than the model assumes.
4. Infectives are diagnosed at a proportional rate γ_J per unit time and isolated. Isolation is imperfect, and there may be transmission of disease by isolated members, with an infectivity factor of ε_J.
5. Quarantined members are monitored, and when they develop symptoms at rate κ_Q they are isolated immediately.
6. Infectives leave the infective class at rate α_I and isolated members leave the isolated class at rate α_J.

These assumptions lead to the $SEQIJR$ model [11]

$$\begin{aligned}
S' &= -\frac{a}{N} S[\varepsilon_E E + \varepsilon_E \varepsilon_Q Q + I + \varepsilon_J J], \\
E' &= \frac{a}{N} S[\varepsilon_E E + \varepsilon_E \varepsilon_Q Q + I + \varepsilon_J J] - (\kappa_E + \gamma_Q) E, \\
Q' &= \gamma_Q E - \kappa_J Q, \\
I' &= \kappa_E E - (\alpha_I + \gamma_J) I, \\
J' &= \kappa_Q Q + \gamma_J I - \alpha_J J.
\end{aligned} \tag{1.11}$$

The model before control measures are begun is the special case

$$\gamma_Q = \gamma_J = \kappa_Q = \alpha_J = 0, \;\; Q = J = 0,$$

of (1.11). It is the same as (1.8).

A flow chart is shown in Figure 1.5.

We define the *control reproduction number* $\mathcal{R}_c$ to be the number of secondary infections caused by a single infective in a population consisting essentially only of susceptibles with the control measures in place. It is analogous to the basic reproduction number, but instead of describing the very beginning of the disease outbreak it describes the beginning of

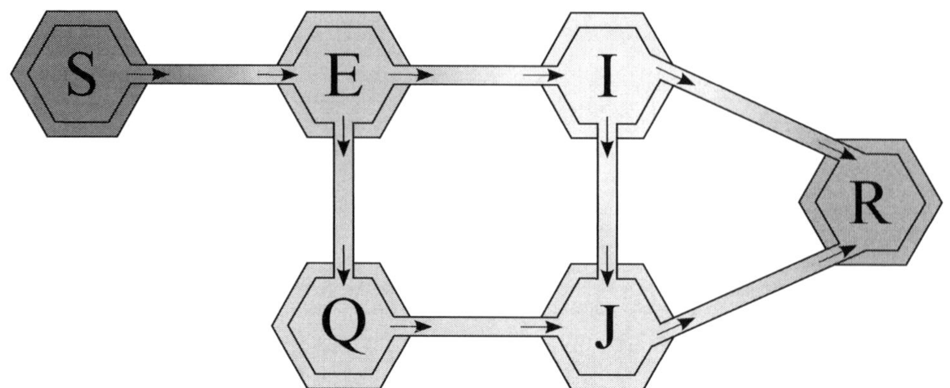

Figure 1.5. *Flow chart for the SEQIJR model.*

the recognition of the epidemic. The basic reproduction number is the value of the control reproduction number with

$$\gamma_Q = \gamma_J = \kappa_Q = \alpha_J = 0.$$

We have already calculated $\mathcal{R}_0$ for (1.8), and we may calculate $\mathcal{R}_c$ in the same way but using the full model with quarantined and isolated classes. We obtain

$$\mathcal{R}_c = \frac{\varepsilon_E a}{D_1} + \frac{a\kappa_E}{D_1 D_2} + \frac{\varepsilon_Q \varepsilon_E a \gamma_Q}{D_1 \kappa_Q} + \frac{\varepsilon_J a \kappa_E \gamma_J}{\alpha_J D_1 D_2} + \frac{\varepsilon_J a \gamma_Q}{\alpha_J D_1},$$

where $D_1 = \gamma_Q + \kappa_E$, $D_2 = \gamma_J + \alpha_I$.

Each term of $\mathcal{R}_c$ has an epidemiological interpretation. The mean duration in E is $1/D_1$ with contact rate $\varepsilon_E \frac{a}{N}$, giving a contribution to $\mathcal{R}_c$ of $\varepsilon_E a/D_1$. A fraction κ_E/D_1 goes from E to I, with contact rate $\frac{a}{N}$ and mean duration $1/D_2$, giving a contribution of $a\kappa_E/D_1 D_2$. A fraction γ_Q/D_1 goes from E to Q, with contact rate $\varepsilon_E \varepsilon_Q \frac{a}{N}$ and mean duration $1/\kappa_Q$, giving a contribution of $\varepsilon_E \varepsilon_Q a \gamma_Q / D_1 \kappa_Q$. A fraction $\kappa_E \gamma_J / D_1 D_2$ goes from E to I to J, with a contact rate of $\varepsilon_J \frac{a}{N}$ and a mean duration of $1/\alpha_J$, giving a contribution of $\varepsilon_J a \kappa_E \gamma_J / \alpha_J D_1 D_2$. Finally, a fraction γ_Q/D_1 goes from E to Q to J with a contact rate of $\varepsilon_J \frac{a}{N}$ and a mean duration of $1/\alpha_J$, giving a contribution of $\varepsilon_J a \gamma_Q / D_1 \alpha_J$. The sum of these individual contributions gives $\mathcal{R}_c$.

In the model (1.11) the parameters γ_Q and γ_J are *control* parameters which may be chosen in the attempt to manage the epidemic. The parameters ϵ_Q and ϵ_J depend on the strictness of the quarantine and isolation processes and are thus also control measures in a sense. The other parameters of the model are specific to the disease being studied. While they are not variable, their measurements are subject to experimental error.

The linearization of (1.11) at the disease-free equilibrium $(N,0,0,0,0)$ has matrix

$$\begin{bmatrix} \epsilon_E a - (\kappa_E + \gamma_Q) & \varepsilon_E \varepsilon_Q \frac{a}{N} & a & \varepsilon_J a \\ \gamma_Q & -\kappa_Q & 0 & 0 \\ \kappa_E & 0 & -(\alpha_I + \gamma_J) & 0 \\ 0 & \kappa_Q & \gamma_J & -\alpha_J \end{bmatrix}.$$

The corresponding characteristic equation is a fourth degree polynomial equation whose leading coefficient is 1 and whose constant term is a positive constant multiple of $1 - \mathcal{R}_c$, thus positive if $\mathcal{R}_c < 1$ and negative if $\mathcal{R}_c > 1$. If $\mathcal{R}_c > 1$, there is a positive eigenvalue, corresponding to an initial exponential growth rate of solutions of (1.11). If $\mathcal{R}_c < 1$, it is possible to show that all eigenvalues of the coefficient matrix have negative real part, and thus solutions of (1.11) die out exponentially [27].

In order to show that analogues of the relation (1.3) and $S_\infty > 0$ derived for the model (1.2) are valid for the management model (1.11), we begin by integrating the equations for $S+E, Q, I, J$, of (1.11) with respect to t from $t=0$ to $t=\infty$, using the initial conditions

$$S(0)+E(0) = N(0) = N, \qquad Q(0) = I(0) = J(0) = 0.$$

We continue by integrating the equation for S, and then an argument similar to the one used for (1.2) but technically more complicated may be used to show that $S_\infty > 0$ for the treatment model (1.11) and also to establish the final size relation

$$\log \frac{S_0}{S_\infty} = \mathcal{R}_c \left[1 - \frac{S_\infty}{N}\right].$$

Thus the asymptotic behavior of the management model (1.11) is the same as that of the simpler model (1.2).

In the various compartmental models that we have studied, there are significant common features. This suggests that compartmental models can be put into a more general framework. In fact, this general framework is the age of infection epidemic model originally introduced by Kermack and McKendrick in 1927.

1.5 The Age of Infection Epidemic Model

The general epidemic model described by Kermack and McKendrick [15] included a dependence of infectivity on the time since becoming infected (age of infection). We let $S(t)$ denote the number of susceptibles at time t and let $\varphi(t)$ be the total infectivity at time t, defined as the sum of products of the number of infected members with each infection age and the mean infectivity for that infection age. We assume that on average members of the population make a constant number a of contacts in unit time. We let $B(\tau)$ be the fraction of infected members remaining infected at infection age τ and let $\pi(\tau)$ with $0 \le \pi(\tau) \le 1$ be the mean infectivity at infection age τ. Then we let

$$A(\tau) = \pi(\tau)B(\tau),$$

the mean infectivity of members of the population with infection age τ. We assume that there are no disease deaths, so that the total population size is a constant N.

The age of infection epidemic model is

$$\begin{aligned} S' &= -\frac{a}{N} S\varphi, \\ \varphi(t) &= \varphi_0(t) + \int_0^t \frac{a}{N} S(t-\tau)\varphi(t-\tau)A(\tau)d\tau \\ &= \varphi_0(t) + \int_0^t [-S'(t-\tau)]A(\tau)d\tau. \end{aligned} \tag{1.12}$$

The basic reproduction number is

$$\mathcal{R}_0 = a\int_0^\infty A(\tau)d\tau.$$

We write

$$-\frac{S'(t)}{S(t)} = \frac{a}{N}\varphi_0(t) + \frac{a}{N}\int_0^t [-S'(t-\tau)]A(\tau)d\tau.$$

Integration with respect to t from 0 to ∞ gives

$$\begin{aligned}
\log\frac{S_0}{S_\infty} &= \frac{a}{N}\int_0^\infty \varphi_0(t)dt + \frac{a}{N}\int_0^\infty\int_0^t [-S'(t-\tau)]A(\tau)d\tau dt \\
&= \frac{a}{N}\int_0^\infty \varphi_0(t)dt + \frac{a}{N}\int_0^\infty A(\tau)\int_\tau^\infty [-S'(t-\tau)]dtd\tau \\
&= \frac{a}{N}\int_0^\infty \varphi_0(t)dt + [S_0 - S_\infty]\int_0^\infty A(\tau)d\tau \qquad (1.13) \\
&= \frac{a}{N}[N - S_\infty]\int_0^\infty A(\tau)d\tau + \frac{a}{N}\int_0^\infty [\varphi_0(t) - (N - S_0)A(\tau)]d\tau \qquad (1.14) \\
&= \mathcal{R}_0\left[1 - \frac{S_\infty}{N}\right] - \frac{a}{N}\int_0^\infty [(N - S_0)A(t) - \varphi_0(t)]dt.
\end{aligned}$$

Here, $\varphi_0(t)$ is the total infectivity of the initial infectives when they reach age of infection t. If all initial infectives have infection age zero at $t = 0$, then $\varphi_0(t) = [N - S_0]A(t)$, and

$$\int_0^\infty [\varphi_0(t) - (N - S_0)A(t)]dt = 0.$$

Then (1.13) takes the form

$$\log\frac{S_0}{S_\infty} = \mathcal{R}_0\left(1 - \frac{S_\infty}{N}\right), \qquad (1.15)$$

and this is the general final size relation. If there are initial infectives with infection age greater than zero, then let $u(\tau)$ be the fraction of these individuals with infection age τ, $\int_0^\infty u(\tau)d\tau = 1$. At time t these individuals have infection age $t + \tau$ and mean infectivity $A(t + \tau)$. Thus

$$\varphi_0(t) = (N - S_\infty)\int_0^\infty u(\tau)A(t+\tau)d\tau$$

and

$$\begin{aligned}
\int_0^\infty \varphi_0(t)dt &= (N - S_\infty)\int_0^\infty\int_0^\infty u(\tau)A(t+\tau)d\tau dt \\
&= (N - S_\infty)\int_0^\infty u(\tau)\left[\int_\tau^\infty A(v)dv\right]d\tau \\
&= (N - S_\infty)\int_0^\infty A(v)\left[\int_0^v u(\tau)d\tau\right]dv \\
&\le (N - S_\infty)\int_0^\infty A(v)dv,
\end{aligned}$$

since $\int_0^v u(\tau)d\tau \le 1$.

Thus, the initial term satisfies

$$\int_0^\infty [(N-S_0)A(t)-\varphi_0(t)]dt \geq 0.$$

The final size relation is sometimes presented in the form

$$\log \frac{S_0}{S_\infty} = \mathcal{R}_0\left(1-\frac{S_\infty}{S_0}\right); \tag{1.16}$$

see, for example, [1, 14]. This form would represent the final size relation for an epidemic started by someone outside the population under study, so that $S_0 = N, I_0 = 0$.

According to [29], the initial exponential growth rate is the solution λ of the equation

$$a\int_0^\infty e^{-\lambda\tau}A(\tau)d\tau = 1. \tag{1.17}$$

The supporting argument given in [29] is not mathematically rigorous as it assumes an exponentially growing population. In fact, a proper justification for the relation (1.17) is obtained by linearizing the system (1.12) about the equilibrium $S = N, \varphi = 0$ and solving the corresponding characteristic equation. The point is that locally there is exponential growth near an unstable equilibrium, and the assumption of exponential growth is superfluous. In the Kermack–McKendrick model formulation, the condition for an epidemic is the instability of a disease-free equilibrium.

In order to find equilibria, we need to use the asymptotic theory of integral equations [16] and use the limit equation of (1.12), which is

$$\begin{aligned} S' &= -\frac{a}{N}S\varphi, \\ \varphi(t) &= \int_0^\infty \frac{a}{N}S(t-\tau)\varphi(t-\tau)A(\tau)d\tau \end{aligned} \tag{1.18}$$

to find equilibria. The linearization at the equilibrium $S = N, \varphi = 0$ is

$$\begin{aligned} u'(t) &= -av(t), \\ v(t) &= a\int_0^\infty v(t-\tau)A(\tau)d\tau. \end{aligned}$$

The characteristic equation is the condition on λ that the linearization have a solution $u = u_0e^{\lambda t}, v = v_0e^{\lambda t}$, and this is just (1.17). Thus the initial exponential growth rate is as claimed in [29]. It should be noted that this calculation depends on the assumption of homogeneous mixing but that the method described here should give a corresponding result for heterogeneous mixing age of infection epidemic models.

The examples studied in Section 1.4 are all included in the age of infection model (1.12) as special cases. However, although the age of infection formulation gives a general structure, calculations involving integrals depending on $A(\tau)$ may be quite complicated.

Example 1. The $SEIR$ model (1.8) can be viewed as an age of infection model with $\varphi = \varepsilon E + I$. In order to use the age of infection interpretation, we need to determine the kernel $A(\tau)$ in order to calculate its integral. We let $u(\tau)$ be the fraction of infected members with infection age τ who are not yet infective and $v(\tau)$ the fraction of infected members who are infective. Then the rate at which members become infective at infection age τ is $\kappa u(\tau)$, and we have

$$\begin{aligned} u'(\tau) &= -\kappa u(\tau), \qquad u(0) = 1, \\ v'(\tau) &= \kappa u(\tau) - \alpha v(\tau), \quad v(0) = 0. \end{aligned}$$

The solution of this system is

$$u(\tau) = e^{-\kappa\tau}, \quad v(\tau) = \frac{\kappa}{\kappa - \alpha}[e^{-\alpha\tau} - e^{-\kappa\tau}].$$

Thus we have

$$A(\tau) = \varepsilon e^{-\kappa\tau} + \frac{\kappa}{\kappa - \alpha}[e^{-\alpha\tau} - e^{-\kappa\tau}],$$

and it is easy to calculate

$$\int_0^\infty A(\tau)d\tau = \frac{1}{\alpha} + \frac{\varepsilon}{\kappa}.$$

This gives the same value for $\mathcal{R}_0$ as was calculated directly.

The age of infection model also includes the possibility of disease stages with nonexponential distributions [9, 10].

For nonexponential period distributions, it is possible to calculate

$$\int_0^\infty A(\tau)d\tau$$

without having to calculate the function $A(\tau)$ explicitly.

Example 2. Consider an $SEIR$ model in which the exposed period has a distribution given by a function Q, and the infective period has a distribution given by a function P. It is necessary to do some preliminary analysis before we can formulate the model. We begin with the equations for S and E,

$$\begin{aligned} S' &= -\frac{a}{N}SI, \\ E(t) &= E_0 Q(t) + \int_0^t [-S'(s)]Q(t-s)ds. \end{aligned}$$

In order to obtain an equation for I, we differentiate the equation for E, obtaining

$$E'(t) = E_0 Q'(t) - S'(t) + \int_0^t [-S'(s)]Q'(t-s)ds.$$

Thus the input to I at time t is

$$E_0 Q'(t) + \int_0^t [-S'(s)]Q'(t-s)ds$$

and

$$I(t) = E_0 \int_0^t Q'(u)P(t-u)du + \int_0^t [-S'(s)]Q'(u-s)ds\,P(t-u)du.$$

The first term in this expression may be written as $I_0(t)$, and the second term may be simplified, using interchange of the order of integration in the iterated integral, to yield

$$\int_0^t \int_0^u [-S'(s)]Q'(u-s)ds\,P(t-u)du = \int_0^t \int_s^t Q'(u-s)du\,P(t-u)[-S'(s)]ds.$$

If we define

$$M(t-s) = \int_s^t Q'(u-s)P(t-u)du = \int_0^{t-s} Q'(t-s-v)P(v)dv$$

or

$$M(\tau) = \int_0^\tau Q'(\tau - v)P(v)dv, \tag{1.19}$$

we obtain

$$I(t) = I_0(t) + \int_0^t [-S'(s)]M(t-s)ds.$$

Then the model is

$$\begin{aligned} S' &= -\frac{a}{N}SI, && (1.20)\\ E(t) &= E_0 Q(t) + \int_0^t [-S'(s)]Q(t-s)ds,\\ I(t) &= I_0(t) + \int_0^t [-S'(s)]M(t-s)ds, \end{aligned}$$

which is in age of infection form with $\varphi = I$ and $A(\tau) = M(\tau)$, and we have an explicit expression for $M(\tau)$. If there is infectivity with a reduction factor ε in the exposed class, we would have $A(\tau) = \varepsilon Q(\tau) + T(\tau)$.

Example 3. Consider the treatment model (1.9) of Section 1.4.3. Then $\mathcal{R}_0$, calculated in Section 1.4.3, is given by (1.10). We now extend this to an age of infection model with general infective and treatment stage distributions. Assume that the distribution of infective periods is given by $P(\tau)$, and the distribution of periods in treatment is given by $Q(\tau)$. Then the $SITR$ model becomes

$$\begin{aligned} S'(t) &= -\frac{a}{N}S(t)[I(t) + \delta T(t)],\\ I(t) &= I_0 P(t) + \int_0^t [-S'(t-\tau)]e^{-\gamma\tau}P(\tau)d\tau, && (1.21)\\ T(t) &= \int_0^t \gamma I(t-\sigma)Q(\sigma)d\sigma. \end{aligned}$$

Then

$$\varphi(t) = I(t) + \delta T(t).$$

We see from the second equation of (1.21) that the contribution to $\mathcal{R}_0$ from $I(t)$ is

$$a\int_0^\infty e^{-\gamma\tau}P(\tau)d\tau.$$

To find the contribution from $T(t)$, we need to write the equation in the form

$$T(t) = T_0(t) + \int_0^t [-S'(t-\tau)]Y(\tau)d\tau,$$

so that the contribution from $T(t)$ would be

$$\delta a \int_0^\infty Y(\tau)d\tau,$$

and we would obtain

$$\mathcal{R}_0 = a\left[\int_0^\infty e^{-\gamma\tau}P(\tau)d\tau + \delta\int_0^\infty Y(\tau)d\tau\right].$$

We rewrite $T(t)$ to find $Y(\tau)$, obtaining

$$\begin{aligned}
T(t) &= \int_0^\infty \gamma I(t-\sigma)Q(\sigma)d\sigma \\
&= \int_0^\infty \gamma\left[\int_0^\infty [-S'(t-u-\sigma)]e^{-\gamma u}P(u)du\right]Q(\sigma)d\sigma \\
&= \int_0^\infty \gamma\left[\int_\sigma^\infty [-S'(t-\tau)]e^{-\gamma(\tau-\sigma)}P(\tau-\sigma)d\tau\right]Q(\sigma)d\sigma \\
&= \int_0^\infty \gamma[-S'(t-\tau)]\int_0^\tau e^{-\gamma(\tau-\sigma)}P(\tau-\sigma)Q(\sigma)d\sigma\, d\tau \\
&= \int_0^\infty [-S'(t-\tau)]B(\tau)d\tau,
\end{aligned}$$

with

$$B(\tau) = \gamma\int_0^\tau e^{-\gamma(\tau-\sigma)}P(\tau-\sigma)Q(\sigma)d\sigma.$$

Now

$$\begin{aligned}
\int_0^\infty B(\tau)d\tau &= \gamma\int_0^\infty\int_0^\tau e^{-\gamma(\tau-\sigma)}P(\tau-\sigma)Q(\sigma)d\sigma\, d\tau \\
&= \gamma\int_0^\infty\int_\sigma^\infty e^{-\gamma(\tau-\sigma)}P(\tau-\sigma)d\tau\, Q(\sigma)d\sigma \\
&= \gamma\int_0^\infty\int_0^\infty e^{-\gamma\omega}P(\omega)d\omega\, Q(v)dv \\
&= \gamma\int_0^\infty e^{-\gamma\omega}P(\omega)d\omega\int_0^\infty Q(\sigma)d\sigma.
\end{aligned} \tag{1.22}$$

Thus,

$$\begin{aligned}
\mathcal{R}_0 &= a\int_0^\infty [A(\tau)+\delta B(\tau)]d\tau \\
&= a\left[\int_0^\infty e^{-\gamma\tau}P(\tau)d\tau + \delta\gamma\int_0^\infty e^{-\gamma\tau}P(\tau)d\tau\int_0^\infty Q(\tau)d\tau\right] \\
&= a\int_0^\infty e^{-\gamma\tau}P(\tau)d\tau\left[1+\delta\gamma\int_0^\infty Q(\tau)d\tau\right].
\end{aligned} \tag{1.23}$$

With exponentially distributed infective and treatment periods, $P(\tau)=e^{-\alpha\tau}$, $Q(\tau)=e^{-\eta\tau}$ we use (1.23) to calculate $\mathcal{R}_0$, obtaining

$$\begin{aligned}\mathcal{R}_0 &= a\int_0^\infty e^{-(\alpha+\gamma)\tau}\,d\tau\left[1+\delta\gamma\int_0^\infty e^{-\eta\tau}\,d\tau\right]\\ &= \frac{a}{\alpha+\gamma}\left[1+\frac{\delta\gamma}{\eta}\right],\end{aligned}$$

the same result as (1.10).

An arbitrary choice of treatment period distribution with mean $1/\eta$ does not affect the quantity $\mathcal{R}_0$, but different infective period distributions may have a significant effect. For example, let us take $\gamma = 1$ and assume the mean infective period is 1. Then, with an exponential distribution, $P(\tau)=e^{-\tau}$,

$$\int_0^\infty e^{-\tau}P(\tau)d\tau = \int_0^\infty e^{-2\tau}\,d\tau = \frac{1}{2}.$$

With an infective period of fixed length 1,

$$\int_0^\infty e^{-\tau}P(\tau)d\tau = \int_0^1 e^{-\tau}\,d\tau = (1-e^{-1}) = 0.632.$$

Thus a model with an infective period of fixed length would lead to a basic reproduction number more than 25% higher than a model with an exponentially distributed infective period that has the same mean.

As suggested by these two examples, there are general methods for calculation of integrals involving $A(\tau)$ without the necessity of calculating the function A explicitly [3, 30].

1.6 Models with Disease Deaths

The assumption in the model (1.2) of a rate of contacts per infective which is proportional to population size N, called *mass-action incidence* or bilinear incidence, was used in all the early epidemic models. However, it is quite unrealistic, except possibly in the early stages of an epidemic in a population of moderate size. It is more realistic to assume a contact rate which is a nonincreasing function of total population size. For example, a situation in which the number of contacts per infective in unit time is constant, called *standard incidence*, is a more accurate description for sexually transmitted diseases. If there are no disease deaths, so that the total population size remains constant, such a distinction is unnecessary.

We generalize the model (1.2) by dropping the assumption (iv) of Section 1.2 and replacing the assumption (i) of Section 1.2 by the assumption that an average member of the population makes $a(N)$ contacts in unit time with $a'(N)\geq 0$ [5, 8], and we define

$$\beta(N) = \frac{a(N)}{N}.$$

It is reasonable to assume $\beta'(N)\leq 0$ to express the idea of saturation in the number of contacts. Then mass-action incidence corresponds to the choice $a(N)=\beta N$, and standard incidence corresponds to the choice $a(N) = \lambda$. The assumptions $a(N) = N\beta(N), a'(N) \geq 0$ imply that

$$\beta(N) + N\beta'(N) \geq 0. \tag{1.24}$$

Some epidemic models [8] have used a Michaelis–Menten type of interaction of the form

$$a(N) = \frac{aN}{1+bN}.$$

Another form based on a mechanistic derivation for pair formation [13] leads to an expression of the form

$$a(N) = \frac{aN}{1+bN+\sqrt{1+2bN}}.$$

Data for diseases transmitted by contact in cities of moderate size [17] suggest that data fit the assumption of a form

$$a(N) = \lambda N^p$$

with $p = 0.05$ quite well. All of these forms satisfy the conditions $a'(N) \geq 0, \beta'(N) \leq 0$.

Because the total population size is now present in the model we must include an equation for total population size. This forces us to make a distinction between members of the population who die of the disease and members of the population who recover with immunity against reinfection. We assume that a fraction f of the αI members leaving the infective class at time t recover and the remaining fraction $(1-f)$ die of disease. We use S, I, and N as variables, with $N = S + I + R$. We now obtain a three-dimensional model:

$$\begin{aligned} S' &= -\beta(N)SI, \\ I' &= \beta(N)SI - \alpha I, \\ N' &= -(1-f)\alpha I. \end{aligned} \tag{1.25}$$

Since N is now a decreasing function, we define $N(0) = N_0 = S_0 + I_0$. We also have the equation $R' = -f\alpha I$, but we need not include it in the model since R is determined when S, I, and N are known. We should note that if $f = 1$, the total population size remains equal to the constant N, and the model (1.25) reduces to the simpler model (1.2) with β replaced by the constant $\beta(N_0)$.

We wish to show that the model (1.25) has the same qualitative behavior as the model (1.2), namely, that there is a basic reproduction number which distinguishes between disappearance of the disease and an epidemic outbreak, and that some members of the population are left untouched when the epidemic passes. These two properties are the central features of all epidemic models.

For the model (1.25) the basic reproduction number is given by

$$\mathcal{R}_0 = \frac{N_0\beta(N_0)}{\alpha},$$

because a single infective introduced into a wholly susceptible population makes $C(N_0) = N_0\beta(N_0)$ contacts in unit time, all of which are with susceptibles and thus produce new infections, and the mean infective period is $1/\alpha$.

We assume that $\beta(0)$ is finite, thus ruling out standard incidence (standard incidence does not appear to be realistic if the total population N approaches zero, and it would be more natural to assume that $C(N)$ grows linearly with N for small N). If we let $t \to \infty$ in the sum of the first two equations of (1.25), we obtain

$$\alpha \int_0^\infty I(s)ds = S_0 + I_0 - S_\infty = N - S_\infty.$$

The first equation of (1.25) may be written as

$$-\frac{S'(t)}{S(t)} = \beta(N(t))I(t).$$

Since

$$\beta(N) \geq \beta(N_0),$$

integration from 0 to ∞ gives

$$\begin{aligned}\log \frac{S_0}{S_\infty} &= \int_0^\infty \beta(N(t))I(t)dt \\ &\geq \beta(N_0) \int_0^\infty I(t)dt \\ &= \frac{\beta(N_0)(N_0 - S_\infty)}{\alpha N_0}.\end{aligned}$$

We now obtain a final size inequality

$$\begin{aligned}\log \frac{S_0}{S_\infty} &= \int_0^\infty \beta(N(t))I(t)dt \\ &\geq \beta(N_0) \int_0^\infty I(t)dt = \mathcal{R}_0 \left[1 - \frac{S_\infty}{N_0}\right].\end{aligned}$$

If the disease death rate is small, the final size inequality is an approximate equality.

It is not difficult to show that $N(t) \geq f N_0$, and then a similar calculation using the inequality $\beta(N) \leq \beta(f N_0) < \infty$ shows that

$$\log \frac{S_0}{S_\infty} \leq \beta(f N_0) \int_0^\infty I(t)dt,$$

from which we may deduce that $S_\infty > 0$.

1.7 Directions for Generalization

A fundamental assumption in the model (1.2) is homogeneous mixing, in which all individuals are equivalent in contacts. A more realistic approach would include separation of the population into subgroups with differences in behavior, and we will describe such models in the third lecture. For example, in many childhood diseases the contacts that transmit infection depend on the ages of the individuals, and a model should include a description of the rate of contact between individuals of different ages. Other heterogeneities that may be important include activity levels of different groups and spatial distribution of populations. Network models may be formulated to include heterogeneity of mixing, or more complicated compartmental models can be developed.

When it is realized that an epidemic has begun, individuals are likely to modify their behavior by avoiding crowds to reduce their contacts and by being more careful about hygiene to reduce the risk that a contact will produce infection.

Many of the important underlying ideas of mathematical epidemiology arose in the study of malaria begun by Ross [25]. Malaria is one example of a disease with vector transmission, the infection being transmitted back and forth between vectors (mosquitoes) and hosts (humans). Other vector diseases include West Nile virus and HIV with heterosexual transmission. Vector transmitted diseases require models that include both vectors and hosts.

Bibliography

[1] Arino, J., F. Brauer, P. van den Driessche, J. Watmough, and J. Wu (2007) *A final size relation for epidemic models*, Math. Biosc. & Eng. **4**: 159–176.

[2] Bansal, S., J. Read, B. Pourbohloul, and L.A. Meyers (2010) *The dynamic nature of contact networks in infectious disease epidemiology*, J. Biol. Dyn. **4**: 478–489.

[3] Brauer, F., C. Castillo-Chavez, and Z. Feng (2010) *Discrete epidemic models*, Math. Biosc. Eng. **7**: 1–15.

[4] Callaway, D.S., M.E.J. Newman, S.H. Strogatz, and D.J. Watts (2000) *Network robustness and fragility: Percolation on random graphs*, Phys. Rev. Letters **85**: 5468–5471.

[5] Castillo-Chavez, C., K. Cooke, W. Huang, and S.A. Levin (1989) *The role of long incubation periods in the dynamics of HIV/AIDS. Part 1: Single populations models*, J. Math. Biol. **27**: 373–398.

[6] Diekmann, O. and J.A.P. Heesterbeek (2000) *Mathematical Epidemiology of Infectious Diseases: Model Building, Analysis and Interpretation*, John Wiley, New York.

[7] Diekmann, O., J.A.P. Heesterbeek, and J.A.J. Metz (1990) *On the definition and the computation of the basic reproductive ratio $\mathcal{R}_0$ in models for infectious diseases in heterogeneous populations*, J. Math. Biol. **28**: 365–382.

[8] Dietz, K. (1982) *Overall patterns in the transmission cycle of infectious disease agents*, in Population Biology of Infectious Diseases, R.M. Anderson and R.M. May, eds., Life Sciences Research Report **25**, Springer-Verlag, Berlin, Heidelberg, New York: 87–102.

[9] Feng, Z. (2007) *Final and peak epidemic sizes for $SEIR$ models with quarantine and isolation*, Math. Biosc. & Eng. **4**: 675–686.

[10] Feng, Z. D., Xu, and W. Zhao (2007) *Epidemiological models with non-exponentially distributed disease stages and applications to disease control*, Bull. Math. Biol. **69**: 1511–1536.

[11] Gumel, A., S. Ruan, T. Day, J. Watmough, P. van den Driessche, F. Brauer, D. Gabrielson, C. Bowman, M.E. Alexander, S. Ardal, J. Wu, and B.M. Sahai (2004) *Modeling strategies for controlling SARS outbreaks based on Toronto, Hong Kong, Singapore and Beijing experience*, Proc. Roy. Soc. London **271**: 2223–2232.

[12] Heesterbeek, J.A.P. (1992) R_0, CWI, Amsterdam.

[13] Heesterbeek, J.A.P. and J.A.J Metz (1993) *The saturating contact rate in marriage and epidemic models*, J. Math. Biol. **31**: 529–539.

[14] Heffernan, J.M., R.J. Smith, and L.M. Wahl (2005) *Perspectives on the basic reproductive ratio*, J. Roy. Soc. Interface **2**: 281–293.

[15] Kermack, W.O. and A.G. McKendrick (1927) *A contribution to the mathematical theory of epidemics*, Proc. Roy. Soc. London **115**: 700–721.

[16] Levin, J.J. and D.F. Shea (1972) *On the asymptotic behavior of the bounded solutions of some integral equations, I, II, III*, J. Math. Anal. & Appl. **37**: 42–82, 288–326, 537–575.

[17] Mena-Lorca, J. and H.W. Hethcote (1992) *Dynamic models of infectious diseases as regulators of population size*, J. Math. Biol. **30**: 693–716.

[18] Meyers, L.A. (2007) *Contact network epidemiology: Bond percolation applied to infectious disease prediction and control*, Bull. Am. Math. Soc. **44**: 63–86.

[19] Meyers, L.A., M.E.J. Newman, and B. Pourbohloul (2006) *Predicting epidemics on directed contact networks*, J. Theor. Biol. **240**: 400–418.

[20] Miller, J.C. (2011) *A note on a paper by Erik Volz: SIR dynamics in random networks*, J. Math. Biol. **62**: 349–358.

[21] Miller, J.C. and E. Volz (2012) *Model hierarchies in edge-based compartmental modeling for infectious disease spread*, J. Math. Biol., DOI:10.1007/SO0285-012-0572-3.

[22] Newman, M.E.J. (2002) *The spread of epidemic disease on networks*, Phys. Rev. E **66**: 016128.

[23] Newman, M.E.J. (2003) *The structure and function of complex networks*, SIAM Rev. **45**: 167–256.

[24] Newman, M.E.J., S.H. Strogatz, and D.J. Watts (2001) *Random graphs with arbitrary degree distributions and their applications*, Phys. Rev. E **64**: 026118.

[25] Ross, R. (1911) *The Prevention of Malaria*, 2nd ed. (with Addendum), John Murray, London.

[26] Strogatz, S.H. (2001) *Exploring complex networks*, Nature **410**: 268–276.

[27] Van den Driessche, P. and J. Watmough (2002) *Reproduction numbers and subthreshold endemic equilibria for compartmental models of disease transmission*, Math. Biosc. **180**: 29–48.

[28] Volz, E. (2008) *SIR dynamics in random networks with heterogeneous connectivity*, J. Math. Biol. **56**: 293–310.

[29] Wallinga, J. and M. Lipsitch (2007) *How generation intervals shape the relationship between growth rates and reproductive numbers*, Proc. Roy. Soc. B **274**: 599–604.

[30] Yang, C.K. and F. Brauer (2008) *Calculation of $\mathcal{R}_0$ for age-of-infection models*, Math. Biosc. & Eng. **5**: 585–599.

Lecture 2

Models for Endemic Diseases

2.1 A Model for Diseases with No Immunity

We have been studying SIR models, in which the transitions are from susceptible to infective to removed, with the removal coming through recovery with full immunity (as in measles) or through death from the disease (as in plague, rabies, and many other animal diseases). Another type of model is an SIS model in which infectives return to the susceptible class on recovery because the disease confers no immunity against reinfection. Such models are appropriate for most diseases transmitted by bacterial or helminth agents and most sexually transmitted diseases (including gonorrhea, but not such diseases as AIDS, from which there is no recovery). One important way in which SIS models differ from SIR models is that there is a continuing flow of new susceptibles, namely recovered infectives. In the next section we will study models that include demographic effects, namely, births and deaths, another way in which a continuing flow of new susceptibles may arise.

The simplest SIS model, due to Kermack and McKendrick [13], is

$$\begin{aligned} S' &= -a\frac{S}{N}I + \alpha I, \\ I' &= a\frac{S}{N}I - \alpha I. \end{aligned} \tag{2.1}$$

This differs from the SIR model only in that the recovered members return to the class S at a rate αI instead of passing to the class R. The total population $N = S + I$ is a constant, since $(S+I)' = 0$. Sometimes population size is measured using N as the unit so that the total population size is one. We may reduce the model to a single differential equation by replacing S by $N - I$ to give the single differential equation

$$\begin{aligned} I' &= a\frac{N-I}{N}I - \alpha I = (a-\alpha)I - \frac{a}{N}I^2 \\ &= (a-\alpha)I\left(1 - \frac{I}{N - \frac{\alpha N}{a}}\right). \end{aligned} \tag{2.2}$$

As (2.2) is a logistic differential equation of the form

$$I' = rI\left(1 - \frac{I}{K}\right),$$

with $r = a - \alpha$ and with $K = N - \alpha N/a$, our qualitative result tells us that if $a - \alpha < 0$ or $a/\alpha < 1$, then all solutions of the model (2.2) with nonnegative initial values except the constant solution $I = K$ approach the limit zero as $t \to \infty$, while if $a\alpha > 1$, then all solutions with nonnegative initial values except the constant solution $I = 0$ approach the limit $K = N(1 - \alpha/a) > 0$ as $t \to \infty$. Thus there is always a single limiting value for I, but the value of the quantity $a\alpha$ determines which limiting value is approached, regardless of the initial state of the disease. In epidemiological terms this says that if the quantity a/α is less than one, the infection dies out in the sense that the number of infectives approaches zero. For this reason the equilibrium $I = 0$, which corresponds to $S = N$, is called the *disease-free equilibrium*. On the other hand, if the quantity $a/\alpha N$ exceeds one, the infection persists. The equilibrium $I = N(1 - \alpha/a)$, which corresponds to $S = \alpha N/a$, is called an *endemic* equilibrium.

As we have seen in epidemic models, the dimensionless quantity a/α is called the basic reproduction number or contact number for the disease, and it is usually denoted by $\mathcal{R}_0$. In studying an infectious disease, the determination of the basic reproduction number is invariably a vital first step. The value one for the basic reproduction number defines a threshold at which the course of the infection changes between disappearance and persistence. Since a is the number of contacts made by an average infective per unit time and $1/\alpha$ is the mean infective period, $\mathcal{R}_0$ represents the average number of secondary infections caused by each infective over the course of the infection. Thus, it is intuitively clear that if $\mathcal{R}_0 < 1$, the infection should die out, while if $\mathcal{R}_0 > 1$, the infection should establish itself. In more highly structured models than the simple one we have developed here the calculation of the basic reproduction number may be much more complicated, but the essential concept of the basic reproduction number as the number of secondary infections caused by an average infective over the course of the disease remains. However, there is a difference from the behavior of epidemic models. Here, the basic reproduction number determines whether the infection establishes itself or dies out, whereas in the SIR epidemic model the basic reproduction number determines whether there will be an epidemic or not.

We were able to reduce the system of two differential equations (2.1) to the single equation (2.2) because of the assumption that the total population $S + I$ is constant. If there are deaths due to the disease, this assumption is violated, and it would be necessary to use a two-dimensional system as a model. We shall consider this in a more general context in the next section.

For models in which there are births and deaths, so that the total population size is not constant, it is more convenient to use the per-capita contact rate $\beta(N) = a(N)/N$ rather than the contact rate $a(N)$. A model for a disease from which infectives recover with no immunity against reinfection and that includes births and deaths is

$$\begin{aligned} S' &= \Lambda(N) - \beta(N)SI - \mu S + f\alpha I, \\ I' &= \beta(N)SI - \alpha I - \mu I, \end{aligned} \tag{2.3}$$

describing a population with a density-dependent birth rate $\Lambda(N)$ per unit time, a density-dependent contact rate, a proportional death rate μ in each class, and with a rate α of departure from the infective class through recovery or disease death and with a fraction f of infectives recovering with no immunity against reinfection. In this model, if $f < 1$, the total population size is not constant and K represents a *carrying capacity*, or maximum possible population size, rather than a constant population size.

In the absence of disease the total population size N satisfies the differential equation

$$N' = \Lambda(N) - \mu N.$$

The *carrying capacity* of the population is the limiting population size K, satisfying

$$\Lambda(K) = \mu K, \qquad \Lambda'(K) < \mu.$$

The condition $\Lambda'(K) < \mu$ assures the asymptotic stability of the equilibrium population size K. It is reasonable to assume that K is the only positive equilibrium, so that

$$\Lambda(N) > \mu N$$

for $0 \leq N \leq K$. For most population models,

$$\Lambda(0) = 0, \qquad \Lambda''(N) \leq 0.$$

However, if $\Lambda(N)$ represents recruitment into a behavioral class, as would be natural for models of sexually transmitted diseases, it would be plausible to have $\Lambda(0) > 0$, or even to consider $\Lambda(N)$ to be a constant function. If $\Lambda(0) = 0$, we require $\Lambda'(0) > \mu$ because if this requirement is not satisfied, there is no positive equilibrium and the population would die out even in the absence of disease.

It is easy to verify that for (2.3)

$$\mathcal{R}_0 = \frac{K\beta(K)}{\mu + \alpha}.$$

If we add the two equations of (2.3), and use $N = S + I$, we obtain

$$N' = \Lambda(N) - \mu N - (1 - f)\alpha I.$$

We will carry out the analysis of the SIS model only in the special case $f = 1$, so that N approaches the constant K. In this case, the system (2.3) is asymptotically autonomous and its asymptotic behavior is the same as that of the single differential equation

$$I' = \beta(K)I(K - I) - (\alpha + \mu)I, \tag{2.4}$$

where S has been replaced by $K - I$. But (2.4) is a logistic equation which is easily solved analytically by separation of variables or qualitatively by an equilibrium analysis. We find that $I \to 0$ if $K\beta(K) < (\mu + \alpha)$, or $\mathcal{R}_0 < 1$ and $I \to I_\infty > 0$ with

$$I_\infty = K - \frac{\mu + \alpha}{\beta(K)} = K\left(1 - \frac{1}{\mathcal{R}_0}\right)$$

if $K\beta(K) > (\mu + \alpha)$ or $\mathcal{R}_0 > 1$.

The endemic equilibrium, which exists if $\mathcal{R}_0 > 1$, is always asymptotically stable. If $\mathcal{R}_0 < 1$, the system has only the disease-free equilibrium, and this equilibrium is asymptotically stable. The verification of these properties remains valid if there are no births and deaths. This suggests that a requirement for the existence of an endemic equilibrium is a flow of new susceptibles either through recovery without immunity against reinfection or through births.

2.2 The SIR Model with Births and Deaths

Epidemics that sweep through a population attract much attention and arouse a great deal of concern. We have omitted births and deaths in our description of epidemic models because the time scale of an epidemic is generally much shorter than the demographic time scale. In effect, we have used a time scale on which the number of births and deaths in unit time is negligible.

However, there are diseases that are endemic in many parts of the world and cause millions of deaths each year. To model a disease that may be endemic we need to think on a longer time scale and include births and deaths. A reference describing the properties of many endemic diseases is [1]. For diseases that are endemic in some region, public health physicians would like to be able to estimate the number of infectives at a given time as well as the rate at which new infections arise. The effects of quarantine or vaccine in reducing the number of victims are of importance, just as in the treatment of epidemics. In addition, the possibility of defeating the endemic nature of the disease and thus controlling or even eradicating the disease in a population is worthy of study.

The model of Kermack and McKendrick [13] includes births in the susceptible class proportional to the total population size and a death rate in each class proportional to the number of members in the class. This model allows the total population size to grow exponentially or die out exponentially if the birth and death rates are unequal. It is applicable to such questions as whether a disease will control the size of a population that would otherwise grow exponentially. We shall return to this topic, which is important in the study of many diseases in less developed countries with high birth rates. To formulate a model in which total population size remains bounded we could follow the approach suggested by Hethcote [9] in which the total population size K is held constant by making birth and death rates equal. Such a model is

$$\begin{aligned} S' &= -\beta SI + \mu(K - S), \\ I' &= \beta SI - \alpha I - \mu I, \\ R' &= \alpha I - \mu R. \end{aligned}$$

Because $S + I + R = K$, we can view R as determined when S and I are known and consider the two-dimensional system

$$\begin{aligned} S' &= -\beta SI + \mu(K - S), \\ I' &= \beta SI - \alpha I - \mu I. \end{aligned}$$

We shall examine a more general SIR model with births and deaths for a disease that may be fatal to some infectives. For such a disease the class R of removed members should contain only recovered members, not members removed by death from the disease. It is not possible to assume that the total population size remains constant if there are deaths due to disease; a plausible model for a disease that may be fatal to some infectives must allow the total population to vary in time.

With a general contact rate and a density-dependent birth rate we would have a model

$$\begin{aligned} S' &= \Lambda(N) - \beta(N)SI - \mu S, \\ I' &= \beta(N)SI - \mu I - \alpha I, \\ N' &= \Lambda(N) - (1 - f)\alpha I - \mu N. \end{aligned} \tag{2.5}$$

If $f = 1$, so that there are no disease deaths, the equation for N is

$$N' = \Lambda(N) - \mu N,$$

so that $N(t)$ approaches a limiting population size K. The theory of *asymptotically autonomous systems* [5, 15, 17, 18] implies that if N has a constant limit, then the system is equivalent to the system in which N is replaced by this limit. Then the system (2.5) is the same as the system

$$\begin{aligned} S' &= \Lambda - \beta SI - \mu S, \\ I' &= \beta SI - \mu I - \alpha I, \\ N' &= \Lambda - \mu N, \end{aligned} \tag{2.6}$$

with $\beta = \beta(N) = a(N)/N$, $\Lambda = \Lambda(N)$. In this model the total population size approaches a limit $K = \Lambda/\mu$ and K is the carrying capacity of the population. Since the system (2.6) is asymptotically autonomous, we may consider N as a constant and describe the model by the first two equations of (2.6).

We shall analyze the model (2.6) qualitatively. In view of the remark above, our analysis will also apply to the more general model (2.5) if there are no disease deaths. Analysis of the system (2.5) with $f < 1$ is much more difficult. We will confine our study of (2.5) to a description without details.

The first stage of the analysis is to note that the model (2.6) is a properly posed problem. That is, since $S' \geq 0$ if $S = 0$ and $I' \geq 0$ if $I = 0$, we have $S \geq 0, I \geq 0$ for $t \geq 0$ and since $N' \leq 0$ if $N = K$ we have $N \leq K$ for $t \geq 0$. Thus the solution always remains in the biologically realistic region $S \geq 0, I \geq 0, 0 \leq N \leq K$ if it starts in this region. By rights, we should verify such conditions whenever we analyze a mathematical model, but in practice this step is frequently overlooked.

Our approach will be to identify equilibria (constant solutions) and then to determine the asymptotic stability of each equilibrium. Asymptotic stability of an equilibrium means that a solution starting sufficiently close to the equilibrium remains close to the equilibrium and approaches it as $t \to \infty$, while instability of the equilibrium means that there are solutions starting arbitrarily close to the equilibrium that do not approach it. To find equilibria (S_∞, I_∞) we set the right side of each of the two equations equal to zero. The second of the resulting algebraic equations factors, giving two alternatives. The first alternative is $I_\infty = 0$, which will give a disease-free equilibrium, and the second alternative is $\beta S_\infty = \mu + \alpha$, which will give an endemic equilibrium, provided $\beta S_\infty = \mu + \alpha < \beta K$. If $I_\infty = 0$, the other equation gives $S_\infty = K = \Lambda/\mu$. For the endemic equilibrium the first equation gives

$$I_\infty = \frac{\Lambda}{\mu + \alpha} - \frac{\mu}{\beta}. \tag{2.7}$$

We linearize about an equilibrium (S_∞, I_∞) by letting $y = S - S_\infty$, $z = I - I_\infty$, writing the system in terms of the new variables y and z and retaining only the linear terms in a Taylor expansion. We obtain a system of two linear differential equations,

$$\begin{aligned} y' &= -(\beta I_\infty + \mu)y - \beta S_\infty z, \\ z' &= \beta I_\infty y + (\beta S_\infty - \mu - \alpha)z. \end{aligned}$$

The coefficient matrix of this linear system is

$$\begin{bmatrix} -\beta I_\infty - \mu & -\beta S_\infty \\ \beta I_\infty & \beta S_\infty - \mu - \alpha \end{bmatrix}.$$

We then look for solutions whose components are constant multiples of $e^{\lambda t}$; this means that λ must be an eigenvalue of the coefficient matrix. The condition that all solutions of the linearization at an equilibrium tend to zero as $t \to \infty$ is that the real part of every eigenvalue of this coefficient matrix is negative. At the disease-free equilibrium the matrix is

$$\begin{bmatrix} -\mu & -\beta K \\ 0 & \beta K - \mu - \alpha \end{bmatrix},$$

which has eigenvalues $-\mu$ and $\beta K - \mu - \alpha$. Thus, the disease-free equilibrium is asymptotically stable if $\beta K < \mu + \alpha$ and unstable if $\beta K > \mu + \alpha$. Note that this condition for instability of the disease-free equilibrium is the same as the condition for the existence of an endemic equilibrium.

In general, the condition that the eigenvalues of a 2×2 matrix have negative real part is that the determinant be positive and the trace (the sum of the diagonal elements) be negative. Since $\beta S_\infty = \mu + \alpha$ at an endemic equilibrium, the matrix of the linearization at an endemic equilibrium is

$$\begin{bmatrix} -\beta I_\infty - \mu & -\beta S_\infty \\ \beta I_\infty & 0 \end{bmatrix}, \tag{2.8}$$

and this matrix has positive determinant and negative trace. Thus, the endemic equilibrium, if there is one, is always asymptotically stable. If the quantity

$$\mathcal{R}_0 = \frac{\beta K}{\mu + \alpha} = \frac{K}{S_\infty} \tag{2.9}$$

is less than one, the system has only the disease-free equilibrium and this equilibrium is asymptotically stable. In fact, it is not difficult to prove that this asymptotic stability is *global*, that is, that every solution approaches the disease-free equilibrium. If the quantity $\mathcal{R}_0$ is greater than one, then the disease-free equilibrium is unstable, but there is an endemic equilibrium that is asymptotically stable. Again, the quantity $\mathcal{R}_0$ is the basic reproduction number. It depends on the particular disease (determining the parameter α) and on the rate of contacts, which may depend on the population density in the community being studied. The disease model exhibits a *threshold* behavior: If the basic reproduction number is less than one, the disease will die out, but if the basic reproduction number is greater than one, the disease will be endemic. Just as for the epidemic models of Lecture 1, the basic reproduction number is the number of secondary infections caused by a single infective introduced into a wholly susceptible population because the number of contacts per infective in unit time is βK, and the mean infective period (corrected for natural mortality) is $1/(\mu + \alpha)$.

There are two aspects of the analysis of the model (2.5) that are more complicated than the analysis of (2.6). The first is in the study of equilibria. Due to the dependence of $\Lambda(N)$ and $\beta(N)$ on N, it is necessary to use two of the equilibrium conditions to solve for S and I in terms of N and then substitute into the third condition to obtain an equation for N. Then by comparing the two sides of this equation for $N = 0$ and $N = K$ it is possible to show that there must be an endemic equilibrium value of N between 0 and K if $\mathcal{R}_0 > 1$.

The second complication is in the stability analysis. Since (2.5) is a three-dimensional system that cannot be reduced to a two-dimensional system, the coefficient matrix of its linearization at an equilibrium is a 3×3 matrix and the resulting characteristic equation is a cubic polynomial equation of the form

$$\lambda^3 + a_1\lambda^2 + a_2\lambda + a_3 = 0.$$

The *Routh–Hurwitz* conditions

$$a_1 > 0, \qquad a_1a_2 > a_3 > 0$$

are necessary and sufficient conditions for all roots of the characteristic equation to have negative real part. A technically complicated calculation is needed to verify that these conditions are satisfied at an endemic equilibrium for the model (2.5).

The asymptotic stability of the endemic equilibrium means that the compartment sizes approach a steady state. If the equilibrium had been unstable, there would have been a possibility of sustained oscillations. Oscillations in a disease model mean fluctuations in the number of cases to be expected, and if the oscillations have long period, this could also mean that experimental data for a short period would be quite unreliable as a predictor of the future. Epidemiological models that incorporate additional factors may exhibit oscillations. A variety of such situations is described in [11, 12].

The epidemic models of the previous chapter also exhibited a threshold behavior of a slightly different kind. For these models, which were SIR models without births or natural deaths, the threshold distinguished between a dying out of the disease and an epidemic or short-term spread of disease.

From the third equation of (2.6) we obtain

$$N' = \Lambda - \mu N - (1-f)\alpha I,$$

where $N = S + I + R$. From this we see that at the endemic equilibrium $N = K - (1-f)\alpha I/\mu$, and the reduction in the population size from the carrying capacity K is

$$(1-f)\frac{\alpha}{\mu}I_\infty = (1-f)\left[\frac{\alpha K}{\mu+\alpha} - \frac{\alpha}{\beta}\right].$$

The parameter α in the SIR model may be considered as describing the pathogenicity of the disease. If α is large, it is less likely that $\mathcal{R}_0 > 1$. If α is small, then the total population size at the endemic equilibrium is close to the carrying capacity K of the population. Thus, the maximum population decrease caused by disease will be for diseases of intermediate pathogenicity.

Numerical simulations indicate that the approach to endemic equilibrium for an SIR model is like a rapid and severe epidemic if the epidemiological and demographic time scales are very different. The same happens in the SIS model. If there are few disease deaths, the number of infectives at endemic equilibrium may be substantial, and there may be damped oscillations of large amplitude about the endemic equilibrium. For both the SIR and SIS models we may write the differential equation for I as

$$I' = I[\beta(N)S - (\mu+\alpha)] = \beta(N)I[S - S_\infty],$$

which implies that whenever S exceeds its endemic equilibrium value S_∞, I is increasing and epidemic-like behavior is possible. If $\mathcal{R}_0 < 1$ and $S < K$, it follows that $I' < 0$, and thus I is decreasing. Thus, if $\mathcal{R}_0 < 1$, I cannot increase and no epidemic can occur.

Next, we will turn to some applications of SIR and SIS models.

2.3 Some Applications

2.3.1 Herd immunity

In order to prevent a disease from becoming endemic it is necessary to reduce the basic reproduction number $\mathcal{R}_0$ below one. This may sometimes be achieved by immunization. If a fraction p of the Λ newborn members per unit time of the population is successfully immunized, the effect is to replace K by $K(1-p)$, and thus to reduce the basic reproduction number to $\mathcal{R}_0(1-p)$. The requirement $\mathcal{R}_0(1-p) < 1$ gives $1-p < 1/\mathcal{R}_0$, or

$$p > 1 - \frac{1}{\mathcal{R}_0}.$$

A population is said to have *herd immunity* if a large enough fraction has been immunized to assure that the disease cannot become endemic. The only disease for which this has actually been achieved worldwide is smallpox, for which $\mathcal{R}_0$ is approximately 5, so that 80 percent immunization does provide herd immunity.

For measles, epidemiological data in the United States indicate that $\mathcal{R}_0$ for rural populations ranges from 5.4 to 6.3, requiring vaccination of 81.5% to 84.1% of the population. In urban areas $\mathcal{R}_0$ ranges from 8.3 to 13.0, requiring vaccination of 88.0% to 92.3% of the population. In Great Britain, $\mathcal{R}_0$ ranges from 12.5 to 16.3, requiring vaccination of 92% to 94% of the population. The measles vaccine is not always effective, and vaccination campaigns are never able to reach everyone. As a result, herd immunity against measles has not been achieved (and probably never can be). Since smallpox is viewed as more serious and requires a lower percentage of the population be immunized, herd immunity was attainable for smallpox. In fact, smallpox has been eliminated; the last known case was in Somalia in 1977, and the virus is maintained now only in laboratories. The eradication of smallpox was actually more difficult than expected because high vaccination rates were achieved in some countries but not everywhere, and the disease persisted in some countries. The eradication of smallpox was possible only after an intensive campaign for worldwide vaccination [10].

2.3.2 Vertical transmission

In some diseases, notably Chagas disease, HIV/AIDS, hepatitis B, and rinderpest (in cattle), infection may be transferred not only horizontally (by contact between individuals) but also vertically (from an infected parent to a newly born offspring) [4]. We formulate an SIR model with vertical transmission by assuming that a fraction q of the offspring of infective members of the population are infective at birth. For simplicity, we assume that there are no disease deaths so that the total population size N is constant, and our model is based on (2.6). The birth rate in this model is $\Lambda = \mu N$, and we assume that births are distributed proportionally among compartments. Thus the rate of births to infectives is μI, and thus the rate of newborn infectives is $q\mu I$ and the rate of newborn susceptibles is $\mu N - q\mu I$. This leads to the model

$$\begin{aligned} S' &= \mu N - q\mu I - \beta S I - \mu S, \\ I' &= q\mu I + \beta S I - \mu I - \alpha I. \end{aligned} \tag{2.10}$$

From the second equation we see that equilibrium requires either $I = 0$ (disease-free) or $\beta S = \mu(1-q) + \alpha$. At the disease-free equilibrium, $S = N, I = 0$, and the matrix of the linearization is

$$\begin{bmatrix} -\mu & -q\mu - \beta N \\ 0 & \beta N - \mu(1-q) - \alpha \end{bmatrix}.$$

Thus the disease-free equilibrium is asymptotically stable if and only if

$$\beta N < \mu(1-q) + \alpha.$$

This suggests that

$$\mathcal{R}_0 = \frac{\beta N + \mu q}{\mu + \alpha}.$$

To see that this is indeed correct, we note that the term $\beta N/(\mu+\alpha)$ represents horizontally transmitted infections at rate βN over a death-adjusted infective period $1/(\mu+\alpha)$, and the term $\frac{\mu q}{\mu+\alpha}$ represents vertically transmitted infections per infective. It is not difficult to verify that the endemic equilibrium, which exists if and only if $\mathcal{R}_0 > 1$, is asymptotically stable.

2.4 The SIS Model with Births and Deaths

In order to describe a model for a disease from which infectives recover with immunity against reinfection and that includes births and deaths as in the model (2.6), we may modify the model (2.6) by removing the equation for R' and moving the term αI describing the rate of recovery from infection to the equation for S'. This gives the model

$$\begin{aligned} S' &= -\beta SI + \mu(K - S) + f\alpha I, \\ I' &= \beta SI - \alpha I - \mu I \end{aligned} \tag{2.11}$$

describing a population with a constant number of births μK per unit time, a proportional death rate μ in each class, and with a rate α of infectives leaving the infective class, with a fraction f recovering with no immunity against reinfection. In this model, if $f < 10$, the total population size is not constant and K represents a carrying capacity rather than a constant population size. The analysis of the model (2.11) is very similar to that of the SIR model (2.6), except that there is no equation for R' to be eliminated.

The only difference is the additional term $f\alpha I$ in the equation for S', and this does not change any of the qualitative results. As in the SIR model we have a basic reproductive number

$$\mathcal{R}_0 = \frac{\beta K}{\mu + \alpha} = \frac{K}{S_\infty},$$

and if $\mathcal{R}_0 < 1$, the disease-free equilibrium $S = K, I = 0$ is asymptotically stable, while if $\mathcal{R}_0 > 1$, there is an endemic equilibrium (S_∞, I_∞) with $\beta S_\infty = \mu + \alpha$ and I_∞ given by (2.7), which is asymptotically stable. There are, however, differences that are not disclosed by the qualitative analysis. If the epidemiological and demographic time scales are very different, for the SIR model we may observe that the approach to endemic equilibrium is like a rapid and severe epidemic. The same happens in the SIS model, especially if there is a significant number of deaths due to disease. If there are few disease deaths, the number of infectives at endemic equilibrium may be substantial, and there may be oscillations of large amplitude about the endemic equilibrium.

For both the SIR and SIS models we may write the differential equation for I as

$$I' = I\big[\beta S - (\mu + \alpha)\big] = \beta I[S - S_\infty],$$

which implies that whenever S exceeds its endemic equilibrium value, I is increasing and epidemic-like behavior is possible. If $\mathcal{R}_0 < 1$ and $S < K$, it follows that $I' < 0$, and thus I is decreasing. Thus, if $\mathcal{R}_0 < 1, I$ cannot increase and no epidemic can occur.

2.5 A Vaccination Model: Backward Bifurcations

In compartmental models for the transmission of communicable diseases there is usually a basic reproductive number $\mathcal{R}_0$, representing the mean number of secondary infections caused by a single infective introduced into a susceptible population. If $\mathcal{R}_0 < 1$, there is a disease-free equilibrium that is asymptotically stable, and the infection dies out. If $\mathcal{R}_0 > 1$, the usual situation is that there is an endemic equilibrium that is asymptotically stable, and the infection persists. Even if the endemic equilibrium is unstable, the instability commonly arises from a Hopf bifurcation and the infection still persists but in an oscillatory manner. More precisely, as $\mathcal{R}_0$ increases through 1 there is an exchange of stability between the disease-free equilibrium and the endemic equilibrium (which is negative as well as unstable and thus biologically meaningless if $\mathcal{R}_0 < 1$). There is a bifurcation, or change in equilibrium behavior, at $\mathcal{R}_0 = 1$, but the equilibrium infective population size depends continuously on $\mathcal{R}_0$. Such a transition is called a forward, or transcritical, bifurcation.

The behavior at a bifurcation may be described graphically by the bifurcation curve, which is the graph of equilibrium infective population size I as a function of the basic reproductive number $\mathcal{R}_0$. For a forward bifurcation, the bifurcation curve is as shown in Figure 2.1.

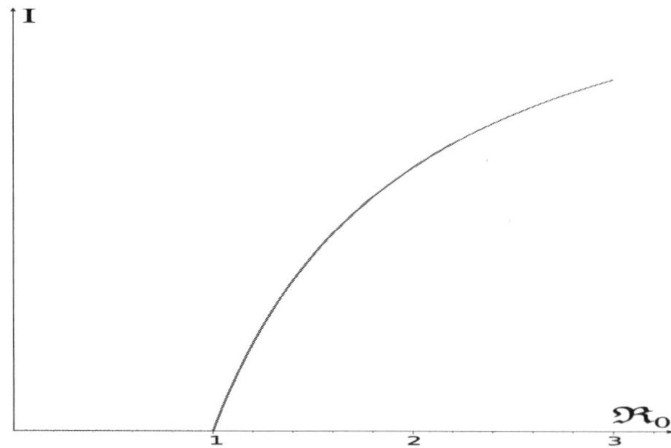

Figure 2.1. *Forward bifurcation.*

It has been noted [6, 7, 8, 14] that in epidemic models with multiple groups and asymmetry between groups or multiple interaction mechanisms it is possible to have a very different bifurcation behavior at $\mathcal{R}_0 = 1$. There may be multiple positive endemic equilibria for values of $\mathcal{R}_0 < 1$ and a backward bifurcation at $\mathcal{R}_0 = 1$. This means that the bifurcation

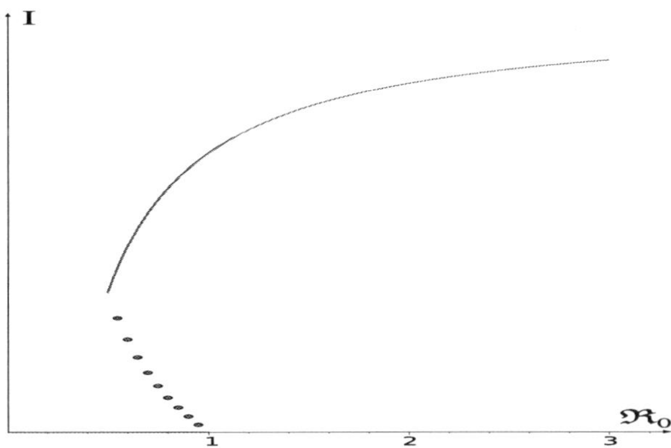

Figure 2.2. *Backward bifurcation.*

curve has the form shown in Figure 2.2 with a broken curve denoting an unstable endemic equilibrium that separates the domains of attraction of asymptotically stable equilibria.

The qualitative behavior of an epidemic system with a backward bifurcation differs from that of a system with a forward bifurcation in at least three important ways. If there is a forward bifurcation at $\mathcal{R}_0 = 1$, it is not possible for a disease to invade a population if $\mathcal{R}_0 < 1$, because the system will return to the disease-free equilibrium $I = 0$ if some infectives are introduced into the population. On the other hand, if there is a backward bifurcation at $\mathcal{R}_0 = 1$ and enough infectives are introduced into the population to put the initial state of the system above the unstable endemic equilibrium with $\mathcal{R}_0 < 1$, the system will approach the asymptotically stable endemic equilibrium.

Other differences are observed if the parameters of the system change to produce a change in $\mathcal{R}_0$. With a forward bifurcation at $\mathcal{R}_0 = 1$ the equilibrium infective population remains zero as long as $\mathcal{R}_0 < 1$ and then increases continuously as $\mathcal{R}_0$ increases. With a backward bifurcation at $\mathcal{R}_0 = 1$, the equilibrium infective population size also remains zero as long as $\mathcal{R}_0 < 1$ but then jumps to the positive endemic equilibrium as $\mathcal{R}_0$ increases through 1. In the other direction, if a disease is being controlled by means that decrease $\mathcal{R}_0$, it is sufficient to decrease $\mathcal{R}_0$ to 1 if there is a forward bifurcation at $\mathcal{R}_0 = 1$, but it is necessary to bring $\mathcal{R}_0$ well below 1 if there is a backward bifurcation.

These behavior differences are important in planning how to control a disease; a backward bifurcation at $\mathcal{R}_0 = 1$ makes control more difficult. One control measure often used is the reduction of susceptibility to infection produced by vaccination. By vaccination we mean either an inoculation that reduces susceptibility to infection or an education program such as encouragement of better hygiene or avoidance of risky behavior for sexually transmitted diseases. Whether vaccination is inoculation or education, typically it reaches only a fraction of the susceptible population and is not perfectly effective. In an apparent paradox, models with vaccination may exhibit backward bifurcations, making the behavior of the model more complicated than the corresponding model without vaccination. It has been argued [2] that a partially effective vaccination program applied to only part of the population at risk may increase the severity of outbreaks of such diseases as HIV/AIDS.

We will give a qualitative analysis of a two-dimensional model for which there is a possibility of a backward bifurcation. The model we will study adds vaccination to the simple SIS model (2.11) with no disease deaths, so that the total population size may be taken as constant [3].

We know that there is a disease-free equilibrium $I = 0$ that is asymptotically stable if

$$\mathcal{R}_0 = \frac{\beta K}{\mu + \alpha} < 1.$$

If $\mathcal{R}_0 > 1$, the disease-free equilibrium is unstable, but there is an endemic equilibrium that is asymptotically stable.

According to the theory of asymptotically autonomous systems, this result extends to the system

$$\begin{aligned} S' &= \Lambda(N) - \beta(N)SI - \mu S + \alpha I, \\ I' &= \beta SI - (\mu + \alpha)I, \end{aligned} \tag{2.12}$$

where the population carrying capacity K is now defined by $\Lambda(K) = \mu K$, $\Lambda'(K) < \mu$ and the contact rate $\beta(N)$ is now a function of total population size with $N\beta(N)$ nondecreasing and $\beta(N)$ nonincreasing.

To the model (2.12) we add the assumption that in unit time a fraction φ of the susceptible class is vaccinated. The vaccination may reduce but not completely eliminate susceptibility to infection. We model this by including a factor σ, $0 \le \sigma \le 1$, in the infection rate of vaccinated members, with $\sigma = 0$ meaning that the vaccine is perfectly effective and $\sigma = 1$ meaning that the vaccine has no effect. We describe the new model by including a vaccinated class V, with

$$\begin{aligned} S' &= \Lambda(N) - \beta(N)SI - (\mu + \varphi)S + \alpha I, \\ I' &= \beta(N)SI + \sigma\beta(N)VI - (\mu + \alpha)I, \\ V' &= \varphi S - \sigma\beta(N)VI - \mu V, \end{aligned} \tag{2.13}$$

and $N = S + I + V$. Again, $N' = \Lambda(N) - \mu N$ and $\lim_{t\to\infty} N(t) = K$ for every choice of initial values, and by the theory of asymptotically autonomous systems we may replace N by K and S by $K - I - V$ to give the qualitatively equivalent system

$$\begin{aligned} I' &= \beta[K - I - (1-\sigma)V]I - (\mu + \alpha)I, \\ V' &= \varphi[K - I] - \sigma\beta VI - (\mu + \varphi)V \end{aligned} \tag{2.14}$$

with $\beta = \beta(K)$. The system (2.14) is the basic vaccination model which we will analyze. We remark that if the vaccine is completely ineffective, $\sigma = 1$, then (2.14) is equivalent to an SIS model. If all susceptibles are vaccinated immediately (formally, $\varphi \to \infty$), the model (2.14) is equivalent to

$$I' = \sigma\beta I(K - I) - (\mu + \alpha)I,$$

which is an SIS model with basic reproductive number

$$\mathcal{R}_0^* = \frac{\sigma\beta K}{\mu + \alpha} = \sigma\mathcal{R}_0 \le \mathcal{R}_0.$$

We will think of the parameters μ, α, φ, and σ as fixed and view β as variable. In practice, the parameter φ is the one most easily controlled, and later we will express our results in terms of an uncontrolled model with parameters β, μ, α, and σ fixed and examine the effect of varying φ. With this interpretation in mind, we will use $\mathcal{R}(\varphi)$ to denote the basic reproductive number of the model (2.14), and we will see that

$$\mathcal{R}_0^* \leq \mathcal{R}(\varphi) \leq \mathcal{R}_0.$$

Equilibria of the model (2.14) are solutions of

$$\begin{aligned} \beta I[K - I - (1-\sigma)V] &= (\mu+\alpha)I, \\ \varphi[K - I] &= \sigma\beta V I + (\mu+\varphi)V. \end{aligned} \tag{2.15}$$

If $I = 0$, then the first of these equations is satisfied and the second leads to

$$V = \frac{\mu}{\mu+\varphi}K, \quad V = \frac{\varphi}{\mu+\varphi}K.$$

This is the disease-free equilibrium.

The matrix of the linearization of (2.14) at an equilibrium (I, V) is

$$\begin{bmatrix} -2\beta I - (1-\sigma)\beta V - (\mu+\alpha) + \beta K & -(1-\sigma)\beta I \\ -(\varphi+\sigma\beta V) & -(\mu+\varphi+\sigma\beta I) \end{bmatrix}.$$

At the disease-free equilibrium this matrix is

$$\begin{bmatrix} -(1-\sigma)\beta V - (\mu+\alpha) + \beta K & 0 \\ -(\varphi+\sigma\beta V) & -(\mu+\varphi) \end{bmatrix},$$

which has negative eigenvalues, implying the asymptotic stability of the disease-free equilibrium, if and only if

$$-(1-\sigma)\beta V - (\mu+\alpha) + \beta K < 0.$$

Using the value of V at the disease-free equilibrium, this condition is equivalent to

$$\mathcal{R}(\varphi) = \frac{\beta K}{\mu+\alpha} \cdot \frac{\mu+\theta+\sigma\varphi}{\mu+\theta+\varphi} = \mathcal{R}_0 \frac{\mu+\theta+\sigma\varphi}{\mu+\theta+\varphi} < 1.$$

The case $\varphi = 0$ is that of no vaccination with $\mathcal{R}(0) = \mathcal{R}_0$, and $\mathcal{R}(\varphi) < \mathcal{R}_0$ if $\varphi > 0$. We note that $\mathcal{R}_0^* = \sigma\mathcal{R}_0 = \lim_{\varphi\to\infty}\mathcal{R}(\varphi) < \mathcal{R}_0$.

If $0 \leq \sigma < 1$, endemic equilibriaare solutions of the pair of equations

$$\begin{aligned} \beta[K - I - (1-\sigma)V] &= \mu+\alpha, \\ \varphi[K - I] &= \sigma\beta V I + (\mu+\varphi)V. \end{aligned} \tag{2.16}$$

We eliminate V using the first equation of (2.16) and substitute into the second equation to give an equation of the form

$$AI^2 + BI + C = 0 \tag{2.17}$$

with

$$
\begin{aligned}
A &= \sigma\beta, \\
B &= (\mu+\theta+\sigma\varphi)+\sigma(\mu+\alpha)-\sigma\beta K, \\
C &= \frac{(\mu+\alpha)(\mu+\theta+\varphi)}{\beta}-(\mu+\theta+\sigma\varphi)K.
\end{aligned}
\tag{2.18}
$$

If $\sigma = 0$, (2.17) is a linear equation with unique solution:

$$
I = K - \frac{(\mu+\alpha)(\mu+\theta+\varphi)}{\beta(\mu+\theta)} = K\left[1-\frac{1}{\mathcal{R}(\varphi)}\right],
$$

which is positive if and only if $\mathcal{R}(\varphi) > 1$. Thus if $\sigma = 0$, there is a unique endemic equilibrium if $\mathcal{R}(\varphi) > 1$ that approaches zero as $\mathcal{R}(\varphi) \to 1+$ and there cannot be an endemic equilibrium if $\mathcal{R}(\varphi) < 1$. In this case it is not possible to have a backward bifurcation at $\mathcal{R}(\varphi) = 1$.

We note that $C < 0$ if $\mathcal{R}(\varphi) > 1$, $C = 0$ if $\mathcal{R}(\varphi) = 1$, and $C > 0$ if $\mathcal{R}(\varphi) < 1$. If $\sigma > 0$, so that (2.17) is quadratic and if $\mathcal{R}(\varphi) > 1$, then there is a unique positive root of (2.17) and thus there is a unique endemic equilibrium. If $\mathcal{R}(\varphi) = 1$, then $C = 0$ and there is a unique nonzero solution of (2.17) $I = -B/A$ which is positive if and only if $B < 0$. If $B < 0$, when $C = 0$ there is a positive endemic equilibrium for $\mathcal{R}(\varphi) = 1$. Since equilibria depend continuously on φ there must then be an interval to the left of $\mathcal{R}(\varphi) = 1$ on which there are two positive equilibria

$$
I = \frac{-B \pm \sqrt{B^2-4AC}}{2A}.
$$

This establishes that the system (2.14) has a backward bifurcation at $\mathcal{R}(\varphi) = 1$ if and only if $B < 0$ when β is chosen to make $C = 0$.

We can give an explicit criterion in terms of the parameters μ, φ, σ for the existence of a backward bifurcation at $\mathcal{R}(\varphi) = 1$. When $\mathcal{R}(\varphi) = 1$, $C = 0$ so that

$$
(\mu+\sigma\varphi)\beta K = (\mu+\alpha)(\mu+\varphi). \tag{2.19}
$$

The condition $B < 0$ is

$$
(\mu+\sigma\varphi)+\sigma(\mu+\alpha) < \sigma\beta K
$$

with βK determined by (2.19), or

$$
\sigma(\mu+\alpha)(\mu+\varphi) > (\mu+\sigma\varphi)[(\mu+\sigma\varphi)+\sigma(\mu+\alpha)],
$$

which reduces to

$$
\sigma(1-\sigma)(\mu+\alpha)\varphi > (\mu+\sigma\varphi)^2. \tag{2.20}
$$

A backward bifurcation occurs at $\mathcal{R}(\varphi) = 1$, with βK given by (2.19) if and only if (2.20) is satisfied. We point out that for an SI model, where $\alpha = 0$, the condition (2.20) becomes

$$
\sigma(1-\sigma)\mu\varphi > (\mu+\sigma\varphi)^2.
$$

But

$$(\mu+\sigma\varphi)^2 = \mu^2+\sigma^2\varphi^2+2\mu\sigma\varphi$$
$$> 2\mu\sigma\varphi > \sigma(1-\sigma)\mu\varphi$$

because $\sigma < 1$. Thus a backward bifurcation is not possible if $\alpha = 0$, that is, for an SI model. Likewise, (2.20) cannot be satisfied if $\sigma = 0$.

If $C > 0$ and either $B \geq 0$ or $B^2 < 4AC$, there are no positive solutions of (2.17) and thus there are no endemic equilibria. Equation (2.17) has two positive solutions, corresponding to two endemic equilibria, if and only if $C > 0$, or $\mathcal{R}(\varphi) < 1$, and $B < 0$, $B^2 > 4AC$, or $B < -2\sqrt{AC} < 0$. If $B = -2\sqrt{AC}$, there is one positive solution $I = -B/2A$ of (2.17).

If (2.20) is satisfied, so that there is a backward bifurcation at $\mathcal{R}(\varphi) = 1$, there are two endemic equilibria for an interval of values of β from

$$\beta K = \frac{(\mu+\alpha)(\mu+\varphi)}{\mu+\sigma\varphi}$$

corresponding to $\mathcal{R}(\varphi) = 1$ to a value β_c defined by $B = -2\sqrt{AC}$. To calculate β_c, we let $x = \mu+\alpha-\beta K$, $U = \mu+\sigma\varphi$ to give $B = \sigma x+U$, $\beta C = \beta KU+(\mu+\alpha)(\mu+\varphi)$. Then $B^2 = 4AC$ becomes

$$(\sigma x+U)^2+4\beta\sigma KU-4\sigma(\mu+\alpha)(\mu+\varphi) = 0,$$

which reduces to

$$(\sigma x)^2-2U(\sigma x)+\left[U^2+4\sigma(1-\sigma)(\mu+\alpha)\varphi\right] = 0$$

with roots

$$\sigma x = U \pm 2\sqrt{\sigma(1-\sigma)(\mu+\alpha)\varphi}.$$

For the positive root $B = \sigma x+U > 0$, and since we require $B < 0$ as well as $B^2-4AC = 0$, we obtain β_c from $\sigma x = U-2\sqrt{\sigma(1-\sigma)(\mu+\alpha)\varphi}$ so that

$$\sigma\beta_c K = \sigma(\mu+\alpha)+2\sqrt{\sigma(1-\sigma)(\mu+\alpha)\varphi}-(\mu+\sigma\varphi). \tag{2.21}$$

Then the critical basic reproductive number $\mathcal{R}_c$ is given by

$$\mathcal{R}_c = \frac{\mu+\sigma\varphi}{\mu+\varphi}\cdot\frac{\sigma(\mu+\alpha)+2\sqrt{\sigma(1-\sigma)(\mu+\alpha)\varphi}-(\mu+\sigma\varphi)}{\sigma(\mu+\alpha)\varphi}$$

and it is easy to verify with the aid of (2.21) that $\mathcal{R}_c < 1$.

2.5.1 The bifurcation curve

In drawing the bifurcation curve (the graph of I as a function of $\mathcal{R}(\varphi)$), we think of β as variable with the other parameters $\mu,\alpha,\sigma,Q,\varphi$ as constant. Then $\mathcal{R}(\varphi)$ is a constant multiple of β and we can think of β as the independent variable in the bifurcation curve.

Implicit differentiation of the equilibrium condition (2.17) with respect to β gives

$$(2AI+B)\frac{dI}{d\beta} = \sigma I(K-I) + \frac{(\mu+\alpha)(\mu+\varphi)}{\beta^2}.$$

It is clear from the first equilibrium condition in (2.16) that $I \leq K$, and this implies that the bifurcation curve has positive slope at equilibrium values with $2AI+B>0$ and negative slope at equilibrium values with $2AI+B<0$. If there is not a backward bifurcation at $\mathcal{R}(\varphi)=1$, then the unique endemic equilibrium for $\mathcal{R}(\varphi)>1$ satisfies

$$2AI+B=\sqrt{B^2-4AC}>0,$$

and the bifurcation curve has positive slope at all points where $I>0$. Thus the bifurcation curve is as shown in Figure 2.1.

If there is a backward bifurcation at $\mathcal{R}(\varphi)=1$, then there is an interval on which there are two endemic equilibria given by

$$2AI+B=\pm\sqrt{B^2-4AC}.$$

The bifurcation curve has negative slope at the smaller of these and positive slope at the larger of these. Thus the bifurcation curve is as shown in Figure 2.2.

The condition $2AI+B>0$ is also significant in the local stability analysis of endemic equilibria. An endemic equilibrium of (2.14) is (locally) asymptotically stable if and only if it corresponds to a point on the bifurcation curve at which the curve is increasing. To prove this, we observe that the matrix of the linearization of (2.14) at an equilibrium (I,V) is

$$\begin{bmatrix} -2\beta I-(1-\sigma)\beta V-(\mu+\alpha)+\beta K & -(1-\sigma)\beta I \\ -(\varphi+\sigma\beta V) & -(\mu+\varphi+\sigma\beta I) \end{bmatrix}.$$

Because of the equilibrium conditions (2.16), the matrix at an endemic equilibrium (I,V) is

$$\begin{bmatrix} -\beta I & -(1-\sigma)\beta I \\ -(\varphi+\sigma\beta V) & -(\mu+\varphi+\sigma\beta I) \end{bmatrix}.$$

This has negative trace, and its determinant is

$$\begin{aligned} &\sigma(\beta I)^2+\beta I(\mu+\varphi)-(1-\sigma)\varphi\beta I-(1-\sigma)\beta V\cdot\sigma\beta I \\ &=\beta I\big[2\sigma\beta I+(\mu+\sigma\varphi)+\sigma(\mu+\alpha)-\sigma\beta K\big] \\ &=\beta I[2AI+B]. \end{aligned}$$

If $2AI+B>0$, that is, if the bifurcation curve has positive slope, then the determinant is positive and the equilibrium is asymptotically stable. If $2AI+B<0$, the determinant is negative and the equilibrium is unstable. In fact, it is a saddle point and its stable separatrices in the (I,V) plane separate the domains of attraction of the other (asymptotically stable) endemic equilibrium and the disease-free equilibrium.

2.6 Temporary Immunity

In the SIR models that we have studied, it has been assumed that the immunity received by recovery from the disease is permanent. This is not always true, as there may be a gradual loss of immunity with time. In addition, there are often mutations in a virus, and as a result the active disease strain is sufficiently different from the strain from which an individual has recovered that the immunity received may wane.

Temporary immunity may be described by an $SIRS$ model in which a rate of transfer from R to S is added to an SIR model. For simplicity, we confine our attention to epidemic models, without including births, natural deaths, and disease deaths, but the analysis of models including births and deaths would lead to the same conclusions. Thus we begin with a model

$$\begin{aligned} S' &= -\beta SI + \theta R, \\ I' &= \beta SI - \alpha I, \\ R' &= \alpha I - \theta R, \end{aligned}$$

with a proportional rate θ of loss of immunity.

Since $N' = (S + I + R)' = 0$, the total population size N is constant, and we may replace R by $N - S - I$ and reduce the model to a two-dimensional system,

$$\begin{aligned} S' &= -\beta SI + \theta(N - S - I), \\ I' &= \beta SI - \alpha I. \end{aligned} \tag{2.22}$$

Equilibria are solutions of the system

$$\begin{aligned} \beta SI + \theta S + \theta I &= \theta N, \\ \alpha I + \theta S + \theta I &= \theta N, \end{aligned}$$

and there is a disease-free equilibrium $S = \alpha/\beta, I = 0$. If $\mathcal{R}_0 = \beta N/\alpha > 1$, there is also an endemic equilibrium with

$$\beta S = \alpha, \quad (\alpha + \theta)I = \theta(N - S).$$

The matrix of the linearization of (2.22) at an equilibrium (S, I) is

$$A = \begin{bmatrix} -(\beta I + \theta) & -(\beta S + \theta) \\ \beta I & \beta S - \alpha \end{bmatrix}.$$

At the disease-free equilibrium A has the sign structure

$$\begin{bmatrix} - & - \\ 0 & \beta N - \alpha \end{bmatrix}.$$

This matrix has negative trace and positive determinant if and only if $\beta N < \alpha$, or $\mathcal{R}_0 < 1$. At an endemic equilibrium, the matrix has sign structure

$$\begin{bmatrix} - & - \\ + & 0 \end{bmatrix},$$

and thus always has negative trace and positive determinant. We see from this that, as in other models studied in this lecture, the disease-free equilibrium is asymptotically stable if and only if the basic reproduction number is less than 1 and the endemic equilibrium, which exists if and only if the basic reproduction number exceeds 1, is always asymptotically stable. However, it is possible for a different $SIRS$ model to have quite different behavior.

We consider an $SIRS$ model, which assumes a constant period of temporary immunity following recovery from the infection in place of an exponentially distributed period of temporary immunity. It will turn out that the endemic equilibrium for this model may be unstable, thus giving an example of a generalization that leads to new possibilities for the behavior of a model.

We add the assumption that there is a temporary immunity period of fixed length ω, after which recovered infectives revert to the susceptible class. The resulting model is described by the system

$$\begin{aligned} S'(t) &= -\beta S(t)I(t) + \alpha I(t-\omega), \\ I'(t) &= \beta S(t)I(t) - \alpha I(t), \\ R'(t) &= \alpha I(t) - \alpha I(t-\omega). \end{aligned}$$

Since $N = S + I + R$ is constant, we may discard the equation for R and use the two-dimensional model

$$\begin{aligned} S'(t) &= -\beta S(t)I(t) + \alpha I(t-\omega), \\ I'(t) &= \beta S(t)I(t) - \alpha I(t). \end{aligned} \tag{2.23}$$

Equilibria are given by $I = 0$ or $\beta S = \alpha$. There is a disease-free equilibrium $S = N, I = 0$. There is also an endemic equilibrium for which $\beta S = \alpha$. However, the two equations for S and I give only a single equilibrium condition. To determine the endemic equilibrium (S_∞, I_∞) we must write the equation for R in the integrated form

$$R(t) = \int_{t-\omega}^{t} \alpha I(x)dx$$

to give $R_\infty = \omega\alpha I_\infty$. We also have $\beta S_\infty = \alpha$, and from $S_\infty + I_\infty + R_\infty = N$ we obtain

$$\beta I_\infty = \frac{\beta N - \alpha}{1 + \omega\alpha}.$$

The characteristic equation at an equilibrium is the condition that the linearization at the equilibrium have a solution whose components are constant multiples of $e^{\lambda t}$. In the ordinary differential equation case this is just the equation that determines the eigenvalues of the coefficient matrix, a polynomial equation, but in the general case it is a transcendental equation. The result on which our analysis depends is that an equilibrium is asymptotically stable if all roots of the characteristic equation have negative real part, or equivalently that the characteristic equation have no roots with real part greater than or equal to zero.

To linearize about an equilibrium (S_∞, I_∞) of (2.23) we substitute

$$S(t) = S_\infty + u(t), \quad I(t) = I_\infty + v(t)$$

and neglect the quadratic term, giving the linearization

$$\begin{aligned} u'(t) &= -\beta I_\infty u(t) - \beta S_\infty v(t) + \alpha v(t-\omega), \\ v'(t) &= \beta I_\infty u(t) + \beta S_\infty v(t) - \alpha v(t). \end{aligned}$$

The characteristic equation is the condition on λ that this linearization have a solution

$$u(t) = u_0 e^{\lambda t}, \quad v(t) = v_0 e^{\lambda t},$$

and this is

$$\begin{aligned}(\beta I_\infty + \lambda)u_0 + (\beta S_\infty - \alpha e^{-\lambda\omega}) &= 0,\\ \beta I_\infty u_0 + (\beta S_\infty - \alpha - \lambda) &= 0,\end{aligned}$$

or

$$\det \begin{bmatrix} \lambda + \beta I_\infty & \beta S_\infty - \alpha e^{\lambda\omega} \\ \beta I_\infty & \beta S_\infty - \alpha - \lambda \end{bmatrix}.$$

This reduces to

$$\beta\alpha I_\infty \frac{1 - e^{-\omega\lambda}}{\lambda} = -[\lambda + \beta S_\infty + \beta I_\infty - \alpha]. \tag{2.24}$$

At the disease-free equilibrium $S_\infty = N$, $I_\infty = 0$, this reduces to a linear equation with a single root $\lambda = \beta N - \alpha$, which is negative if and only if $\mathcal{R}_0 = \beta N/\alpha < 1$.

We think of ω and N as fixed and consider β and α as parameters. If $\alpha = 0$, (2.24) is linear and its only root is $-\beta I_\infty < 0$. Thus, there is a region in the (β, α) parameter space containing the β-axis in which all roots of (2.24) have negative real part. In order to find how large this stability region is we make use of the fact that the roots of (2.24) depend continuously on β and α. A root can move into the right half-plane only by passing through the value zero or by crossing the imaginary axis as β and α vary. Thus, the stability region contains the β-axis and extends into the plane until there is a root $\lambda = 0$ or until there is a pair of pure imaginary roots $\lambda = \pm iy$ with $y > 0$. Since the left side of (2.24) is positive and the right side of (2.24) is negative for real $\lambda \geq 0$, there cannot be a root $\lambda = 0$.

The condition that there is a root $\lambda = iy$ is

$$\alpha\beta I_\infty \frac{1 - e^{-i\omega\alpha}}{iy} = -(\beta I_\infty + iy) \tag{2.25}$$

and separation into real and imaginary parts gives the pair of equations

$$\alpha \frac{\sin \omega y}{y} = -1, \qquad \alpha\beta I_\infty \frac{1 - \cos \omega y}{y} = y. \tag{2.26}$$

To satisfy the first condition it is necessary to have $\omega\alpha > 1$ since $|\sin \omega y| \leq |\omega y|$ for all y. This implies, in particular, that the endemic equilibrium is asymptotically stable if $\omega\alpha < 1$. In addition, it is necessary to have $\sin \omega y < 0$. There is an infinite sequence of intervals on which $\sin \omega y < 0$, the first being $\pi < \omega y < 2\pi$. For each of these intervals equations (2.26) define a curve in the (β, α) plane parametrically with y as parameter. The region in the plane below the first of these curves is the region of asymptotic stability, that is, the set of values of β and α for which the endemic equilibrium is asymptotically stable. This curve is shown for $\omega = 1$, $N = 1$ in Figure 2.3. Since $\mathcal{R}_0 = \beta/\alpha > 1$, only the portion of the (β,α) plane below the line $\alpha = \beta$ is relevant.

The new feature of the model of this section is that the endemic equilibrium is not asymptotically stable for all parameter values. What is the behavior of the model if the

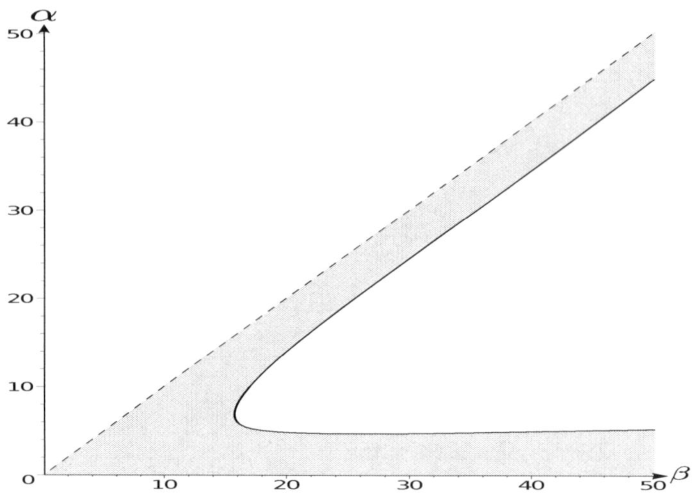

Figure 2.3. *Region of asymptotic stability for endemic equilibria* ($\omega = 1$, $N = 1$).

parameters are such that the endemic equilibrium is unstable? A plausible suggestion is that since the loss of stability corresponds to a root $\lambda = iy$ of the characteristic equation there are solutions of the model behaving like the real part of e^{iyt}, that is, there are periodic solutions. This is exactly what happens according to a very general result called the Hopf bifurcation theorem, which says that when roots of the characteristic equation cross the imaginary axis a stable periodic orbit arises.

From an epidemiological point of view periodic behavior is unpleasant. It implies fluctuations in the number of infectives which makes it difficult to allocate resources for treatment. It is also possible for oscillations to have a long period. This means that if data are measured over only a small time interval, the actual behavior may not be displayed. Thus, the identification of situations in which an endemic equilibrium is unstable is an important problem.

2.7 Diseases in Exponentially Growing Populations

Many parts of the world experienced very rapid population growth in the 18th century. The population of Europe increased from 118 million in 1700 to 187 million in 1800. In the same time period the population of Great Britain increased from 5.8 million to 9.15 million, and the population of China increased from 150 million to 313 million [16]. The population of English colonies in North America grew much more rapidly than this, aided by substantial immigration from England, but the native population, which had been reduced to one-tenth of their previous size by disease following the early encounters with Europeans and European diseases, grew even more rapidly. While some of these population increases may be explained by improvements in agriculture and food production, it appears that an even more important factor was the decrease in the death rate due to diseases. Disease death rates dropped sharply in the 18th century, partly from better understanding of the links between illness and sanitation and partly because the recurring invasions of bubonic plague subsided, perhaps due to reduced susceptibility. One plausible explanation for these population increases is that the bubonic plague invasions served to control the population size, and when this control was removed the population size increased rapidly.

In developing countries it is quite common to have high birth rates and high disease death rates. In fact, when disease death rates are reduced by improvements in health care and sanitation it is common for birth rates to decline as well, as families no longer need to have as many children to ensure that enough children survive to take care of the older generations. Again, it is plausible to assume that population size would grow exponentially in the absence of disease but is controlled by disease mortality.

The SIR model with births and deaths of Kermack and McKendrick [13] includes births in the susceptible class proportional to population size and a natural death rate in each class proportional to the size of the class. Let us analyze a model of this type with birth rate r and a natural death rate $\mu < r$. For simplicity we assume the disease is fatal to all infectives with disease death rate α, so that there is no removed class and the total population size is $N = S + I$. Our model is

$$\begin{aligned} S' &= r(S+I) - \beta SI - \mu S, \\ I' &= \beta SI - (\mu + \alpha)I. \end{aligned} \tag{2.27}$$

From the second equation we see that equilibria are given by either $I = 0$ or $\beta S = \mu + \alpha$. If $I = 0$, the first equilibrium equation is $rS = \mu S$, which implies $S = 0$ since $r > \mu$. It is easy to see that the equilibrium (0,0) is unstable. What actually would happen if $I = 0$ is that the susceptible population would grow exponentially with exponent $r - \mu > 0$. If $\beta S = \mu + \alpha$, the first equilibrium condition gives

$$r\frac{\mu+\alpha}{\beta} + rI - (\mu+\alpha)I - \frac{\mu(\mu+\alpha)}{\beta} = 0,$$

which leads to

$$(\alpha + \mu - r)I = \frac{(r-\mu)(\mu+\alpha)}{\beta}.$$

Thus, there is an endemic equilibrium, provided $r < \alpha + \mu$, and it is possible to show by linearizing about this equilibrium that it is asymptotically stable. On the other hand, if $r > \alpha + \mu$, there is no positive equilibrium value for I. In this case we may add the two differential equations of the model to give

$$N' = (r-\mu)N - \alpha I \geq (r-\mu)N - \alpha N = (r - \mu - \alpha)N,$$

and from this we may deduce that N grows exponentially. For this model we either have an asymptotically stable endemic equilibrium or population size grows exponentially. In the case of exponential population growth we may have either vanishing of the infection or an exponentially growing number of infectives.

If only susceptibles contribute to the birth rate, as may be expected if the disease is sufficiently debilitating, the behavior of the model is quite different. Let us consider the model

$$\begin{aligned} S' &= rS - \beta SI - \mu S = S(r - \mu - \beta I), \\ I' &= \beta SI - (\mu+\alpha)I = I(\beta S - \mu - \alpha), \end{aligned} \tag{2.28}$$

which has the same form as the Lotka–Volterra predator-prey model of population dynamics. This system has two equilibria, obtained by setting the right sides of each of the equations equal to zero, namely, (0,0), and an endemic equilibrium $((\mu+\alpha)/\beta,(r-\mu)/\beta)$. It turns out that the qualitative analysis approach we have been using is not helpful as the equilibrium (0,0) is unstable and the eigenvalues of the coefficient matrix at the endemic equilibrium have real part zero. In this case the behavior of the linearization does not necessarily carry over to the full system. However, we can obtain information about the behavior of the system by a method that begins with the elementary approach of separation of variables for first order differential equations. We begin by taking the quotient of the two differential equations and using the relation

$$\frac{I'}{S'} = \frac{dI}{dS}$$

to obtain the separable first order differential equation

$$\frac{dI}{dS} = \frac{I(\beta S - \mu - \alpha)}{S(r - \beta I)}.$$

Separation of variables gives

$$\int \left(\frac{r}{I} - \beta\right) dI = \int \left(\beta - \frac{\mu+\alpha}{S}\right) dS.$$

Integration gives the relation

$$\beta(S+I) - r\log I - (\mu+\alpha)\log S = c,$$

where c is a constant of integration. This relation shows that the quantity

$$V(S,I) = \beta(S+I) - r\log I - (\mu+\alpha)\log S$$

is constant on each orbit (path of a solution in the (S,I) plane). Each of these orbits is a closed curve corresponding to a periodic solution.

This model is the same as the simple epidemic model of Section 1.2 except for the birth and death terms, and in many examples the time scale of the disease is much faster than the time scale of the demographic process. We may view the model as describing an epidemic initially, leaving a susceptible population small enough that infection cannot establish itself. Then there is a steady population growth until the number of susceptibles is large enough for an epidemic to recur. During this growth stage the infective population is very small and random effects may wipe out the infection, but the immigration of a small number of infectives will eventually restart the process. As a result, we would expect recurrent epidemics. In fact, bubonic plague epidemics did recur in Europe for several hundred years. If we modify the demographic part of the model to assume limited population growth rather than exponential growth in the absence of disease, the effect would be to give behavior like that of the model studied in the previous section, with an endemic equilibrium that is approached slowly in an oscillatory manner if $\mathcal{R}_0 > 1$.

Bibliography

[1] Anderson, R.M. and R.M. May (1991) *Infectious Diseases of Humans*, Oxford University Press, Oxford.

[2] Blower, S.M. and A.R. Mclean (1994) *Prophylactic vaccines, risk behavior change, and the probability of eradicating HIV in San Francisco*, Science **265**: 1451–1454.

[3] Brauer, F. (2004) *Backward bifurcations in simple vaccination models*, J. Math. Anal. & Appl. **298**: 418–431.

[4] Busenberg, S. and K.L. Cooke (1993) *Vertically Transmitted Diseases: Models and Dynamics,* Biomathematics **23**, Springer-Verlag, Berlin, Heidelberg, New York.

[5] Castillo-Chavez, C. and H.R. Thieme (1993) *Asymptotically autonomous epidemic models*, in Mathematical Population Dynamics: Analysis of Heterogeneity, Vol. 1, Theory of Epidemics, O. Arino, D. Axelrod, M. Kimmel, and M. Langlais, eds., Wuerz, Winnipeg: 33–50.

[6] Dushoff, J., W. Huang, and C. Castillo-Chavez (1998) *Backwards bifurcations and catastrophe in simple models of fatal diseases*, J. Math. Biol. **36**: 227–248.

[7] Hadeler, K.P. and C. Castillo-Chavez (1995) *A core group model for disease transmission*, Math Biosc. **128**: 41–55.

[8] Hadeler, K.P. and P. van den Driessche (1997) *Backward bifurcation in epidemic control*, Math. Biosc. **146**: 15–35.

[9] Hethcote, H.W. (1976) *Qualitative analysis for communicable disease models*, Math. Biosc. **28**: 335–356.

[10] Hethcote, H.W. (1978) *An immunization model for a heterogeneous population*, Theor. Pop. Biol. **14**: 338–349.

[11] Hethcote, H.W. and S.A. Levin (1989) *Periodicity in epidemic models*, in Applied Mathematical Ecology, S.A. Levin, T.G. Hallam, and L.J. Gross, eds., Biomathematics **18**, Springer-Verlag, Berlin, Heidelberg, New York: 193–211.

[12] Hethcote, H.W., H.W. Stech, and P. van den Driessche (1981) *Periodicity and stability in epidemic models: A survey*, in Differential Equations and Applications in Ecology, Epidemics and Population Problems, S. Busenberg and K.L. Cooke, eds., Academic Press, New York: 65–82.

[13] Kermack, W.O. and A.G. McKendrick (1932) *Contributions to the mathematical theory of epidemics, part II*, Proc. Roy. Soc. London **138**: 55–83.

[14] Kribs-Zaleta, C.M. and J.X. Velasco-Hernandez (2000), *A simple vaccination model with multiple endemic states*, Math Biosc. **164**: 183–201.

[15] Markus, L. (1956) *Asymptotically autonomous differential systems*, in Contributions to the Theory of Nonlinear Oscillations III, S. Lefschetz, ed., Annals of Mathematics Studies **36**, Princeton University Press, Princeton, NJ: 17–29.

[16] McNeill, W.H. (1976) *Plagues and Peoples,* Doubleday, New York.

[17] Thieme, H.R. (1994) *Asymptotically autonomous differential equations in the plane*, Rocky Mountain J. Math. **24**: 351–380.

[18] Thieme, H.R. and C. Castillo-Chavez (1993) *How may infection-age-dependent infectivity affect the dynamics of HIV/AIDS?*, SIAM J. Appl. Math. **53**: 1447–1479.

Lecture 3

Heterogeneity in Epidemic Models

3.1 Introduction to Heterogeneity

The classical simple epidemic models [1, 2, 3, 11, 20] assume homogeneous mixing of members of the population being studied, and this is certainly unrealistically simple. Members of the population may differ, for example, in rate of contact. In the study of sexually transmitted diseases differences in activity levels are important aspects. Contact rates may be age-dependent, and this would suggest the use of age-structured models. In this lecture we consider heterogeneity in behavior, specifically contact rates. In a later lecture we will look at age structure in disease transmission models.

We begin with an epidemic vaccination model as an example of behavioral heterogeneity introduced into a homogeneous epidemic model.

3.2 A Vaccination Model

To cope with annual seasonal influenza epidemics there is a program of vaccination before the "flu" season begins. Each year a vaccine is produced aimed at protecting against the three influenza strains considered most dangerous for the coming season. We formulate a model to add vaccination to the simple SIR model (1.2) under the assumption that vaccination reduces susceptibility (the probability of infection if a contact with an infected member of the population is made).

We consider a population of total size N and assume that a fraction γ of this population is vaccinated prior to a disease outbreak. Thus we have a subpopulation of size $N_U = (1-\gamma)N$ of unvaccinated members and a subpopulation of size $N_V = \gamma N$ of vaccinated members. We assume that vaccinated members have susceptibility to infection reduced by a factor $\sigma, 0 \leq \sigma \leq 1$, with $\sigma = 0$ describing a perfectly effective vaccine and $\sigma = 1$ describing a vaccine that has no effect. We assume also that vaccinated individuals who are infected have infectivity reduced by a factor δ and may also have a recovery rate α_V, which is different from the recovery rate of infected unvaccinated individuals α_U.

We let S_U, S_V, I_U, I_V denote the number of unvaccinated susceptibles, the number of vaccinated susceptibles, the number of unvaccinated infectives, and the number of vaccinated infectives, respectively.

The resulting model is

$$\begin{aligned} S_U' &= -\beta S_U(I_U+\delta I_V), \\ S_V' &= -\sigma\beta S_V(I_U+\delta I_V), \\ I_U' &= \beta S_U(I_U+\delta I_V)-\alpha_U I_U, \\ I_V' &= \sigma\beta S_V(I_U+\delta I_V)-\alpha_V I_V. \end{aligned} \tag{3.1}$$

The initial conditions prescribe $S_U(0), S_V(0), I_U(0), I_V(0)$, with

$$S_U(0)+I_U(0)=N_U, \quad S_V(0)+I_V(0)=N_V.$$

Since the infection now is beginning in a population which is not fully susceptible, we speak of the *control reproduction number* $\mathcal{R}_c$ rather than the basic reproduction number. However, as we will soon see, calculation of the control reproduction number will require a more general definition and a considerable amount of technical computation. The computation method is applicable to both basic and control reproduction numbers. We will use the term reproduction number to denote either a basic reproduction number or a control reproduction number. We are able to obtain final size relations without knowledge of the reproduction number, but these final size relations do contain information about the reproduction number, and more.

Since S_U and S_V are decreasing nonnegative functions, they have limits $S_U(\infty)$, $S_V(\infty)$, respectively, as $t\to\infty$. The sum of the equations for S_U and I_U in (3.1) is

$$(S_U+I_U)' = -\alpha_U I_U,$$

from which we conclude, just as in the analysis of (1.2), that $I_U(t)\to 0$ as $t\to\infty$, and that

$$\alpha\int_0^\infty I_U(t)dt = N_U - S_U(\infty). \tag{3.2}$$

Similarly, using the sum of the equations for S_V and I_V, we see that $I_V(t)\to 0$ as $t\to\infty$, and that

$$\alpha\int_0^\infty I_V(t)dt = N_V - S_V(\infty). \tag{3.3}$$

Integration of the equation for S_U in (3.1) and use of (3.2), (3.3) gives

$$\begin{aligned} \log\frac{S_U(0)}{S_U(\infty)} &= \beta\left[\int_0^\infty I_U(t)dt + \delta\int_0^\infty I_V(t)dt\right] \\ &= \frac{\beta N_U}{\alpha}\left[1-\frac{S_U(\infty)}{N_U}\right]+\frac{\delta\beta N_V}{\alpha}\left[1-\frac{S_V(\infty)}{N_V}\right]. \end{aligned} \tag{3.4}$$

A similar calculation using the equation for S_V gives

$$\log\frac{S_V(0)}{S_V(\infty)} = \frac{\sigma\beta N_U}{\alpha}\left[1-\frac{S_U(\infty)}{N_U}\right]+\frac{\delta\sigma\beta N_V}{\alpha}\left[1-\frac{S_V(\infty)}{N_V}\right]. \tag{3.5}$$

The two equations (3.4), (3.5) are the final size relations. They make it possible to calculate $S_U(\infty), S_V(\infty)$ if the parameters of the model are known.

It is convenient to define the matrix

$$K = \begin{bmatrix} K_{11} & K_{12} \\ K_{21} & K_{22} \end{bmatrix} = \begin{bmatrix} \frac{\beta N_U}{\alpha_U} & \frac{\delta\beta N_V}{\alpha_V} \\ \frac{\sigma\beta N_U}{\alpha_U} & \frac{\delta\sigma\beta N_V}{\alpha_V} \end{bmatrix}.$$

Then the final size relations (3.4), (3.5) may be written

$$\begin{aligned} \log\frac{S_U(0)}{S_U(\infty)} &= K_{11}\left[1 - \frac{S_U(\infty)}{N_U}\right] + K_{12}\left[1 - \frac{S_V(\infty)}{N_V}\right], \\ \log\frac{S_V(0)}{S_V(\infty)} &= K_{21}\left[1 - \frac{S_U(\infty)}{N_U}\right] + K_{22}\left[1 - \frac{S_V(\infty)}{N_V}\right]. \end{aligned} \tag{3.6}$$

The matrix K is closely related to the reproduction number. In the next section we describe a general method for calculating reproduction numbers that will involve this matrix.

3.3 The Next Generation Matrix

Up to this point, we have calculated reproduction numbers by following the secondary cases caused by a single infective introduced into a population. However, if there are subpopulations with different susceptibility to infection, as in the vaccination model introduced in Section 3.2, it is necessary to follow the secondary infections in the subpopulations separately, and this approach will not yield the reproduction number. It is necessary to give a more general approach to the meaning of the reproduction number, and this is done through the *next generation matrix* [11, 12, 27]. The underlying idea is that we must calculate the matrix whose (i, j) entry is the number of secondary infections caused in compartment i by an infected individual in compartment j.

In a compartmental disease transmission model we sort individuals into compartments based on a single, discrete state variable. A compartment is called a *disease compartment* if the individuals therein are infected. Note that this use of the term disease is broader than the clinical definition and includes stages of infection such as exposed stages in which infected individuals are not necessarily infective. Suppose there are n disease compartments and m nondisease compartments, and let $x \in R^n$ and $y \in R^m$ be the subpopulations in each of these compartments. In the nondisease compartment y_j, we assume that the rate of growth of the compartment size is given by a function g_j. Further, we denote by $\mathcal{F}_i$ the rate at which secondary infections increase the ith disease compartment and by $\mathcal{V}_i$ the rate at which disease progression, death, and recovery decrease the ith compartment. The compartmental model can then be written in the form

$$\begin{aligned} x_i' &= \mathcal{F}_i(x, y) - \mathcal{V}_i(x, y), \quad i = 1, \ldots, n, \\ y_j' &= g_j(x, y), \quad j = 1, \ldots, m. \end{aligned} \tag{3.7}$$

Note that the decomposition of the dynamics into $\mathcal{F}$ and $\mathcal{V}$ and the designation of compartments as infected or uninfected may not be unique; different decompositions correspond to different epidemiological interpretations of the model. The definitions of $\mathcal{F}$ and $\mathcal{V}$ used here differ slightly from those in [27].

The derivation of the basic reproduction number is based on the linearization of the ordinary differential equation model about a disease-free equilibrium. For an epidemic model with a line of equilibria, it is customary to use the equilibrium with all members of the population susceptible. We assume

- $\mathcal{F}_i(0,y)=0$ and $\mathcal{V}_i(0,y)=0$ for all $y \geq 0$ and $i=1,\ldots,n$;
- the disease-free system $y'=g(0,y)$ has a unique equilibrium that is asymptotically stable, that is, all solutions with initial conditions of the form $(0,y)$ approach a point $(0,y_o)$ as $t \to \infty$. We refer to this point as the disease-free equilibrium.

The first assumption says that all new infections are secondary infections arising from infected hosts; there is no immigration of individuals into the disease compartments. It ensures that the disease-free set, which consists of all points of the form $(0,y)$, is invariant. That is, any solution with no infected individuals at some point in time will be free of infection for all time. The second assumption ensures that the disease-free equilibrium is also an equilibrium of the full system.

Next, we assume

- $\mathcal{F}_i(x,y) \geq 0$ for all nonnegative x and y and $i=1,\ldots,n$;
- $\mathcal{V}_i(x,y) \geq 0$ whenever $x_i=0$, $i=1,\ldots,n$;
- $\sum_{i=1}^{n} \mathcal{V}_i(x,y) \geq 0$ for all nonnegative x and y.

The reasons for these assumptions are that the function $\mathcal{F}$ represents new infections and cannot be negative, that each component, $\mathcal{V}_i$, represents a net outflow from compartment i and must be negative (inflow only) whenever the compartment is empty, and that the sum $\sum_{i=1}^{n} \mathcal{V}_i(x,y)$ represents the total outflow from all infected compartments. Terms in the model leading to increases in $\sum_{i=1}^{n} x_i$ are assumed to represent secondary infections and therefore belong in $\mathcal{F}$.

Suppose that a single infected person is introduced into a population originally free of disease. The initial ability of the disease to spread through the population is determined by an examination of the linearization of (3.7) about the disease-free equilibrium $(0,y_o)$. It is easy to see that the assumption $\mathcal{F}_i(0,y)=0, \mathcal{V}_i(0,y)=0$ implies

$$\frac{\partial \mathcal{F}_i}{\partial y_j}(0,y_o)=\frac{\partial \mathcal{V}_i}{\partial y_j}(0,y_o)=0$$

for every pair (i,j). This implies that the linearized equations for the disease compartments, x, are decoupled from the remaining equations and can be written as

$$x'=(F-V)x, \tag{3.8}$$

where F and V are the $n \times n$ matrices with entries

$$F=\frac{\partial \mathcal{F}_i}{\partial x_j}(0,y_o) \qquad \text{and} \qquad V=\frac{\partial \mathcal{V}_i}{\partial x_j}(0,y_o).$$

Because of the assumption that the disease-free system $y'=g(0,y)$ has a unique asymptotically stable equilibrium, the linear stability of the system (3.7) is completely determined by the linear stability of the matrix $(F-V)$ in (3.8).

The number of secondary infections produced by a single infected individual is the product of the expected duration of the infectious period and the rate at which secondary infections occur. For the general model with n disease compartments, these are computed for each compartment for a hypothetical index case. The expected time that an index case spends in each compartment is given by the integral $\int_0^\infty t\phi(t,x_0)\,dt$, where $\phi(t,x_0)$ is the solution of (3.8) with $F=0$ (no secondary infections) and nonnegative initial conditions, x_0, representing an infected index case:

$$x' = -Vx, \qquad x(0) = x_0. \tag{3.9}$$

In effect, this solution shows the path of the index case through the disease compartments from the initial exposure through to death or recovery with the ith component of $\phi(t,x_0)$ interpreted as the probability that the index case (introduced at time $t=0$) is in disease state i at time t. The solution of (3.9) is $\phi(t,x_0)=e^{-Vt}x_0$, where the exponential of a matrix is defined by the Taylor series

$$e^A = I + A + \frac{A^2}{2} + \frac{A^3}{3!} + \cdots + \frac{A^k}{k!} + \cdots.$$

This series converges for all t (see, for example [16]) and can be integrated term by term. Thus

$$\int_0^\infty te^{-Vt}dtx_0 = V^{-1}x_0 \geq 0,$$

and the (i,j) entry of the matrix V^{-1} can be interpreted as the expected time an individual initially introduced into disease compartment j spends in disease compartment i.

The (i,j) entry of the matrix F is the rate at which secondary infections are produced in compartment i by an index case in compartment j. Hence, the expected number of secondary infections produced by the index case is given by

$$\int_0^\infty Fe^{-Vt}x_0\,dt = FV^{-1}x_0.$$

Following [11], we call the matrix $K_L = FV^{-1}$ the *next generation matrix with large domain* for the system at the disease-free equilibrium. The (i,j) entry of K is the expected number of secondary infections in compartment i produced by individuals initially in compartment j, assuming, of course, that the environment seen by the individual remains homogeneous for the duration of its infection.

Shortly, we will describe some results from matrix theory which imply that the matrix, $K_L = FV^{-1}$, is nonnegative and therefore has a nonnegative eigenvalue, $\mathcal{R}_0 = \rho(FV^{-1})$, such that there are no other eigenvalues of K_L with modulus greater than $\mathcal{R}_0$, and there is a nonnegative eigenvector ω associated with $\mathcal{R}_0$ [4, Theorem 1.3.2]. This eigenvector is, in a sense, the distribution of infected individuals that produces the greatest number, $\mathcal{R}_0$, of secondary infections per generation. Thus, $\mathcal{R}_0$ and the associated eigenvector ω suitably define a "typical" infective and the basic reproduction number can be rigorously defined as the spectral radius of the matrix, K_L. The *spectral radius* of a matrix K_L, denoted by $\rho(K_L)$, is the maximum of the moduli of the eigenvalues of K_L. If K_L is irreducible, then $\mathcal{R}_0$ is a simple eigenvalue of K_L and is strictly larger in modulus than all other eigenvalues of K_L. However, if K_L is reducible, which is often the case for diseases with multiple strains, then K_L may have several positive real eigenvectors corresponding to reproduction numbers for each competing strain of the disease.

We have interpreted the reproduction number for a disease as the number of secondary infections produced by an infected individual in a population of susceptible individuals. If the reproduction number $\mathcal{R}_0 = \rho(FV^{-1})$ is consistent with the differential equation model, then it should follow that the disease-free equilibrium is asymptotically stable if $\mathcal{R}_0 < 1$ and unstable if $\mathcal{R}_0 > 1$.

This is shown through a sequence of lemmas.

The *spectral bound* (or abscissa) of a matrix A is the maximum real part of all eigenvalues of A. If each entry of a matrix T is nonnegative, we write $T \geq 0$ and refer to T as a nonnegative matrix. A matrix of the form $A = sI - B$, with $B \geq 0$, is said to have the Z sign pattern. These are matrices whose off-diagonal entries are negative or zero. If, in addition, $s \geq \rho(B)$, then A is called an M-matrix. Note that in this section, I denotes an identity matrix, not a population of infectious individuals. The following lemma is a standard result from [4].

Lemma 3.1. *If A has the Z sign pattern, then $A^{-1} \geq 0$ if and only if A is a nonsingular M-matrix.*

The assumptions we have made imply that each entry of F is nonnegative and that the off-diagonal entries of V are negative or zero. Thus V has the Z sign pattern. Also, the column sums of V are positive or zero, which, together with the Z sign pattern, implies that V is a (possibly singular) M-matrix [4, condition M_{35} of Theorem 6.2.3]. In what follows, it is assumed that V is nonsingular. In this case, $V^{-1} \geq 0$, by Lemma 3.1. Hence, $K_L = FV^{-1}$ is also nonnegative. The matrix K_L is called the *next generation matrix with large domain.*

Lemma 3.2. *If F is nonnegative and V is a nonsingular M-matrix, then $\mathcal{R}_0 = \rho(FV^{-1}) < 1$ if and only if all eigenvalues of $(F - V)$ have negative real parts.*

Proof. Suppose $F \geq 0$ and V is a nonsingular M-matrix. By the proof of Lemma 3.1, $V^{-1} \geq 0$. Thus, $(I - FV^{-1})$ has the Z sign pattern, and by Lemma 3.1, $(I - FV^{-1})^{-1} \geq 0$ if and only if $\rho(FV^{-1}) < 1$. From the equalities $(V - F)^{-1} = V^{-1}(I - FV^{-1})^{-1}$ and $V(V - F)^{-1} = I + F(V - F)^{-1}$, it follows that $(V - F)^{-1} \geq 0$ if and only if $(I - FV^{-1})^{-1} \geq 0$. Finally, $(V - F)$ has the Z sign pattern, so by Lemma 3.1, $(V - F)^{-1} \geq 0$ if and only if $(V - F)$ is a nonsingular M-matrix. Since the eigenvalues of a nonsingular M-matrix all have positive real parts, this completes the proof. □

Theorem 3.3. *Consider the disease transmission model given by* (3.7). *The disease-free equilibrium of* (3.7) *is locally asymptotically stable if $\mathcal{R}_0 < 1$, but unstable if $\mathcal{R}_0 > 1$.*

Proof. Let F and V be as defined as above, and let J_{21} and J_{22} be the matrices of partial derivatives of g with respect to x and y evaluated at the disease-free equilibrium. The Jacobian matrix for the linearization of the system about the disease-free equilibrium has the block structure

$$J = \begin{bmatrix} F - V & 0 \\ J_{21} & J_{22} \end{bmatrix}.$$

The disease-free equilibrium is locally asymptotically stable if the eigenvalues of the Jacobian matrix all have negative real parts. Since the eigenvalues of J are those of $(F-V)$ and J_{22}, and the latter all have negative real parts by assumption, the disease-free equilibrium is locally asymptotically stable if all eigenvalues of $(F-V)$ have negative real parts. By the assumptions on $\mathcal{F}$ and $\mathcal{V}$, F is nonnegative and V is a nonsingular M-matrix. Hence, by Lemma 3.2 all eigenvalues of $(F-V)$ have negative real parts if and only if $\rho(FV^{-1})<1$. It follows that the disease-free equilibrium is locally asymptotically stable if $\mathcal{R}_0=\rho(FV^{-1})<1$.

Instability for $\mathcal{R}_0>1$ can be established by a continuity argument. If $\mathcal{R}_0\leq 1$, then for any $\epsilon>0$, $((1+\epsilon)I-FV^{-1})$ is a nonsingular M-matrix and, by Lemma 3.1, $((1+\epsilon)I-FV^{-1})^{-1}\geq 0$. By the proof of Lemma 3.2, all eigenvalues of $((1+\epsilon)V-F)$ have positive real parts. Since $\epsilon>0$ is arbitrary, and eigenvalues are continuous functions of the entries of the matrix, it follows that all eigenvalues of $(V-F)$ have nonnegative real parts. To reverse the argument, suppose all the eigenvalues of $(V-F)$ have nonnegative real parts. For any positive ϵ, $(V+\epsilon I-F)$ is a nonsingular M-matrix, and by the proof of Lemma 3.2, $\rho(F(V+\epsilon I)^{-1})<1$. Again, since $\epsilon>0$ is arbitrary, it follows that $\rho(FV^{-1})\leq 1$. Thus, $(F-V)$ has at least one eigenvalue with positive real part if and only if $\rho(FV^{-1})>1$, and the disease-free equilibrium is unstable whenever $\mathcal{R}_0>1$. □

These results validate the extension of the definition of the reproduction number to more general situations. In the vaccination model (3.1) of the previous section we calculated a pair of final size relations which contained the elements of a matrix K. This matrix is precisely the next generation matrix with large domain $K_L=FV^{-1}$ that has been introduced in this section.

Example 1. Consider the $SEIR$ model with infectivity in the exposed stage,

$$\begin{aligned} S' &= -\beta S(I+\varepsilon E), \\ E' &= \beta S(I+\varepsilon E)-\kappa E, \\ I' &= \kappa E-\alpha I, \\ R' &= \alpha I. \end{aligned} \tag{3.10}$$

Here the disease states are E and I,

$$\mathcal{F}=\begin{bmatrix} \varepsilon E\beta N+I\beta N \\ 0 \end{bmatrix}$$

and

$$F=\begin{bmatrix} \varepsilon\beta N & \beta N \\ 0 & 0 \end{bmatrix}, \quad V=\begin{bmatrix} \kappa & 0 \\ -\kappa & \alpha \end{bmatrix}, \quad V^{-1}=\begin{bmatrix} \frac{1}{\kappa} & 0 \\ \frac{1}{\alpha} & \frac{1}{\alpha} \end{bmatrix}.$$

Then we may calculate

$$K_L=FV^{-1}=\begin{bmatrix} \frac{\varepsilon\beta N}{\kappa}+\frac{\beta N}{\alpha} & \frac{\beta N}{\alpha} \\ 0 & 0 \end{bmatrix}.$$

Since FV^{-1} has rank 1, it has only one nonzero eigenvalue, and since the trace of the matrix is equal to the sum of the eigenvalues, it is easy to see that

$$\mathcal{R}_0 = \frac{\varepsilon\beta N}{\kappa} + \frac{\beta N}{\alpha},$$

the element in the first row and first column of FV^{-1}. If all new infections are in a single compartment, as is the case here, the basic reproduction number is the trace of the matrix FV^{-1}.

In general, it is possible to reduce the size of the next generation matrix to the number of *states at infection* [11]. The states at infection are those disease states in which there can be new infections. Suppose that there are n disease states and k states at infection with $k < n$. Then we may define an auxiliary $n \times k$ matrix E in which each column corresponds to a state at infection and has 1 in the corresponding row and 0 elsewhere. Then the next generation matrix is the $k \times k$ matrix

$$K = E^T K_L E.$$

It is easy to show, using the fact that $EE^T K_L = K_L$, that the $n \times n$ matrix K_L and the $k \times k$ matrix K have the same nonzero eigenvalues and therefore the same spectral radius. Construction of the next generation matrix which has lower dimension than the next generation matrix with large domain may simplify the calculation of the basic reproduction number.

In Example 1 above, the only disease state at infection is E, the matrix A is

$$\begin{bmatrix} 1 \\ 0 \end{bmatrix},$$

and the next generation matrix K is the 1×1 matrix

$$K = \begin{bmatrix} \frac{\varepsilon\beta N}{\kappa} + \frac{\beta N}{\alpha} \end{bmatrix}.$$

Example 2. Consider the vaccination model (3.1). The disease states are I_U and I_V. Then

$$\mathcal{F} = \begin{bmatrix} \beta N_U(I_U + \delta I_V) \\ \sigma\beta N_V(I_U + \delta I_V \end{bmatrix}$$

and

$$F = \begin{bmatrix} \beta N_U & \delta\beta N_U \\ \sigma\beta N_V & \sigma\delta\beta N_V \end{bmatrix}, \quad V = \begin{bmatrix} \alpha_U & 0 \\ 0 & \alpha_V \end{bmatrix}.$$

It is easy to see that the next generation matrix with large domain is the matrix K calculated in the vaccination section. Since each disease state is a disease state at infection, the next generation matrix is K, the same as the next generation matrix with large domain. As in Example 1, the determinant of K is zero and K has rank 1. Thus the control reproduction number is the trace of K,

$$\mathcal{R}_c = \frac{\beta N_U}{\alpha_U} + \frac{\delta\sigma N_V}{\alpha_V}.$$

3.4 Vector Transmission

Many of the important underlying ideas of mathematical epidemiology arose in the study of malaria begun by Ross [26]. Malaria is one example of a disease with vector transmission, the infection being transmitted back and forth between vectors (mosquitoes) and hosts (humans). It kills nearly 1,000,000 people annually, mostly children and mostly in poor countries in Africa. Among communicable diseases, only tuberculosis causes more deaths. Other vector diseases include West Nile virus and HIV with heterosexual transmission.

Vector-transmitted diseases require models that include both vectors and hosts. For most diseases transmitted by vectors, the vectors are insects, with a much shorter life span than the hosts, which may be humans as for malaria or animals as for West Nile virus. For heterosexually transmitted human diseases, transmission goes back and forth between males and females rather than between two different species, but a model still requires two separate groups.

The compartmental structure of the disease may be different in host and vector species; for many diseases with insects as vectors an infected vector remains infected for life so that the disease may have an SI structure in the vectors and an SIR or SIS structure in the hosts. We will describe a vector model with SIR structure in both species, but the analysis of other types of vector transmitted diseases is similar.

Consider a host population with birth rate Λ_h and death rate μ_h and a vector population with birth rate Λ_v and death rate μ_v. We assume mass-action contact with contact rates β_h, β_v and recovery rates α_h, α_v, respectively. For simplicity, we assume that there are no disease deaths of either hosts or vectors so that the two populations have constant total sizes N_h, N_v, respectively. The resulting model is

$$\begin{aligned} S_h' &= \Lambda_h - \beta_h S_h I_v - \mu_h S_h, \\ I_h' &= \beta_h S_h I_v - (\mu_h + \alpha_h) I_h, \\ S_v' &= \Lambda_v - \beta_v S_v I_h - \mu_v S_v, \\ I_v' &= \beta_v S_v I_h - (\mu_v + \alpha_v) I_v. \end{aligned} \tag{3.11}$$

There is always a disease-free equilibrium $(N_h, 0, N_v, 0)$, and there may also be an endemic equilibrium with both species infective population sizes positive. At an endemic equilibrium,

$$\begin{aligned} \beta_h S_h I_v &= (\alpha_h + \mu_h) I_v, \\ \beta_v S_v I_h &= (\alpha_v + \mu_v) I_h, \\ \Lambda_h &= S_h(\mu_h + \beta_h I_v), \\ \Lambda_v &= S_v(\mu_v + \beta_v I_h). \end{aligned}$$

In applying the next generation matrix approach to determine the basic reproduction number we obtain

$$F = \begin{bmatrix} 0 & \beta_h N_h \\ \beta_v N_v & 0 \end{bmatrix}, \quad V = \begin{bmatrix} \alpha_h + \mu_h & 0 \\ 0 & \alpha_v + \mu_v \end{bmatrix}.$$

This leads to

$$FV^{-1} = \begin{bmatrix} 0 & \frac{\beta_h N_h}{\alpha_v + \mu_v} \\ \frac{\beta_v N_v}{\alpha_h + \mu_h} & 0 \end{bmatrix}.$$

This would imply that

$$\mathcal{R}_0 = \sqrt{\frac{\beta_h \beta_v N_h N_v}{(\alpha_v + \mu_v)(\alpha_h + \mu_h)}}.$$

However, this approach views the transition from host to vector to host as two generations, and it may be more reasonable to say that

$$\mathcal{R}_0 = \frac{\beta_h \beta_v N_h N_v}{(\alpha_v + \mu_v)(\alpha_h + \mu_h)}. \tag{3.12}$$

With either choice, the transition is at $\mathcal{R}_0 = 1$. Since a single infectious host infects

$$\frac{\beta_v N_v}{\mu_h + \alpha_h}$$

vectors in a completely susceptible vector population, and each of these infects

$$\frac{\beta_h N_h}{\mu_v + \alpha_v}$$

hosts in a completely susceptible host population, thus the number of secondary host infections caused by an infective host (and also the number of secondary vector infections caused by an infective vector) is given by (3.12), and this is the correct choice for $\mathcal{R}_0$.

By linearizing the system (3.11) at an equilibrium it is possible to show that the disease-free equilibrium is asymptotically stable if and only if $\mathcal{R}_0 < 1$ and that the endemic equilibrium exists only if $\mathcal{R}_0 > 1$ and is asymptotically stable. Because (3.11) is a four-dimensional system, this requires showing that the roots of a fourth degree polynomial have negative real parts, and this is technically complicated.

Ross received the second Nobel Prize in Medicine for demonstrating the vector transmission nature of malaria, and then constructed a model in 1909 that predicted the possibility of controlling malaria by decreasing the mosquito population below a threshold. This prediction was borne out in practice, but controlling mosquito populations is a very difficult problem because of mosquitoes' ability to adapt to pesticides. Malaria remains a very dangerous disease.

3.5 Heterogeneous Mixing

In disease transmission models not all members of the population make contacts at the same rate. In sexually transmitted diseases there is often a "core" group of very active members who are responsible for most of the disease cases, and control measures aimed at this core group have been very effective in control [15]. In epidemics there are often "super-spreaders," who make many contacts and are instrumental in spreading disease, and in general some members of the population make more contacts than others. Recently there has been a move to complicated network models for simulating epidemics [13, 14, 17, 18, 19, 21]. These assume knowledge of the mixing patterns of groups of members of the population and make predictions based on simulations of a stochastic model. A basic description of network models may be found in [25]. While network models can give very detailed predictions, they have some serious disadvantages. For a detailed network model, simulations take long enough to make it difficult to examine a significant range of parameter values, and it is difficult to estimate the sensitivity with respect to parameters of the model. The theoretical analysis of network models is a very active and rapidly developing field [21, 22, 23].

However, it is possible to consider models more realistic than simple compartmental models but simpler to analyze than detailed network models. To model heterogeneity in mixing we may assume that the population is divided into subgroups with different activity levels. We will analyze an SIR model in which there are two groups with different contact rates. The approach extends easily to models with more compartments, such as exposed periods or a sequence of infective stages and also to models with an arbitrary number of activity levels. In this way, we may hope to provide models that are intermediate between the too simple compartmental models with homogeneous mixing and the too complicated full network models.

In this section, we describe the formulation of models for two groups with different activity levels and give the main results for the simplest compartmental epidemic models. The analysis of models of the same type with more complicated compartmental structure is given in [8] and the analysis of models with more groups is given in [9].

Consider two subpopulations of constant sizes N_1, N_2, respectively, each divided into susceptibles, infectives, and removed members with subscripts to identify the subpopulation. Suppose that group i members make a_i contacts in unit time and that the fraction of contacts made by a member of group i that is with a member of group j is p_{ij} $(i, j = 1,2)$. Then

$$p_{11} + p_{12} = p_{21} + p_{22} = 1.$$

Suppose the mean infective period in group i is $1/\alpha_i$. We assume that there are no disease deaths, so that the population size of each group is constant.

The two-group SIR epidemic model is

$$\begin{aligned} S_1' &= -\left[p_{11}a_1\frac{S_1 I_1}{N_1} + p_{12}a_1\frac{S_1 I_2}{N_2}\right], \\ I_1' &= \left[p_{11}a_1\frac{S_1 I_1}{N_1} + p_{12}a_1\frac{S_1 I_2}{N_2}\right] - \alpha_1 I_1, \\ S_2' &= -\left[p_{21}a_2\frac{S_2 I_1}{N_1} + p_{22}a_2\frac{S_2 I_2}{N_2}\right], \\ I_2' &= \left[p_{21}a_2\frac{S_2 I_1}{N_1} + p_{22}a_2\frac{S_2 I_2}{N_2}\right] - \alpha_2 I_2. \end{aligned} \tag{3.13}$$

As initial conditions, we prescribe $S_1(0), I_1(0), S_2(0), I_2(0)$ with

$$S_1(0) + I_1(0) = N_1, \quad S_2(0) + I_2(0) = N_2.$$

The two-group model includes two possibilities. It may describe a population with groups differing by activity levels and possibly by vulnerability to infection. It may also describe a population with one group which has been vaccinated against infection, so that the two groups have the same activity level but different disease model parameters.

It is easy to show [8] that just as for a one-group model [7],

$$S_1 \to S_1(\infty) > 0, \quad S_2 \to S_2(\infty) > 0,$$

as $t \to \infty$.

It is not possible to calculate the reproduction number for the two-group model (3.13) directly by counting secondary infections. It is necessary to use the next generation matrix approach of [27] and calculate the reproduction number as the largest eigenvalue of the matrix FV^{-1}, where

$$F = \begin{bmatrix} p_{11}a_1 & p_{12}a_1 \\ p_{21}a_2 & p_{22}a_2 \end{bmatrix}, \quad V = \begin{bmatrix} \alpha_1 & 0 \\ 0 & \alpha_2 \end{bmatrix}.$$

Then

$$FV^{-1} = \begin{bmatrix} \frac{p_{11}a_1}{\alpha_1} & \frac{p_{12}a_1}{\alpha_2} \\ \frac{p_{21}a_2}{\alpha_1} & \frac{p_{22}a_2}{\alpha_2} \end{bmatrix}.$$

The eigenvalues of the matrix FV^{-1} are the roots of the quadratic equation

$$\lambda^2 - \left(\frac{p_{11}a_1}{\alpha_1} + \frac{p_{22}a_2}{\alpha_2}\right)\lambda + (p_{11}p_{22} - p_{12}p_{21})\frac{a_1a_2}{\alpha_1\alpha_2} = 0. \tag{3.14}$$

The basic reproduction number $\mathcal{R}_0$ is the larger of these two eigenvalues,

$$\mathcal{R}_0 = \frac{\frac{p_{11}a_1}{\alpha_1} + \frac{p_{22}a_2}{\alpha_2} + \sqrt{\left(\frac{p_{11}a_1}{\alpha_1} - \frac{p_{22}a_2}{\alpha_2}\right)^2 + 4\frac{p_{12}p_{21}a_1a_2}{\alpha_1\alpha_2}}}{2}.$$

In order to obtain a more useful expression for $\mathcal{R}_0$, it is necessary to make some assumptions about the nature of the mixing between the two groups. The mixing is determined by the two quantities p_{12}, p_{21} since $p_{11} = 1 - p_{12}$ and $p_{22} = 1 - p_{21}$. However, these quantities are not completely arbitrary. The total number of contacts made in unit time by members of group 1 with members of group 2 is $a_1 p_{12} N_1$, and because this must equal the total number of contacts by members of group 2 with members of group 1, we have a balance relation

$$\frac{p_{12}a_1}{N_2} = \frac{p_{21}a_2}{N_1}.$$

There has been much study of mixing patterns; see, for example, [5, 6, 10]. One possibility is proportionate mixing, that is, that the number of contacts between groups is proportional to the relative activity levels. In other words, mixing is random but constrained by the activity levels [24]. Under the assumption of proportionate mixing,

$$p_{ij} = \frac{a_j N_j}{a_1 N_1 + a_2 N_2},$$

and we may write

$$p_{11} = p_{21} = p_1, \quad p_{12} = p_{22} = p_2,$$

with $p_1 + p_2 = 1$. In particular,

$$p_{11}p_{22} - p_{12}p_{21} = 0,$$

and thus

$$\mathcal{R}_0 = \frac{p_1 a_1}{\alpha_1} + \frac{p_2 a_2}{\alpha_2}.$$

Another possibility is preferred mixing [24], in which a fraction π_i of each group mixes randomly with its own group and the remaining members mix proportionately. Thus, preferred mixing is given by

$$\begin{aligned} p_{11} &= \pi_1 + (1-\pi_1)p_1, \quad p_{12} = (1-\pi_1)p_2, \\ p_{21} &= (1-\pi_2)p_1, \quad p_{22} = \pi_2 + (1-\pi_2)p_2, \end{aligned} \tag{3.15}$$

with

$$p_i = \frac{(1-\pi_i)a_i N_i}{(1-\pi_1)a_1 N_1 + (1-\pi_2)a_2 N_2}.$$

Proportionate mixing is the special case of preferred mixing with $\pi_1 = \pi_2 = 0$.

It is also possible to have like-with-like mixing, in which members of each group mixes only with members of the same group. This is the special case of preferred mixing with $\pi_1 = \pi_2 = 1$. For like-with-like mixing,

$$p_{11} = p_{22} = 1, \quad p_{12} = p_{21} = 0.$$

Then the roots of (3.14) are a_1/α_1 and a_2/α_2, and the reproduction number is

$$\mathcal{R}_0 = \max\left[\frac{a_1}{\alpha_1}, \frac{a_2}{\alpha_2}\right].$$

By calculating the partial derivatives of $p_{11}, p_{12}, p_{21}, p_{22}$ with respect to π_1, π_2, we may show that p_{11} and p_{22} increase when either π_1 or π_2 is increased, while p_{12} and p_{21} decrease when either π_1 or π_2 is increased. From this, we may see from the general expression for $\mathcal{R}_0$ that increasing either of the preferences π_1, π_2 increases the basic reproduction number.

3.6 The Final Size Relation

For a one-group epidemic model there is a final size relation that makes it possible to calculate the size of the epidemic from the reproduction number [7, 20]. There is a corresponding final size relation for the two-group model (3.13), established in much the same way. This relation does not involve the reproduction number explicitly but still makes it possible to calculate the size of the epidemic from the model parameters.

The final size relation is the pair of equations

$$\begin{aligned} \log\frac{S_1(0)}{S_1(\infty)} &= a_1\left[\frac{p_{11}}{\alpha_1}\left(1-\frac{S_1(\infty)}{N_1}\right) + \frac{p_{12}}{\alpha_2}\left(1-\frac{S_2(\infty)}{N_2}\right)\right], \\ \log\frac{S_2(0)}{S_2(\infty)} &= a_2\left[\frac{p_{21}}{\alpha_1}\left(1-\frac{S_1(\infty)}{N_1}\right) + \frac{p_{22}}{\alpha_2}\left(1-\frac{S_2(\infty)}{N_2}\right)\right]. \end{aligned} \tag{3.16}$$

The final size relation makes it possible to calculate $S_1(\infty)$ and $S_2(\infty)$ and thence the number of disease cases

$$[N_1 - S_1(\infty)] + [N_2 - S_2(\infty)].$$

The final size relation takes a simpler form if the mixing is proportionate. With proportionate mixing, since

$$p_{11} = p_{21} = p_1, \quad p_{12} = p_{22} = p_2,$$

(3.16) implies

$$a_2 \log \frac{S_1(0)}{S_1(\infty)} = a_1 \log \frac{S_2(0)}{S_2(\infty)},$$

and we may write the final size relations as

$$\log \frac{S_1(0)}{S_1(\infty)} = \frac{a_1 p_1}{\alpha_1}\left[1 - \frac{S_1(\infty)}{N_1}\right] + \frac{a_1 p_2}{\alpha_2}\left[1 - \frac{S_2(\infty)}{N_2}\right],$$
$$\left[\frac{S_1(\infty)}{S_1(0)}\right]^{a_2} = \left[\frac{S_2(\infty)}{S_2(0)}\right]^{a_1}. \tag{3.17}$$

We recall that in the case of proportionate mixing

$$\mathcal{R}_0 = \frac{p_1 a_1}{\alpha_1} + \frac{p_2 a_2}{\alpha_2},$$

and the final size relation is expressed in terms of the components of $\mathcal{R}_c$.

The second equation of (3.17) implies that if $a_1 > a_2$, then

$$1 - \frac{S_1(\infty)}{S_1(0)} > 1 - \frac{S_2(\infty)}{S_2(0)},$$

that is, the attack ratio is greater in the more active group.

It is not difficult to show that the final size relations (3.17) give a unique set of final numbers of susceptibles in each group. The final size relation can also be obtained in a similar way for more complicated compartmental models [1, 2, 3].

3.7 Heterogeneous Mixing Age of Infection Models

Just as with homogeneous mixing epidemic models, there is a general setting that includes many different compartmental structures. In this section, we describe an age of infection model dividing the population into two subgroups with different contact rates. Our description generalizes easily to any finite number of subgroups and even to a continuous distribution of subgroups [9], but we restrict ourselves to two subgroups for simplicity and clarity.

A two-group age of infection model with general mixing would be

$$\begin{aligned}
S_1'(t) &= -a_1 S_1 \left[p_{11} \frac{\varphi_1(t)}{N_1} + p_{12} \frac{\varphi_2(t)}{N_2} \right], \\
\varphi_1(t) &= \varphi_1^{(0)}(t) + \int_0^t [-S_1'(t-\tau)] A_1(\tau) d\tau, \\
S_2'(t) &= -a_2 S_2 \left[p_{21} \frac{\varphi_1(t)}{N_1} + p_{22} \frac{\varphi_2(t)}{N_2} \right], \\
\varphi_2(t) &= \varphi_2^{(0)}(t) + \int_0^t [-S_2'(t-\tau)] A_2(\tau) d\tau,
\end{aligned} \tag{3.18}$$

where $\varphi_i(t)$ is the infectivity in group i at time t, $\varphi_i^{(0)}(t)$ is the infectivity at time t of members of group i who were infected at time 0, and $A_i(\tau)$ is the average infectivity of members of group i with infection age τ.

The infectivity of an infected member of group 2 with infection age τ towards a susceptible member of group 1 is

$$a_1 p_{12} A_2(\tau).$$

One type of mixing between groups is proportionate mixing, that is, the number of contacts between groups is proportional to the relative activity levels. In other words, mixing is random but constrained by the activity levels [24]. With proportionate mixing p_{ij} is independent of i and we may write

$$p_{ij} = p_j, \quad p_1 + p_2 = 1.$$

The assumption of proportionate mixing implies that the next generation operator in the sense of [11, 12] is separable and the basic reproduction number is

$$\mathcal{R}_0 = p_1 a_1 \int_0^\infty A_1(\tau) d\tau + p_2 a_2 \int_0^\infty A_2(\tau) d\tau.$$

If the mixing is not proportionate, the next generation operator is not separable and the calculation of $\mathcal{R}_0$ is much more difficult. However, it is still possible to obtain a system of final size relations.

Integration of the equation for $S_i'(t)/S_i(t)$ in (3.18) gives

$$\begin{aligned}
\log \frac{S_i(0)}{S_i(\infty)} &= a_i \int_0^\infty \sum_{j=1}^2 p_{ij} \frac{\varphi_j(t)}{N_j} dt \\
&= a_i \int_0^\infty \sum_{j=1}^2 p_{ij} \frac{\varphi_j^{(0)}(t) + \int_0^t [-S_j'(t-\tau)] A_j(\tau) d\tau}{N_j} dt \\
&= a_i \int_0^\infty \sum_{j=1}^2 p_{ij} \frac{\varphi_j(t)}{N_j} dt \\
&\quad + a_i \int_0^\infty \sum_{j=1}^2 p_{ij} \frac{\int_0^t [-S_j'(t-\tau)] A_j(\tau) d\tau}{N_j} dt.
\end{aligned} \tag{3.19}$$

If all initial infectives have infection age zero at time $t = 0$,

$$\varphi_j^{(0)}(t) = A_j(t)[N_j - S_j(0)],$$

and the first term on the right side of (3.19) is

$$a_i \int_0^\infty \sum_{j=1}^{2} p_{ij} A_j(t) \left[1 - \frac{S_j(0)}{N_j}\right] dt.$$

The second term on the right side of (3.19) is

$$\begin{aligned}
& a_i \int_0^\infty \sum_{j=1}^{2} \frac{p_{ij}}{N_j} \int_0^t [-S_j'(t-\tau)] A_j(\tau) d\tau dt \\
&= a_i \int_0^\infty \sum_{j=1}^{2} \frac{p_{ij}}{N_j} \int_\tau^\infty [-S_j'(t-\tau)] A_j(\tau) dt d\tau \\
&= a_i \int_0^\infty \sum_{j=1}^{2} p_{ij} \left[\frac{S_j(0) - S_j(\infty)}{N_j}\right] A_j(\tau) d\tau \\
&= a_i \sum_{j=1}^{2} p_{ij} \left[1 - \frac{S_j(\infty)}{N_j}\right] \hat{A}_j - a_i \sum_{j=1}^{2} p_{ij} \left[1 - \frac{S_j(0)}{N_j}\right].
\end{aligned}$$

Thus we may rewrite (3.19) as the final size system

$$\log \frac{S_i(0)}{S_i(\infty)} = a_i \sum_{j=1}^{2} p_{ij} \left[1 - \frac{S_j(\infty)}{N_j}\right] \int_0^\infty A_j(\tau) d\tau, \quad i = 1, 2, \ldots, n. \tag{3.20}$$

If there are initial infectives with positive infection age, the final size system contains an initial term and takes the form

$$\log \frac{S_i(0)}{S_i(\infty)} = a_i \sum_{j=1}^{2} p_{ij} \left[1 - \frac{S_j(\infty)}{N_j}\right] \int_0^\infty A_j(\tau) d\tau - \Gamma_i, \tag{3.21}$$

with

$$\Gamma_i = a_i \sum_{j=1}^{2} \frac{p_{ij}}{N_j} \int_0^\infty \left[A_j(t)\left(N_j - S_j(0)\right) - \varphi_j^{(0)}(t)\right] dt \geq 0.$$

The system of equations (3.21) has a unique solution $(S_1(\infty), S_2(\infty))$.

In order to prove the existence of a unique solution of (3.21), we define

$$\begin{aligned}
g_1(x_1, x_2) &= \log \frac{S_1(0)}{x_1} - a_1 \sum_{j=1}^{2} p_{1j} \left[1 - \frac{x_j}{N_j}\right] \int_0^\infty A_j(\tau) d\tau - \Gamma_1, \\
g_2(x_1, x_2) &= \log \frac{S_1(0)}{x_2} - a_2 \sum_{j=1}^{2} p_{1j} \left[1 - \frac{x_j}{N_j}\right] \int_0^\infty A_j(\tau) d\tau - \Gamma_2.
\end{aligned}$$

A solution of (3.21) is a solution (x_1, x_2) of the system

$$g_1(x_1, x_2) = 0, \quad g_2(x_1, x_2) = 0.$$

For each $x_2, g_1(0+, x_2) > 0, g_1(S_1(0), x_2) < 0$. Also, as a function of $x_1, g_1(x_1, x_2)$ either decreases or decreases initially and then increases to a negative value when $x_1 = S_1(0)$. Thus for each $x_2 < S_2(0)$, there is a unique $x_1(x_2)$ such that $g_1(x_1(x_2), x_2) = 0$. In addition, since $g_1(x_1, x_2)$ is an increasing function of x_2, the function $x_1(x_2)$ is increasing. Now, since $g_2(x_1, 0+) > 0, g_2(x_1, S_2(0)) < 0$, there exists x_2 such that $g_2(x_1(x_2), x_2) = 0$. Also, $g_2(x_1(x_2), x_2)$ either decreases monotonically or decreases initially and then increases to a negative value when $x_2 = S_2(0)$. Therefore this solution is also unique. This implies that

$$(x_1(x_2), x_2)$$

is the unique solution of the final size relations.

The final size relation takes a simpler form if the mixing is proportionate. With proportionate mixing, since p_{ij} is independent of i,

$$\frac{1}{a_i} \log \frac{S_i(0)}{S_i(\infty)} = \frac{1}{a_j} \log \frac{S_j(0)}{S_j(\infty)}.$$

This enables us to write $S_2(\infty)$ on the right side of the final size relation in terms of $S_1(\infty)$, and gives the final size system as an equation for $S_1(\infty)$. Then we obtain the epidemic final size by solving a single equation for $S_1(\infty)$ and using the expression for $S_2(\infty)$ in terms of $S_1(\infty)$.

3.8 Extensions

As we have already indicated, the model can be extended easily in several directions. Extension to models with an arbitrary number of groups with different activity levels, models with more stages in the progression through compartments, and models in which there are differences between groups in susceptibility is straightforward. For example, influenza has two characteristics not included in the model (3.13) that are of importance. There is a latent period between infection and the development of infectivity and influenza symptoms. Also, only a fraction of latent members develop symptoms, while the remainder go through an asymptomatic stage in which there is some infectivity.

In particular, the age of infection model may include treatment, which could be directed at either group or both groups, and could be used for making decisions on how to target groups for treatment. We suggest that in advance planning for a pandemic, the number of groups to be considered for different treatment rates should determine the number of groups to be used in the model. On the other hand, the number of groups to be considered should also depend on the amount and reliability of data, and these two criteria may be contradictory. A model with fewer groups and parameters chosen as weighted averages of the parameters for a model with more groups may give predictions that are quite similar to those of the more detailed models. We suggest also that use of the final size relations for a model with total population size assumed constant is a good time-saving procedure for making predictions if the disease death rate is small.

Bibliography

[1] Arino, J., F. Brauer, P. van den Driessche, J. Watmough, and J. Wu (2006) *Simple models for containment of a pandemic*, J. Roy. Soc. Interface **3**: 453–457.

[2] Arino, J., F. Brauer, P. van den Driessche, J. Watmough, and J. Wu (2007) *A final size relation for epidemic models*, Math. Biosc. & Eng. **4**: 159–176.

[3] Arino, J., F. Brauer, P. van den Driessche, J. Watmough, and J. Wu (2008) *A model for influenza with vaccination and antiviral treatment*, Theor. Pop. Biol. **253**: 118–130.

[4] Berman, A. and R.J. Plemmons (1970) *Nonnegative Matrices in the Mathematical Sciences*, Academic Press; Classics in Applied Mathematics, SIAM, Philadelphia (1994).

[5] Blythe, S.P., S. Busenberg, and C. Castillo-Chavez (1995) *Affinity and paired-event probability*, Math. Biosc. **128**: 265–284.

[6] Blythe, S.P., C. Castillo-Chavez, J. Palmer, and M. Cheng (1991) *Towards a unified theory of mixing and pair formation*, Math. Biosc. **107**: 379–405.

[7] Brauer, F. (2005) *The Kermack-McKendrick epidemic model revisited*, Math. Biosc. **198**: 119–131.

[8] Brauer, F. (2008) *Epidemic models with treatment and heterogeneous mixing*, Bull. Math. Biol. **70**: 1869–1885.

[9] Brauer, F. and J. Watmough (2009), *Age of infection models with heterogeneous mixing*, J. Biol. Dyn. **3**: 324–330.

[10] Busenberg, S. and C. Castillo-Chavez (1989) *Interaction, pair formation and force of infection terms in sexually transmitted diseases*, in Mathematical and Statistical Approaches to AIDS Epidemiology, C. Castillo-Chavez, ed., Lect. Notes in Biomath. **83**, Springer-Verlag, Berlin, Heidelberg, New York: 289–300.

[11] Diekmann, O. and J.A.P. Heesterbeek (2000) *Mathematical Epidemiology of Infectious Diseases: Model Building, Analysis and Interpretation*, John Wiley, New York.

[12] Diekmann, O., J.A.P. Heesterbeek, and J.A.J. Metz (1990) *On the definition and the computation of the basic reproductive ratio $\mathcal{R}_0$ in models for infectious diseases in heterogeneous populations*, J. Math. Biol. **28**: 365–382.

[13] Ferguson, N.M., D.A.T. Cummings, S. Cauchemez, C. Fraser, S. Riley, A. Meeyai, S. Iamsirithaworn, and D.S. Burke (2005) *Strategies for containing an emerging influenza pandemic in Southeast Asia*, Nature **437**: 209–214.

[14] Gani, R., H. Hughes, T. Griffin, J. Medlock, and S. Leach (2005) *Potential impact of antiviral use on hospitalizations during influenza pandemic*, Emerg. Infect. Dis. **11**: 1355–1362.

[15] Hethcote, H.W. and J.A. Yorke (1984) *Gonorrhea Transmission Dynamics and Control*, Lect. Notes in Biomath. **56**, Springer-Verlag, Berlin, Heidelberg, New York.

[16] Hirsch, M. and S. Smale (1974) *Differential Equations, Dynamical Systems, and Linear Algebra*, Academic Press, Orlando, FL.

[17] Longini, I.M., M.E. Halloran, A. Nizam, and Y. Yang (2004) *Containing pandemic influenza with antiviral agents*, Am. J. Epidem. **159**: 623–633.

[18] Longini, I.M., A. Nizam, S. Xu, K. Ungchusak, W. Hanshaoworakul, D.A.T. Cummings, and M.E. Halloran (2005) *Containing pandemic influenza at the source*, Science **309**: 1083–1087.

[19] Longini, I.M. and M. E. Halloran (2005) *Strategy for distribution of influenza vaccine to high—risk groups and children*, Am. J. Epidem. **161**: 303–306.

[20] Ma, J. and D.J.D. Earn (2006) *Generality of the final size formula for an epidemic of a newly invading infectious disease*, Bull. Math. Biol. **68**: 679–702.

[21] Meyers, L.A. (2007) *Contact network epidemiology: Bond percolation applied to infectious disease prediction and control*, Bull. Am. Math. Soc. **44**: 63–86.

[22] Meyers, L.A., M.E.J. Newman, and B. Pourbohloul (2006) *Predicting epidemics on directed contact networks*, J. Theor. Biol. **240**: 400–418.

[23] Meyers, L.A., B. Pourbohloul, M.E.J. Newman, D.M. Skowronski, and R.C. Brunham (2005) *Network theory and SARS: Predicting outbreak diversity*, J. Theor. Biol. **232**: 71–81.

[24] Nold, A. (1980) *Heterogeneity in disease transmission modeling*, Math. Biosc. **52**: 227–240.

[25] Pourbohloulm P. and J. Miller (2008) *Network Theory and the Spread of Communicable Diseases*, CDM Preprint 2008-03, Center for Disease Modelling, York University.

[26] Ross, R. (1911) *The Prevention of Malaria*, 2nd ed. (with Addendum), John Murray, London.

[27] Van den Driessche, P. and J. Watmough (2002) *Reproduction numbers and subthreshold endemic equilibria for compartmental models of disease transmission*, Math. Biosc. **180**: 29–48.

Lecture 4

Models Structured by Age

4.1 Introduction to Age Structure

Age is one of the most important characteristics in the modeling of populations and infectious diseases. Because age groups frequently mix heterogeneously it may be appropriate to include age structure in epidemiological models. While there are other aspects of heterogeneity in disease transmission models, such as behavioral and spatial heterogeneity, age structure is one of the most important aspects of heterogeneity in disease modeling. As references for the mathematical details, we suggest [3, Chapters 9,13], [31, Part III], [34, Chapter 19], [44, Section 10.9], [53, Chapter 22]. Some applications may be found in [2, 4, 14, 15, 18, 31, 39, 40, 43, 57, 58].

Childhood diseases, such as measles, chicken pox, and rubella, are spread mainly by contacts between children of similar ages. More than half of the deaths attributed to malaria are in children under 5 years of age due to their weaker immune systems. This suggests that in models for disease transmission in an age-structured population it may be advisable to allow the contact rates between two members of the population to depend on the ages of both members.

Sexually transmitted diseases (STDs) are spread through partner interactions with pair formations, and the pair formations are age-dependent in most cases. For example, most AIDS cases occur in the group of young adults. More instances of age dependence may be found in [3].

Mixing models of the type considered in the previous lecture could be used for disease transmission in age-structured models if the time span under consideration is short enough that changes in age of individuals in the population can be neglected. It was assumed in these models that individuals remain in the same activity group. However, for long-term models in which births and natural deaths are included and endemic states are possible it must be recognized that the ages of individuals change and therefore that activity levels of an individual may change.

A description of age-structured disease transmission models requires an introduction to age-structured population models. In fact, the first models for age-structured populations [41] were designed for the study of disease transmission in such populations.

Therefore, we begin this lecture with a brief description of some aspects of age-structured population models.

With the advent of substantial intercontinental air travel, it is possible for diseases to move from one location to a completely separate location very rapidly. This was an essential aspect of modeling SARS during the epidemic of 2002–2003 and has become a very important part of the study of the spread of epidemics. Mathematically, it has led to the study of metapopulation models or models with patchy environments and movement between patches [5, 6, 7, 8, 48, 56].

The mathematical analysis of spatial spread of a disease in a single patch because of the (continuous) motion of individuals is based on partial differential equations of reaction-diffusion type. It is technically complicated and requires substantial mathematical background; we will not explore this topic in these lectures. As references for some of the mathematical details, we suggest [13, Chapter 5], [20, Chapters 9–11], [34, Chapters 15–18], [44, Chapters 11 and 13], [45, Chapters 1 and 2].

An introduction to models for the spatial spread of epidemics in a single location may be found in other references such as [2, 14, 17, 25, 55]. One characteristic feature of such models is the appearance of traveling waves, which have been observed frequently in the spread of epidemics through Europe from medieval times to the more recent studies of fox rabies [1, 33, 38, 46]. The asymptotic speed of spread of disease is the minimum wave speed [9, 16, 42, 47, 51, 59]. Models describing spatial spread and including age of infection are analyzed in [22, 23, 27, 45].

4.2 Linear Age-Structured Models

It was a physician, Lt. Col. A.G. McKendrick who first introduced age structure into the dynamics of a one-sex population [41]. The McKendrick model assumes that the female population can be described by a function of two variables: age and time. Let $\rho(a,t)$ denote the *density* of individuals of age a at time t; that is, the number of individuals with ages between a and $a+\Delta a$ at time t is approximately $\rho(a,t)\Delta a$. Then the total population at time t is approximately $\sum_a \rho(a,t)\Delta a$, whose "limit as $\Delta a \to 0$" is $\int_0^\infty \rho(a,t)da$, and we define the total population

$$P(t) = \int_0^\infty \rho(a,t)da.$$

In practice, it is reasonable to expect that $\rho(a,t) = 0$ for all sufficiently large a, so that this integral is not necessarily an infinite integral.

Age and time are related. For the *cohort* of members of the population born at the same time, say c, $da/dt = 1$, and $a = t - c$. More generally, if a represents some physiological measure such as size, $da/dt = g(a)$. The cohort born at c has size $\rho(0,c)$. It proceeds along the *characteristic* $a = t - c$ and is altered only by deaths as no new members can join the cohort. If $da/dt = g(a)$, the characteristics are the solution curves of

$$\frac{da}{dt} = g(a).$$

We will assume that members leave the population only through death, and that there is an age-dependent death rate $\mu(a)$. This means that over the time interval from t to $t+\Delta t$ a fraction $\mu(a)\Delta t$ of the members with ages between a and $a+\Delta a$ at time t die.

At time t there are $\rho(a,t)\Delta a$ individuals with ages between a and $a+\Delta a$. Between the times t and $t+\Delta t$ the number of deaths from this age cohort is $\rho(a,t)\Delta a\mu(a)\Delta t$, and the remainder survive, having ages between $a+\Delta t$ and $a+\Delta t+\Delta a$ at time $t+\Delta t$. Thus,

$$\rho(a+\Delta t,t+\Delta t)\Delta a \approx \rho(a,t)\Delta a - \rho(a,t)\mu(a)\Delta a\Delta t.$$

Division by $\Delta a\Delta t$ gives

$$\frac{\rho(a+\Delta t,t+\Delta t)-\rho(a,t)}{\Delta t} + \mu(a)\rho(a,t) \approx 0.$$

We then let $\Delta t \to 0$. If $\rho(a,t)$ is a differentiable function of a and t, we have

$$\begin{aligned}\lim_{\Delta t\to 0}\frac{\rho(a+\Delta t,t+\Delta t)-\rho(a,t)}{\Delta t} &= \lim_{\Delta t\to 0}\frac{\rho(a+\Delta t,t+\Delta t)-\rho(a,t+\Delta t)}{\Delta t}\\ &\quad + \lim_{\Delta t\to 0}\frac{\rho(a,t+\Delta t)-\rho(a,t)}{\Delta t}\\ &= \lim_{\Delta t\to 0}\left(\rho_a(a,t+\Delta t)+\rho_t(a,t)\right)\\ &= \rho_a(a,t)+\rho_t(a,t).\end{aligned}$$

Thus we obtain the *McKendrick equation* (1926)

$$\rho_a(a,t)+\rho_t(a,t)+\mu(a)\rho(a,t)=0. \tag{4.1}$$

This equation is also known as the *von Foerster* equation, because the same equation arises in cellular biology. The function $\mu(a)\geq 0$ is called the *mortality function* or *death modulus*. If $y(\alpha)$ is the number of individuals starting at age a who survive to age α, then

$$y(\alpha+\Delta\alpha)-y(\alpha)\approx -\mu(\alpha)y(\alpha)\Delta\alpha.$$

If we divide by $\Delta\alpha$ and let $\Delta\alpha\to 0$, we obtain $y'(\alpha)=-\mu(\alpha)y(\alpha)$, and this implies $y(a_2)=y(a_1)e^{-\int_{a_1}^{a_2}\mu(\alpha)d\alpha}$. Thus the probability that an individual of age a_1 will survive to age a_2 is $e^{-\int_{a_1}^{a_2}\mu(\alpha)d\alpha}$. In particular,

$$\pi(a)=e^{-\int_0^a\mu(\alpha)d\alpha}$$

is the probability of survival from birth to age a.

Next, we assume that the birth process is governed by a function $\beta(a)$ called the *birth modulus*, that is, that $\beta(a)\Delta t$ is the number of offspring produced by members with ages between a and $a+\Delta a$ in the time interval from t to $t+\Delta t$. Thus, the total number of births between time t and time $t+\Delta t$ is $\Delta t\sum\beta(a)\rho(a,t)\Delta a$, which "tends as $\Delta a\to 0$" to $\Delta t\int_0^\infty\beta(a)\rho(a,t)da$. As this quantity must also be $\rho(0,t)\Delta t$, we obtain the *renewal condition*

$$B(t)=\rho(0,t)=\int_0^\infty\beta(a)\rho(a,t)da.$$

Observe that if we know $B(t)$, then we can calculate $\rho(a,t)$ as the number of births at time $t-a$ multiplied by the survival fraction to age a plus the number of survivors from the initial population born before time $t-a$ and surviving to time t. The upper triangle of the first quadrant of the (a,t) plane represents members of the population who were already alive at time $t = 0$.

In order to complete the model we must specify an initial age distribution (at time zero)

$$\rho(a,0) = \varphi(a).$$

Then the full model consists of a partial differential equation and two auxiliary conditions, one of which is an integral condition. The full model is

$$\begin{aligned} \rho_a(a,t) + \rho_t(a,t) + \mu(a)\rho(a,t) &= 0, \\ \rho(0,t) &= \int_0^\infty \beta(a)\rho(a,t)da, \\ \rho(a,0) &= \phi(a). \end{aligned} \tag{4.2}$$

The solution of the model (4.2) is carried out using the *method of characteristics*.

4.3 The Method of Characteristics

In order to transform the problem (4.2) into a more manageable form, we will integrate along characteristics of the partial differential equation. The characteristics are the lines $t = a + c$. Their importance lies in the fact that the value of the function ρ at a point (a,t) is determined by the values of ρ on the characteristic through (a,t) because a member of the population of age a at time t must have been of age $a - \alpha$ at time $t - \alpha$ for every $\alpha \geq 0$ such that $\alpha \leq a$ and $\alpha \leq t$. In other words, the points on a given characteristic $t = a + c$ all correspond to the same age cohort.

If $t \geq a$, $\rho(a,t)$ is just the number of survivors to age a of the $\rho(0,t-a)$ members born at time $(t-a)$. Since the fraction surviving to age a is $\pi(a)$, we have $\rho(a,t) = \rho(0,t-a)\pi(a)$ if $t \geq a$. If $t < a$, $\rho(a,t)$ is just the number of survivors to age a of the $\phi(a-t)$ members who were of age $(a-t)$ at time zero. Since the fraction surviving from age $(a-t)$ to age a is $\pi(a)/\pi(a-t)$, we have $\rho(a,t) = \phi(a-t)\pi(a)/\pi(a-t)$ if $t < a$. Thus

$$\rho(a,t) = \begin{cases} \rho(0,t-a)\pi(a) & \text{for } t \geq a, \\ \phi(a-t)\pi(a)/\pi(a-t) & \text{for } t < a. \end{cases} \tag{4.3}$$

In terms of μ, we may write this as

$$\begin{aligned} \rho(a,t) &= \rho(0,t-a)e^{-\int_0^a \mu(\alpha)d\alpha} && \text{for } t \geq a, \\ \rho(a,t) &= \phi(a-t)e^{-\int_{a-t}^a \mu(\alpha)d\alpha} && \text{for } t < a. \end{aligned}$$

We have defined the function $B(t)$ representing the number of births in unit time t by

$$B(t) = \rho(0,t).$$

Then the original problem is

$$\begin{aligned} \rho_a(a,t) + \rho_t(a,t) + \mu(a)\rho(a,t) &= 0, \\ B(t) &= \int_0^\infty \beta(a)\rho(a,t)da, \\ \rho(a,0) &= \phi(a), \end{aligned}$$

and we have obtained the representation

$$\rho(a,t) = B(t-a)e^{-\int_0^a \mu(\alpha)d\alpha} \qquad \text{for } t \geq a,$$
$$\rho(a,t) = \phi(a-t)e^{-\int_{a-t}^a \mu(\alpha)d\alpha} \qquad \text{for } t < a.$$

We let $\psi(t)$ be the rate of births from members who were present in the population at time zero. From (4.1) and (4.3) we have

$$\begin{aligned}
\rho(0,t) &= \int_0^\infty \beta(a)\rho(a,t)\,da \\
&= \int_0^t \beta(a)\rho(a,t)\,da + \int_t^\infty \beta(a)\rho(a,t)\,da \\
&= \int_0^t \beta(a)\rho(0,t-a)e^{-\int_0^a \mu(\alpha)d\alpha}\,da + \int_t^\infty \beta(a)\phi(a-t)e^{-\int_{a-t}^a \mu(\alpha)d\alpha}\,da \\
&= \int_0^t \beta(a)e^{-\int_0^a \mu(\alpha)d\alpha}B(t-a)\,da + \int_t^\infty \beta(a)\phi(a-t)e^{-\int_{a-t}^a \mu(\alpha)d\alpha}\,da.
\end{aligned}$$

Thus, we may evaluate ψ in terms of the birth and death moduli and the initial age distribution

$$\begin{aligned}
\psi(t) &= \int_t^\infty \beta(a)\phi(a-t)e^{-\int_{a-t}^a \mu(\alpha)d\alpha}\,da \\
&= \int_0^\infty \beta(t+s)\phi(s)e^{-\int_s^{s+t} \mu(\alpha)d\alpha}\,ds.
\end{aligned} \tag{4.4}$$

We also write $\pi(a) = e^{-\int_0^a \mu(\alpha)d\alpha}$, and we see that $B(t)$ is a solution of the *renewal equation*

$$B(t) = \psi(t) + \int_0^t \beta(a)\pi(a)B(t-a)da,$$

a linear Volterra integral equation of convolution type with kernel $\beta(a)\pi(a)$. Conversely, if $B(t)$ is a solution of the renewal equation, then we have a solution of the original problem given by

$$\rho(a,t) = \begin{cases} B(t-a)e^{-\int_0^a \mu(\alpha)d\alpha} = B(t-a)\pi(a) & \text{for } t \geq a, \\ \phi(a-t)e^{-\int_{a-t}^a \mu(\alpha)d\alpha} & \text{for } t < a. \end{cases}$$

The problem which now faces us is to describe the behavior of solutions of the renewal equation under the assumptions that $\phi(t) \to 0$ as $t \to \infty$, and, in fact, $\int_0^\infty \phi(t)dt < \infty$ and $R = \int_0^\infty \beta(a)\pi(a)da < \infty$. The number R is the expected number of offspring for each individual over a lifetime, being the sum over all ages a of probability of survival to age a multiplied by number of offspring at age a. This analysis can be carried out, and it may be shown that asymptotically (as $t \to \infty$) every age distribution tends to a stable age distribution.

A *stable age distribution* (or *persistent age distribution*) is defined to be a solution $\rho(a,t)$ of the form $\rho(a,t) = A(a)T(t)$. We may shift a constant factor between $A(a)$ and $T(t)$ and thus assume $\int_0^\infty A(a)da = 1$; then we have

$$P(t) = \int_0^\infty \rho(a,t)da = T(t)\int_0^\infty A(a)da = T(t).$$

Thus $\rho(a,t) = P(t)A(a)$, and in a stable age distribution the proportion $\rho(a,t)/P(t)$ of age a is $A(a)$, independent of time.

Substitution of the form $\rho(a,t) = A(a)P(t)$ into the McKendrick equation (4.1) gives

$$A'(a)P(t) + A(a)P'(t) + \mu(a)A(a)P(t) = 0,$$

or

$$-\mu(a) - \frac{A'(a)}{A(a)} = \frac{P'(t)}{P(t)}.$$

Here primes denote derivatives with respect to the appropriate variable. Because the left side of this equation is a function of a only, while the right side is a function of t only, each side must be equal to a constant p_0 (as yet undetermined). Thus we have two separate ordinary differential equations:

$$P'(t) - p_0 P(t) = 0,$$

with solution

$$P(t) = P(0)e^{p_0 t},$$

and

$$A'(a) + (\mu(a) + p_0)A(a) = 0,$$

with solution

$$A(a) = A(0)e^{-p_0 a}e^{-\int_0^a \mu(\alpha)d\alpha} = A(0)e^{-p_0 a}\pi(a).$$

To satisfy the renewal condition $\rho(0,t) = \int_0^\infty \beta(a)\rho(a,t)da$ we must have

$$\begin{aligned} P(t)A(0) &= \int_0^\infty \beta(a)A(a)P(t)da \\ &= P(t)\int_0^\infty \beta(a)A(0)e^{-p_0 a}\pi(a)da \end{aligned}$$

or

$$\int_0^\infty \beta(a)\pi(a)e^{-p_0 a}da = 1,$$

which is known as the *Lotka–Sharpe equation* [37] for p_0. As we have already remarked, this has a unique real root, which is positive if $R = \int_0^\infty \beta(a)\pi(a)da > 1$, zero if $R = 1$, and negative if $R < 1$. In a stable age distribution,

$$\rho(a,t) = ce^{p_0 t}e^{-p_0 a}\pi(a) = ce^{p_0(t-a)}\pi(a),$$

and, as we have remarked earlier, asymptotically every age distribution tends to a stable age distribution.

If $R = 1$, then the total population size $P(t)$ is constant,

$$\rho(a,t) = B\pi(a),$$

and the birth rate is also a constant,

$$B(t) = \int_0^\infty \beta(a)P(0)A(0)\pi(a)da = P(0)A(0)\int_0^\infty \beta(a)\pi(a)da = P(0)A(0).$$

In this case we have an *equilibrium age distribution*. It is easy to see that, conversely, if the total population size is constant, then the birth rate is also constant and $\rho(a,t)$ is independent of t.

Example 1. In the "genesis" model we assume $\phi(a) = \delta(a)$, the Dirac delta function with $\delta(a) = 0$ for $a \neq 0$, $\int_0^\infty \delta(a)da = 1$. Thus the initial population is all at age zero. Let us assume also that the birth modulus $\beta(a)$ and the death modulus $\mu(a)$ are both constants, β and μ, respectively. Then the renewal equation takes the form

$$B(t) = \phi(t) + \int_0^t \beta e^{-\int_0^a \mu d\alpha} B(t-a)da,$$

with

$$\begin{aligned}\psi(t) &= \int_0^\infty \beta\phi(s)e^{-\int_s^{s+t}\mu d\alpha} ds \\ &= \int_0^\infty \delta(s)e^{-\mu t}ds = \beta e^{-\mu t}.\end{aligned}$$

Also

$$\beta e^{-\int_0^a \mu d\alpha} = \beta e^{-\mu a}.$$

Thus, $B(t)$ satisfies

$$\begin{aligned}B(t) &= \beta e^{-\mu t} + \beta\int_0^t e^{-\mu a}B(t-a)da \\ &= \beta e^{-\mu t} + \beta\int_0^t e^{-\mu(t-s)}B(s)ds \\ &= \beta e^{-\mu t} + \beta e^{-\mu t}\int_0^t e^{\mu s}B(s)ds.\end{aligned}$$

Differentiation gives

$$\begin{aligned}B'(t) &= -\mu\beta e^{-\mu t} + \beta e^{-\mu t}e^{\mu t}B(t) - \beta\mu e^{-\mu t}\int_0^t e^{\mu s}B(s)ds \\ &= -\mu\left(\beta e^{-\mu t} + \beta e^{-\mu t}\int_0^t e^{\mu s}B(s)ds\right) + \beta B(t) \\ &= -\mu B(t) + \beta B(t) = (\beta - \mu)B(t).\end{aligned}$$

From the renewal equation with $t = 0$ we see that $B(0) = \beta$. Now $B'(t) = (\beta - \mu)B(t)$, $B(0) = \beta$ implies $B(t) = \beta e^{(\beta-\mu)t}$, and this gives the age distribution function

$$\rho(a,t) = \begin{cases}\beta e^{(\beta-\mu)(t-a)-\mu a} & \text{for } t \geq a, \\ \delta(a-t)e^{-\mu t} & \text{for } t < a.\end{cases}$$

The total population size is

$$\begin{aligned}
P(t) &= \int_0^\infty \rho(a,t)da = \int_0^t \rho(a,t)da + \int_t^\infty \rho(a,t)da \\
&= \int_t^0 \beta e^{(\beta-\mu)t} e^{-\beta a} da + \int_t^\infty \delta(a-t)e^{-\mu t} da \\
&= \beta e^{(\beta-\mu)t} \int_0^t e^{-\beta a} da + e^{-\mu t} \\
&= e^{(\beta-\mu)t}(1-e^{-\beta t}) + e^{-\mu t} = e^{(\beta-\mu)t}.
\end{aligned}$$

4.4 Nonlinear Age-Structured Models

In the previous section, the birth and death rates were linear, and this implies that total population size either grows exponentially, dies out exponentially, or remains constant. In studying models without age structure, we considered situations in which populations have a carrying capacity that is approached as $t \to \infty$. In order to allow this possibility for age-structured models we must assume some nonlinearity. We now consider the possibility of birth and death moduli of the form $\beta(a, P(t))$ and $\mu(a, P(t))$, depending on total population size. A variant, which can be developed by analogous methods, would be to allow the birth modulus (and possibly also the death modulus) to depend on $\rho(a,t)$, the number of members in the same age cohort. We will consider only the continuous case because the methods of linear algebra methods used to treat the linear discrete case have no direct adaptation to the nonlinear discrete model.

If the birth and death moduli are allowed to depend on total population size, the description of the model must include the definition of $P(t)$. Thus, the full model is now

$$\begin{aligned}
\rho_a(a,t) + \rho_t(a,t) + \mu(a, P(t))\rho(a,t) &= 0, \\
B(t) = \rho(0,t) &= \int_0^\infty \beta(a, P(t))\rho(a,t)da, \\
P(t) &= \int_0^\infty \rho(a,t)da, \\
\rho(a,0) &= \phi(a).
\end{aligned} \tag{4.5}$$

We can transform the problem just as in the linear case by integrating along characteristics. If we define

$$\mu^*(\alpha) = \mu(\alpha, P(t-a+\alpha)),$$

the same calculations give

$$\rho(a,t) = \begin{cases} B(t-a)e^{-\int_0^a \mu^*(\alpha)d\alpha} & \text{for } t \geq a, \\ \phi(a-t)e^{-\int_{a-t}^a \mu^*(\alpha)d\alpha} & \text{for } t < a. \end{cases} \tag{4.6}$$

When we substitute these expressions into (4.5) and (4.6) we obtain a pair of functional equations for $B(t)$ and $P(t)$, whose solution gives an explicit solution for $\rho(a,t)$, namely,

$$B(t) = b(t) + \int_0^t \beta(a, P(t)) e^{-\int_0^a \mu^*(\alpha) d\alpha} B(t-a) da,$$

$$P(t) = p(t) + \int_0^t e^{-\int_0^a \mu^*(\alpha) d\alpha} B(t-a) da,$$

where

$$\mu^*(\alpha) = \mu(\alpha, P(t-a+\alpha)),$$

$$b(t) = \int_t^\infty \beta(a, P(t)) \phi(a-t) e^{-\int_{a-t}^a \mu^*(\alpha) d\alpha} da,$$

$$p(t) = \int_t^\infty \phi(a-t) e^{-\int_{a-t}^a \mu^*(\alpha) d\alpha} da.$$

It is reasonable to assume that $\int_0^\infty \phi(a) da < \infty$ and that the functions $\beta(a, P), \mu(a, P)$ are continuous and nonnegative. Under these hypotheses it is easy to verify that $b(t)$ and $p(t)$ are continuous and nonnegative and tend to zero as $t \to \infty$, and that $b(0) > 0$, $p(0) > 0$. Without additional assumptions it is not necessarily true that the pair of functional equations has a solution for $0 \le t < \infty$ but is possible to prove that if $\sup_{a \ge 0, P \ge 0} \beta(a, P) < \infty$, then there is a unique continuous nonnegative solution on $0 \le t < \infty$. This model is due to Gurtin and MacCamy [26].

A solution $\rho(a,t)$ that is independent of t is called an *equilibrium* age distribution. If $\rho(a,t) = \rho(a)$ is an equilibrium age distribution, then both $P(t) = \int_0^\infty \rho(a) da$ and $B(t) = \int_0^\infty \beta(a, P(t)) \rho(a) da$ are constant. Conversely, if $P(t)$ and $B(t)$ are constant, then $\rho(a,t)$ is independent of t and thus is an equilibrium age distribution.

If $\rho(a)$ is an equilibrium age distribution, the McKendrick equation becomes an ordinary differential equation $\rho'(a) + \mu(a, P)\rho(a) = 0$, with initial condition $\rho(0) = B$, whose solution is

$$\rho(a) = B e^{-\int_0^a \mu(\alpha, P) d\alpha}.$$

If we define

$$\pi(a, P) = e^{-\int_0^a \mu(\alpha, P) d\alpha}, \tag{4.7}$$

the probability of survival from birth to age a when the population size is the constant P, then

$$\rho(a) = B\pi(a, P).$$

From $P = \int_0^\infty \rho(a) da$, we obtain

$$P = B \int_0^\infty \pi(a) da,$$

and from $B = \int_0^\infty \beta(a, P) \rho(a) da$, we obtain

$$P = B \int_0^\infty \beta(a, P) \pi(a, P) da.$$

Thus, for an equilibrium age distribution with birth rate B and population size P, P must satisfy the equation

$$R(P) = \int_0^\infty \beta(a,P)\pi(a,P)da = 1,$$

and then B is given by

$$B = \frac{P}{\int_0^\infty \pi(a,P)da}.$$

Then $1/\int_0^\infty \pi(a,P)da$ is the average life expectancy and the equilibrium age distribution is $\rho(a) = B\pi(a,P)$. $R(P)$, called the *reproductive number*, is the expected number of offspring that an individual has over its lifetime, when the total population size is P.

Example 2. Suppose that β is independent of age and is a function of P only. Then

$$\begin{aligned} B(t) &= \int_0^\infty \beta(P(t))\rho(a,t)da = \beta(P(t))\int_0^\infty \rho(a,t)da \\ &= P(t)\beta(P(t)), \end{aligned} \tag{4.8}$$

and the problem is reduced to a single functional equation for $P(t)$ together with this explicit formula for $B(t)$. If we define $g(P) = P\beta(P)$, the equation for $P(t)$ is

$$P(t) = p(t) + \int_0^t e^{-\int_0^a \mu^*(\alpha)d\alpha} g(P(t-a))da.$$

Example 3. Suppose that β is independent of age and in addition that μ is independent of population size and is a function of age only. Then, instead of $\mu^*(\alpha) = \mu(\alpha, P(t-a+\alpha))$, we have $\mu(\alpha)$, and the equation for $P(t)$ is a Volterra integral equation called the *nonlinear renewal equation*:

$$\begin{aligned} P(t) &= p(t) + \int_0^t e^{-\int_0^a \mu(\alpha)d\alpha} g(P(t-a))da \\ &= p(t) + \int_0^t \pi(\alpha)g(P(t-a))da. \end{aligned} \tag{4.9}$$

In order to analyze (4.9), we first apply a theorem of Levin and Shea [35] which states that the asymptotic behavior of (4.9) is the same as that of the *limit equation*

$$P(t) = \int_0^\infty \pi(\alpha)g(P(t-a))da = \int_{-\infty}^t \pi(t-u)g(P(u))da. \tag{4.10}$$

In other words, the particular choice

$$p(t) = \int_t^\infty g(P(t-a))\pi(a)da$$

of initial function is general.

It is possible to prove [36] that every bounded solution of (4.10) approaches a limit P_∞ as $t \to \infty$ with

$$P_\infty = g(P_\infty)\int_0^\infty \pi(a)da,$$

or

$$\beta(P_\infty)\int_0^\infty \pi(a)da = 1.$$

If we differentiate the integral equation after writing

$$\int_0^t \pi(a)g(P(t-a))da = \int_0^t \pi(t-\tau)g(P(\tau))d\tau$$

and using the relation

$$\begin{aligned}\frac{d}{dt}\int_0^t \pi(t-\tau)g(P(\tau))d\tau &= \pi(0)g(P(t)) + \int_0^t \pi'(t-\tau)g(P(\tau))d\tau \\ &= \pi(0)g(P(t)) + \int_0^t \pi'(a)g(P(t-a))da,\end{aligned}$$

we obtain the integro-differential equation

$$P'(t) = p'(t) + \pi(0)g(P(t)) + \int_0^t g(P(t-a))\pi'(a)da,$$

whose linearization about the equilibrium P_∞ is

$$u'(t) = \pi(0)g'(P_\infty)u(t) + g'(P_\infty)\int_0^t u(t-a)\pi'(a)da.$$

We recall that for the linear integro-differential equation $u'(t) = \alpha u(t) + \beta\int_0^t u(t-a)k(a)da$ with $\int_0^\infty k(a)da = 1$ if $\alpha+\beta \geq 0$ then solutions do *not* tend to zero [12, Section 3.4]. Here $\alpha = \pi(0)g'(P_\infty)$,

$$k(a) = \frac{\pi'(a)}{\int_0^\infty \pi'(a)da} = \frac{\pi'(a)}{\pi(0)},$$

so that $\beta = g'(P_\infty)\int_0^\infty \pi'(a)da = -g(P_\infty)\pi(0)$ and $\alpha+\beta = 0$. Thus, the "equilibrium" P_∞ of the nonlinear renewal equation cannot be asymptotically stable. However, it can be shown [10, 11] that if $g'(P_\infty)\int_0^\infty \pi(a)da < 1$, the equilibrium P_∞ is stable in a weaker sense, namely, that small disturbances do not alter the solution very much, while if

$$g'(P_\infty)\int_0^\infty \pi(a)da > 1,$$

solutions tend away from P_∞. Thus, the condition $g'(P_\infty)\int_0^\infty \pi(a)da < 1$ is necessary for the limit P_∞ to be meaningful biologically. Since

$$g'(P_\infty) = \beta(P_\infty) + P_\infty\beta'(P_\infty)$$

and $\beta(P_\infty)\int_0^\infty \pi(a)da = 1$, this condition is equivalent to $\beta'(P_\infty) < 0$.

For age-structured populations with μ a function of age only and β a function of population size only, we have shown that every solution tends to an equilibrium age distribution, and we have

$$\lim_{t\to\infty} P(t) = P_\infty, \qquad \lim_{t\to\infty} B(t) = P_\infty \beta(P_\infty),$$

while

$$\rho(a,t) = B(t-a)\pi(a) \sim P_\infty \beta(P_\infty)\pi(a).$$

Such models are more realistic than models described by ordinary differential equations in which age dependence is ignored completely.

In the special case of a constant death rate

$$\pi(a) = e^{-\mu a},$$

differentiation of (4.10) gives

$$P'(t) = g(P(t)) - \mu P(t),$$

an ordinary differential model with a density-dependent birth rate.

4.5 Age-Structured Epidemic Models

The fundamental assumption in age-structured disease transmission models is that the number of susceptible, infective, and removed members of the population are stratified by age. That is, we assume that if u represents a compartment, then $u(a,t)$ represents the *density* of individuals of age a at time t; that is, the number of individuals with ages between a and $a+k$ at time t is approximately $u(a,t)k$. Then the total population of the compartment at time t is approximately $\sum_a u(a,t)k$, whose "limit as $k \to 0$" is $\int_0^\infty u(a,t)da$, and we define the total compartment size

$$U(t) = \int_0^\infty u(a,t)da.$$

In practice, it is reasonable to expect that there is a maximum attainable age, so that $u(a,t) = 0$ for all sufficiently large a and this integral is not necessarily an infinite integral.

Our first task is to determine how the function $u(a,t)$ changes as a function of t, and we may calculate that this is

$$u_a(a,t) + u_t(a,t).$$

We will assume that if members leave the compartment through natural death, there is an age-dependent death rate $\mu(a)$. This means that over the time interval from t to $t+h$ a fraction $\mu(a)h$ of the members with ages between a and $a+k$ at time t die. If $y(a)$ is the number of individuals who survive to age a, then

$$y'(a) = -\mu(a)y(a),$$

and this implies $y(a) = y(0)e^{-\int_0^a \mu(\alpha)d\alpha}$. Thus

$$\pi(a) = e^{-\int_0^a \mu(\alpha)d\alpha}$$

is the probability of survival from birth to age a.

Suppose that we have an age-structured population in which there is an infectious disease of SIR type. We introduce functions $s(t,a), i(t,a), r(t,a)$ representing the age distribution at time t of susceptible, infective, and removed members, respectively, so that the total numbers of susceptible, infective, and removed members in the population are

$$S(t) = \int_0^\infty s(a,t)da, \quad I(t) = \int_0^\infty i(a,t)da, \quad R(t) = \int_0^\infty r(a,t)da,$$

respectively. The age-distributed population is given by

$$s(a,t) + i(a,t) + r(a,t) = \rho(a,t),$$

and the total population size is

$$P(t) = S(t) + I(t) + R(t) = \int_0^\infty \rho(a,t)da.$$

As we have seen, the rate of change in time of a function $u(a,t)$ of time and age is

$$u_t(a,t) + u_a(a,t).$$

Thus we may write a system of equations

$$\begin{aligned}
s_t(a,t) + s_a(a,t) &= -(\mu(a) + \lambda(a,t))s(t,a), \\
i_t(a,t) + i_a(a,t) &= \lambda(a,t)s(a,t) - (\mu(a) + \gamma(a))i(a,t), \\
r_t(a,t) + r_a(a,t) &= -\mu(a)r(a,t) + \gamma(a)i(a,t)
\end{aligned}$$

to describe the transmission dynamics of the disease in the age-structured population. Here $\mu(a)$ is the natural death rate in each class, $\gamma(a)$ is the recovery rate, and $\lambda(a,t)$ represents the infection rate. To this system of partial differential equations we must add the initial conditions

$$s(a,0) = \Phi(a), \quad i(a,0) = \Psi(a), \quad r(a,0) = 0, \tag{4.11}$$

where Φ and Ψ are the initial distributions of susceptibles and infectives, respectively. In addition there is the birth or renewal condition, assuming that the age-dependent birth rate $\beta(a,P(t))$ (which may also depend on the total population size $P(t)$) does not depend on disease status and that all newborns are in the susceptible class

$$s(0,t) = \int_0^\infty \beta(a,P(t))\rho(a,t)da. \tag{4.12}$$

Further analysis requires some assumption on the nature of the infection term $\lambda(a,t)$. One possibility is *intracohort* mixing,

$$\lambda(a,t) = f(a)i(a,t),$$

corresponding to the assumption that infection can be transmitted only between individuals of the same age. Another possibility is *intercohort* mixing,

$$\lambda(a,t) = \int_0^\infty b(a,\alpha)i(\alpha,t)d\alpha,$$

with $b(a,\alpha)$ giving the rate of infection from contacts between an infective of age α with a susceptible of age a. For intercohort mixing it is necessary to make further assumptions on the mixing, that is, on the nature of the function $b(a,\alpha)$. One possibility here would be separable pair formation,

$$b(a,\alpha) = b_1(a)b_2(\alpha).$$

The analysis of an age-structured disease transmission model begins with a search for an endemic equilibrium. An endemic equilibrium is a nontrivial equilibrium age distribution, which is a solution of the model that is independent of t and is a function of a only. Endemic equilibria are solutions of systems of ordinary differential equations. The analysis of the stability of an equilibrium age distribution is usually quite complicated. Threshold results can be established for the existence of endemic states [15, 32]. The incorporation of age structure leads to possibilities of behavior that are not possible without the age dependence, such as sustained oscillations [4, 49, 52]. However, there is no indication of period-doubling or chaotic behavior unless seasonal variation of contacts is assumed [19, 21]. Age structure is an important aspect of the transmission of childhood diseases [24], e.g., for pertussis [29], rubella [30], varicella [50], and must be included in models designed to suggest realistic vaccination strategies. Optimal ages of vaccination are considered in [28, 43]. Age structure can also be incorporated as the time since becoming infected (age of infection) [60]. This is an important characteristic of HIV/AIDS models [54]. Rather than pursuing the analysis further here, we refer the reader to more advanced references such as [32].

Bibliography

[1] Anderson, R.M., H.C. Jackson, R.M. May, and A.M. Smith (1981) *Population dynamics of fox rabies in Europe*, Nature **289**: 765–771.

[2] Anderson, R.M. and R.M. May (1979) *Population biology of infectious diseases* I, Nature **280**: 361–367.

[3] Anderson, R.M. and R.M. May (1991) *Infectious Diseases of Humans*, Oxford University Press, Oxford.

[4] Andreasen, V. (1995) *Instability in an SIR-model with age dependent susceptibility*, in Mathematical Population Dynamics: Analysis of Heterogeneity, Vol. 1, Theory of Epidemics, O. Arino, D. Axelrod, M. Kimmel, and M. Langlais, eds., Wuerz, Winnipeg: 3–14.

[5] Arino, J., R. Jordan, and P. van den Driessche (2007) *Quarantine in a multispecies epidemic model with spatial dynamics*, Math. Biosc. **206**: 46–60.

[6] Arino, J. and P. van den Driessche (2003) *The basic reproduction number in a multi-city compartmental epidemic model*, Lecture Notes in Control and Information Science **294**: 135–142.

[7] Arino, J. and P. van den Driessche (2003) *A multi-city epidemic model*, Mathematical Population Studies **10**: 175–93.

[8] Arino, J. and P. van den Driessche (2006) *Metapopulation epidemic models*, Fields Institute Communications **48**: 1–13.

[9] Aronson, D.G. (1977) *The asymptotic spread of propagation of a simple epidemic*, in Nonlinear Diffusion, W.G. Fitzgibbon and H.F. Walker, eds., Research Notes in Mathematics **14**, Pitman, London.

[10] Brauer, F. (1976) *Perturbations of the nonlinear renewal equation*, Adv. in Math. **22**: 32–51.

[11] Brauer, F. (1987) *A class of Volterra integral equations arising in delayed-recruitment population models*, Nat. Res. Modeling **2**: 259–278.

[12] Brauer, F. and C. Castillo-Chavez (2012) *Mathematical Models in Population Biology and Epidemiology*, 2nd ed., Texts in Applied Mathematics **40**, Springer-Verlag, Berlin, Heidelberg.

[13] Britton, N.F. (2003) *Essentials of Mathematical Biology*, Springer-Verlag, Berlin, Heidelberg.

[14] Capasso, V. (1993) *Mathematical Structures of Epidemic Systems*, Lect. Notes in Biomath. **83**, Springer-Verlag, Berlin, Heidelberg, New York.

[15] Cha, Y., M. Ianelli, and F. Milner (1998) *Existence and uniqueness of endemic states for the age-structured S-I-R epidemic model*, Math. Biosc. **150**: 177–190.

[16] Diekmann, O. (1978) *Run for your life. A note on the asymptotic speed of propagation of an epidemic*, J. Diff. Eqns. **33**: 58–73.

[17] Diekmann, O. and J.A.P. Heesterbeek (2000) *Mathematical Epidemiology of Infectious Diseases: Model Building, Analysis and Interpretation*, John Wiley, New York.

[18] Dietz, K. (1975) *Transmission and control of arbovirus diseases*, in Epidemiology, D. Ludwig and K.L. Cooke, eds., SIAM, Philadelphia: 104–121.

[19] Earn, D.J.D., P. Rohani, B.M. Bolker, and B.T. Grenfell (2000) *A simple model for complex dynamical transitions in epidemics*, Science **287**: 667–670.

[20] Edelstein-Keshet, L. (2005) *Mathematical Models in Biology*, Classics in Applied Mathematics **46**, SIAM, Philadelphia.

[21] Ellner, S., R. Gallant, and J. Theiler (1995) *Detecting nonlinearity and chaos in epidemic data*, in Epidemic Models: Their Structure and Relation to Data, D. Mollison, ed., Cambridge University Press, Cambridge: 229–247.

[22] Fitzgibbon, W.E., M.E. Parrott, and G.F. Webb (1995) *Diffusive epidemic models with spatial and age-dependent heterogeneity*, Discrete Contin. Dyn. Syst. **1**: 35–57.

[23] Fitzgibbon, W.E., M.E. Parrott, and G.F. Webb (1996) *A diffusive age-structured SEIRS epidemic model*, Methods Appl. Anal. **3**: 358–369.

[24] Greenhalgh, D. (1990) *Vaccination campaigns for common childhood diseases*, Math. Biosc. **100**: 201–240.

[25] Grenfell, B.T. and A. Dobson, eds. (1995) *Ecology of Infectious Diseases in Natural Populations*, Cambridge University Press, Cambridge.

[26] Gurtin, M.L. and R.C. MacCamy (1974) *Nonlinear age dependent population dynamics*, Arch. Rat. Mech. Analysis **54**: 281–300.

[27] Hadeler, K.P. (2003) *The role of migration and contact distributions in epidemic spread*, in Bioterrorism: Mathematical Modeling Applications in Homeland Security, H. T. Banks and C. Castillo-Chavez, eds., SIAM, Philadelphia: 199–210.

[28] Hadeler, K.P. and J. Müller (1996) *Optimal vaccination patterns in age-structured populations II: Optimal strategies*, in Models for Infectious Human Diseases: Their Structure and Relation to Data, V. Isham and G. Medley, eds., Cambridge University Press, Cambridge: 102–114.

[29] Hethcote, H.W. (1997) *An age structured model for pertussis transmission*, Math. Biosc. **145**: 89–136.

[30] Hethcote, H.W. (2000) *The mathematics of infectious diseases*, SIAM Rev. **42**: 599–653.

[31] Hoppensteadt, F. (1975) *Mathematical Theories of Populations: Demographics, Genetics, and Epidemics*, SIAM, Philadelphia.

[32] Iannelli, M. (1995) *Mathematical Theory of Age-Structured Population Dynamics*, Appl. Mathematical Monographs, C.N.R., Giardini Editori e Stampatori, Pisa.

[33] Källén, A., P. Arcuri, and J.D. Murray (1985) *A simple model for the spatial spread and control of rabies*, J. Theor. Biol. **116**: 377–393.

[34] Kot, M. (2001) *Elements of Mathematical Ecology*, Cambridge University Press, Cambridge.

[35] Levin, J.J. and D.F. Shea (1972) *On the asymptotic behavior of the bounded solutions of some integral equations, I, II, III*, J. Math. Anal. & Appl. **37**: 42–82, 288–326, 537–575.

[36] Londen, S.-O. (1974) *On the asymptotic behavior of the bounded solutions of a nonlinear Volterra equation*, SIAM J. Math. Anal., **5**: 849–875.

[37] Lotka, A.J. and F.R. Sharpe (1923) *Contributions to the analysis of malaria epidemiology*, Am. J. Hygiene, **3** (Suppl.): 1–21.

[38] MacDonald, D.W. (1980) *Rabies and Wildlife. A Biologist's Perspective*, Oxford University Press, Oxford.

[39] May, R.M. (1986) *Population biology of macroparasitic infections*, in Mathematical Ecology; An Introduction, T.G. Hallam and S.A. Levin, eds., Biomathematics **18**, Springer-Verlag, Berlin, Heidelberg, New York: 405–442.

[40] May, R.M. and Anderson, R.M. (1979) *Population biology of infectious diseases II*, Nature **280**: 455–461.

[41] McKendrick, A.G. (1926) *Applications of mathematics to medical problems*, Proc. Edinburgh Math. Soc. **44**: 98–130.

[42] Mollison, D. (1977) *Spatial contact models for ecological and epidemic spread*, J. Roy. Stat. Soc. Ser. B **39**: 283–326.

[43] Müller, J. (1998) *Optimal vaccination patterns in age-structured populations*, SIAM J. Appl. Math. **59**: 222–241.

[44] Murray, J.D. (2002) *Mathematical Biology, Vol. I*, Springer-Verlag, Berlin, Heidelberg, New York.

[45] Murray, J.D. (2002) *Mathematical Biology, Vol. II*, Springer-Verlag, Berlin, Heidelberg, New York.

[46] Murray, J.D., E.A. Stanley, and D.L. Brown (1986) *On the spatial spread of rabies among foxes*, Proc. Roy. Soc. Lond. B **229**: 111–150.

[47] Radcliffe, J. and L. Rass (1986) *The asymptotic spread of propagation of the deterministic non-reducible n-type epidemic*, J. Math. Biol. **23**: 341–359.

[48] Sattenspiel, L. and K. Dietz (1995) *A structured epidemic model incorporating geographic mobility among regions*, Math. Biosc. **128**: 71–91.

[49] Schenzle, D. (1984) *An age-structured model of pre- and post-vaccination measles transmission*, IMA J. Math. Med. Biol. **1**: 169–191.

[50] Schuette, M.C. and H.W. Hethcote (1999) *Modeling the effects of varicella vaccination programs on the incidence of chickenpox and shingles*, Bull. Math. Biol. **61**: 1031–1064.

[51] Thieme, H.R. (1979) *Asymptotic estimates of the solutions of nonlinear integral equations and asymptotic speeds for the spread of populations*, J. Reine Angew. Math. **306**: 94–121.

[52] Thieme, H.R. (1990) *Stability change of the endemic equilibrium in age-structured models for the spread of S-I-R type infectious diseases*, in Differential Equations Models in Biology, Epidemiology and Ecology, S. Busenberg and M. Martelli, eds., Lect. Notes in Biomath. **92**, Springer-Verlag, Berlin, Heidelberg, New York: 139–158.

[53] Thieme, H.R. (2003) *Mathematics in Population Biology*, Princeton University Press, Princeton, NJ.

[54] Thieme, H.R. and C. Castillo-Chavez (1993) *How may infection-age-dependent infectivity affect the dynamics of HIV/AIDS?*, SIAM J. Appl. Math. **53**: 1447–1479.

[55] Van den Bosch, F., J.A.J. Metz, and O. Diekmann (1990) *The velocity of spatial population expansion*, J. Math. Biol. **28**: 529–565.

[56] Van den Driessche, P. (2008) *Spatial structure: Patch models*, in Mathematical Epidemiology, F. Brauer, P. van den Driessche, and J. Wu, eds., Lecture Notes in Math. **1945**, Springer-Verlag, Berlin, Heildelberg, New York: 179–189.

[57] Waltman, P. (1974) *Deterministic Threshold Models in the Theory of Epidemics*, Lect. Notes in Biomath. **1**, Springer-Verlag, Berlin, Heidelberg, New York.

[58] Webb, G.F. (1985) *Theory of Nonlinear Age-Dependent Population Dynamics*, Marcel Dekker, New York.

[59] Weinberger, H.F. (1981) *Some deterministic models for the spread of genetic and other alterations*, in Biological Growth and Spread, W. Jaeger, H. Rost, and P. Tautu, eds., Lect. Notes in Biomath. **38**, Springer-Verlag, Berlin, Heidelberg, New York: 320–333.

[60] Zhou, Y., B. Song, and Z. Ma (2002) *The global stability analysis for an SIS model with age and infection age structure*, in Mathematical Approaches for Emerging and Re-emerging Diseases: Models, Methods, and Theory, C. Castillo-Chavez, with S. Blower, P. van den Driessche, D. Kirschner, and A.-A. Yakubu, eds., Springer-Verlag, Berlin, Heidelberg, New York: 313–335.

Lecture 5

Models for Diseases in Highly Mobile Populations

5.1 Introduction to Models for Mobile Populations

Classical demography [76, 77, 80] has rarely paid explicit attention to the study of social dynamics. Furthermore, mathematical demography has often bypassed the modeling difficulties associated with pairing (two-sex models). Instead, it has focused on the study of models that assume a 50-50 sex ratio. This simplifying assumption has reduced the study of reproduction and aging dynamics to the analysis of a single-sex framework [76, 77]. The dynamics of Leslie's single-sex model [76, 77] *eventually* settles in what is referred to as the *stable age* distribution (no growth or exponential growth or decay with age proportions remaining fixed). A large percentage of the applications of mathematics to human demography have been carried out in populations that have reached this distribution.

Theoretical work that incorporates *population-level mating structures* has been carried out with the aid of *marriage* functions pioneered by Kendall and Keyfitz in the late 1940s [70, 71], later extended by a group of researchers that include Fredrickson [45], McFarland [81], Parlett [85], and Pollard [86]. The use of marriage functions in the study of the dynamics of pairing has been carried out primarily in the context of multigroup differential or partial differential (structured populations) equation models.

Advances in the study of the dynamics of social interactions in demography and epidemiology had been rather limited until the emergence of HIV [2, 3, 19, 20, 48, 55, 59, 60, 62, 63, 65, 73]. In the context of sexually transmitted diseases (STDs), Dietz [41] and Dietz and Hadeler [42] introduced models that included the processes of pair formation and dissolution. We, a generic "we" that includes many collaborators, cited throughout the text, have developed and explored population-level mathematical mating/mixing frameworks built under rather general assumptions [10, 11, 13, 17, 18, 21, 22, 25, 26, 27, 49, 58, 64, 83]. Furthermore, efforts to ground this theoretical mixing/contact mathematical research on data have been carried out as well. For example, "we" have gathered mixing/contact data [12, 35, 89] as part of past efforts aimed at connecting "mixing" (social dynamics) and disease transmission [20, 23, 25, 26, 47, 58, 62, 63, 83].

In this lecture, we revisit the mixing framework introduced in [10, 11, 13, 17, 18, 21, 22, 25, 26, 27, 49, 58, 64, 83] and apply it to the study of the role of individuals' mobility on the transmission dynamics of communicable diseases, like smallpox. The rest of the chapter is organized as follows: Section 5.2 revisits the basic contact/social/mixing structure formalism and states basic theoretical results; Section 5.3 introduces a model that is used to address the dynamics of communicable diseases in multilayer mixing communities; Section 5.4 highlights the complexities associated with analyzing realistic models with emphasis on the computation of the basic reproduction number; Section 5.5 focuses on the dynamics of a *potential* deliberate release of smallpox in a resident-tourist scenario in an urban center; and Section 5.6 summarizes results and revisits some the themes discussed in this chapter.

5.2 Contact Structures Framework

The mass-action law has played a central role in the development of stochastic and deterministic models for the transmission dynamics and control of diseases (see [1, 3, 6, 14, 15] and the references therein). The assumption that the rate of new infections (the incidence) is proportional to the product of susceptible and infective individuals, while useful, has its limitations, particularly when it is modeled exclusively using mass-action terms. Limitations become evident when factors like disease-induced mortality (selection) play a role. Mass-action epidemiological models would usually require the knowledge of parameters, typically assumed to be constant on populations of fixed size. These parameters may now have to be considered functions of a dynamic total population size. In the literature this issue is bypassed by declaring a priori whether or not the mass-action or the so-called standard incidence nonlinear terms are used in the model at hand, typically without addressing the implications of making either assumption. The use of both modeling formalisms have, for example, generated discrepancies in the estimated values of important quantities like the basic reproduction number. Clarifying, a priori, the nature of the nonlinearities associated with the interactions or contacts between individuals of different types, would make an excellent modeling practice. Dealing with mixing (who interacts with whom) in structured populations or in models involving interacting subpopulations adds additional challenges. Some efforts carried out in this direction include [10, 11, 13, 17, 18, 21, 22, 27, 49, 83] and the references therein.

Soon after the start of the HIV/AIDS epidemic it became obvious that quantifying the contact social structure of a population, heterogeneous mixing, was central to the study of the transmission dynamics of potentially fatal diseases like HIV [19, 20, 57]. In the context of malaria, the importance of heterogeneous contact processes was already clearly recognized by Ross [87]. Ross's insights motivated the extensions that we have carried out over the past couple of decades that will be briefly discussed in the next section (see [10, 11, 13, 17, 18, 21, 22, 27, 49, 64, 83]).

5.2.1 Two-sex age-structured mixing functions

A general approach used to model age-dependent contact or mixing processes, that is, our way of describing who mixes or pairs with whom, is described below following the work in [13, 17, 18, 19, 21, 22, 24, 27]. We formulate this framework for two-sex age-structured populations (two-sex models are discussed, in the modeling of STDs, in this monograph). We let $M(a,t)$ denote the density of males of age a who are not in pairs at time t ("singles") and $F(a,t)$ denote the density of females of age a who are also single at time t. The process of pairing (or mixing) is defined using the following mixing definitions and assumptions:

- $p(a,a',t)$ denotes the proportion of partnerships (contacts) of males of age a with females of age a' at time t, given that they formed a partnership (made a contact);
- $q(a,a',t)$ denotes the proportion of partnerships of females of age a with males of age a' at time t, given that they formed a partnership (made a contact);
- $C(a,t)$ expected or average age-specific number of partners (contacts) involving males of age a at time t per unit time;
- $D(a,t)$ expected or average age-specific number of partners of females of age a at time t per unit time.

Definition 5.1. *The following conditions (axioms or properties) are used to characterize mixing functions:*

(i) $p,q \geq 0$;

(ii) $\int_0^\infty p\left(a,a',t\right)da' = \int_0^\infty q\left(a',a,t\right)da = 1$;

(iii) $p\left(a,a',t\right)C\left(a,t\right)M\left(a,t\right) = q\left(a',a,t\right)D\left(a',t\right)F\left(a',t\right)$;

(iv) $C\left(a,t\right)M\left(a,t\right)D\left(a',t\right)F\left(a',t\right) = 0 \Rightarrow p\left(a,a',t\right) = q\left(a',a,t\right) = 0$.

Condition (ii) is due to the fact that p and q can be thought of as conditional probabilities. Condition (iii) simply states that the total rate of pair formation between males of age a and females of age a' equals the total rate of pair formation between females of age a' and males of age a (all per unit time and age). Condition (iv) states that there is no mixing in the age and activity levels where there are no active individuals; that is, on the set $\mathcal{L}(t) = \{(a,a',t):\ C(r,a,t)M(a,t)D(a,t)F(a,t) = 0\}$.

The pair (p,q) is called a *two-sex mixing function* as long as it satisfies axioms (i)–(iv). What would some special solutions look like? A two-sex mixing function is *separable* if and only if

$$p\left(a,a',t\right) = p_1\left(a,t\right)p_2\left(a',t\right) \quad \text{and} \quad q\left(a,a',t\right) = q_1\left(a,t\right)q_2\left(a',t\right).$$

Defining

$$h_p\left(a,t\right) = C\left(a,t\right)M\left(a,t\right)$$

and

$$h_q\left(a,t\right) = D\left(a,t\right)F\left(a,t\right),$$

then omitting t to simplify the notation, one can immediately verified the result established in [18, 21, 22, 27], namely, the following result.

Result 1. The only two-sex separable mixing function satisfying conditions (i)–(iv) is given by the Ross solution $(\hat{p},\hat{q})$, where

$$\hat{p}(a') = \frac{h_q(a')}{\int_0^\infty h_p(u)du},$$

$$\hat{q}(a) = \frac{h_p(a)}{\int_0^\infty h_q(u)du}.$$

This solution was named the *Ross solution* (see [21, 22, 26, 27]) as soon as it became clear, after reading Ross's paper [87], that he was already aware of the importance and necessity of Axiom (iii) in his efforts to model the transmission dynamics of malaria. Ross also noted the potential use of his modeling framework on the study of the dynamics of STDs. Axiom (iii) was also identified by Lotka [78] in his review of Ross's work on malaria models. In [17, 18, 21, 22, 26]), we also established the following result.

Result 2. Any solution of axioms (i)–(iv) can be written as a multiplicative perturbation of the Ross solution $(\hat{p}, \hat{q})$. These perturbations are a measure of the deviation from random or proportionate mixing among subpopulations (given by the Ross solutions) and can be parametrized by matrices that estimate the affinities/preferences of individuals.

Methods to connect these functions to data and surveys tied in to "dating" and "sexual activity" in college populations have been carried out was well (see [12, 35, 62, 63, 83, 89]).

5.2.2 Discrete multigroup mixing functions

The framework put in place in [17, 18, 11] has provided an axiomatic approach for the formulation of the process of mixing within structured populations. It works just as well in the modeling of mixing involving multiple subpopulations, a fixed number of interacting groups. The mixing of a fixed number of interacting dynamic subpopulations will be described in terms of a conditional *"probability"* matrix, here called P, with entries P_{ij} that depend on the state variables of the system. Each (P_{ij}) models the fraction of contacts that individuals from group or subpopulation i have with individuals in group or subpopulation j given that members from group i had contacts. Since, we have primarily applied these models using deterministic models (see, however, [79]), the subpopulations involved are large, each with size denoted by N_i, $i = 1, 2, \ldots, L$. In order to complete the setup, we let C_i $(i = 1, 2, \ldots, L)$ denote the per-capita average contact rates, assumed constant. The mixing matrix $(P_{ij}; i, j \text{ in } \{1, 2, \ldots, L\})$ is now assumed to satisfy the properties or mixing axioms stated in the previous section (omitting the last one), namely,

$$0 \le P_{ij} \le 1, \quad \text{all} \quad i, j, \tag{5.1}$$

$$\sum_{j=1}^{L} P_{ij} = 1, \quad \text{all} \quad i, \tag{5.2}$$

$$C_i N_i P_{ij} = C_j N_j P_{ji}, \quad \text{all} \quad i, j. \tag{5.3}$$

Here, we assume that all $P_{ij} > 0$ and observe that from the first two conditions, it follows that P is a stochastic matrix. The third condition arises from the natural assumption that the average total contact *rates* between pairs of groups must be balanced. It was shown (see [11, 12, 17, 18]) that the only separable solution to the mixing axioms is *proportionate* mixing. This important solution is represented as

$$P_{ij} = \bar{P}_j = \frac{C_j N_j}{\sum_l C_l N_l}.$$

In the above references, it was also shown that matrices P_{ij} satisfying the above three mixing axioms can be generated as multiplicative perturbations of proportionate mixing with the aid of symmetric "preference" matrix Φ. The explicit result states the following.

Result 3 (see [11, 17, 18].) The solution to the mixing axioms is given by $P_{ij} = \bar{P}_j[\frac{R_i R_j}{V} + \phi_{ij}]$, where $R_i = 1 - \sum_k \bar{P}_k \phi_{ik}$, $V = \sum_k \bar{P}_k R_k$, and $\Phi = (\phi_{ij})$ is an $L \times L$ symmetric matrix, that is, $\phi_{ij} = \phi_{ji}$, for all $i,\, j \in \{1,2,\ldots,L\}$.

Efforts to interpret the symmetric matrix $\Phi = (\phi_{ij})$ as group affinities can be found in [10, 13, 17, 23, 49, 62, 83]. In the next section, we make use of a modified form of proportionate mixing to model a multilevel mixing environment that is later used to highlight some of the possible outcomes that emerge from deliberate releases of smallpox scenarios (or similar infectious agents).

5.3 Modeling Epidemics in Urban Centers

The role of individual mobility, most often just the result of routine activities, like the use of mass transportation systems, on disease dynamics has been addressed by a number of researchers in the context of communicable and sexually transmitted diseases. Pioneer modeling efforts to connect epidemic patterns to transportation systems are found in [8, 90]. In the case of influenza A, the role of airline transportation epidemic patterns in the U.S. has been addressed [61, 72]. The role of airline traffic on the 2009 global influenza A/H1N1 pandemic was explored, for example, in [72], while the role of bus transportation in the context of this pandemic in Mexico was studied in [54]. Past modeling efforts include those associated with smallpox dynamics [31], tuberculosis [32], HIV [68], and influenza [54]. Consequently, modeling frameworks have been built to capture multicity or multiregion effects on disease dynamics (see, for example, [5, 8, 28, 31, 54, 61, 90]). Less specific (detailed) modeling approaches have been advanced to study the role of host mobility on the dynamics of STDs as well [33, 74, 68].

5.3.1 Deliberate releases of biological agents

The increased interest in studying ways of protecting our populations against bioterrorism, here defined as the deliberate release of biological agents and their consequences [29], has become, after the World Trade Center attacks in New York City on September 11, 2001, a fundamental component of national security policies across the world. In the First National Symposium on Medical and Public Health Response to Bioterrorism held on February 16–17, 1999, in Arlington, VA, Henderson noted [50]: *"What is the possible aftermath of an act of biological terrorism? Which biological threats warrant the most concern?"* As observed in [31], this symposium

> was motivated, in part, by the 1995 sarin gas attack by a Japanese religious cult, which actually attempted to aerosolize anthrax in the Tokyo area; the establishment of Russia's bioweapons research program; and the emigration of a large number of scientists after the crash of [the] former Soviet Union....
>
> *Bioterrorism* is now defined as the deliberate release of biological agents and their consequences.... This is not a novel activity. Smallpox was used as a weapon

> by British forces during the French and Indian Wars via the distribution of smallpox-infected blankets before cowpox vaccination against smallpox took practice in 1796.... Biological weapons have been recently utilized by Iraq in its wars with Iran and local Kurds. The distribution of anthrax spores through the US mail in 2001 has shown that the type and number of channels for bioterrorist activities is so extensive that efforts to address the source of such attacks (individuals) must become a priority....

Smallpox was officially declared "eradicated " in 1980, but official repositories were left at the Centers for Disease Control and Prevention (CDC) in Atlanta (U.S.) and the State Research Center of Virology and Biotechnology in Koltsovo, Novosibirsk (Russia). However, there are serious concerns regarding the possibility of the existence of additional sites housing smallpox [94]. After September 11, 2001, the idea of building a stockpile of smallpox vaccine for the 300 million individuals living in the U.S. was carried out in record time. There were roughly 50 million vaccine doses worldwide prior to September 11, 2001, and now there are at least 300×10^6 in the U.S. alone [34].

5.3.2 Smallpox epidemiology, vaccine, and treatment

Smallpox is a viral communicable disease that is passed from person to person, with transmission likely whenever an individual is within a seven-foot radius of an infectious individual. Airborne transmission is also possible [16, 92, 94, 66]. The following (as noted in an earlier lecture) not-quite-standard epidemiological definitions are used throughout: the *latent period* is the time from the acquisition of infection to the time when the host becomes infectious; the *infectious period* is the time during which the infected individual is capable of transmitting the disease; the *incubation period* is the time interval between the point of acquisition of infection and the appearance of symptoms. Following exposure to the smallpox virus, there is an initial asymptomatic (infectious) period lasting on the average 12 to 14 days, followed by a symptomatic period, the prodrome phase, where transmission is less efficient. Infected persons are most contagious two to three days after the prodrome state, and this period of infectiousness lasts about four days (see [51]).

Effective smallpox treatment is *essentially unavailable*, and therefore it can be *primarily* prevented by vaccinating individuals *before exposure or within* 3–4 *days following exposure*, a policy that has been estimated to generate protection at the 97% level (among vaccinated individuals). It has been estimated that acquired immunity may last up to 5 years. Since the vaccination of the U.S. population stopped 40 years ago, we must all be (differentially) susceptible to smallpox.

The World Health Organization (WHO) carried out a successful smallpox eradication campaign using a ring or trace vaccination (TV) model (requiring the exclusive vaccination of those who have had direct contact with smallpox infected individuals). Naturally, the CDC recommended the use of this tested strategy in the event of a smallpox outbreak. An alternative strategy, mass vaccination (MV), was proposed by Kaplan [67] as better suited to the context of interest, namely, the deliberate release of smallpox. Randy Larsen considered the stockpiling of vaccines and the training of medical professionals essential [37] and noted, in response to a "dark winter" [36] scenario, that vaccinating all individuals would not be a viable option, given the high number of people in the U.S. population with compromised immune systems or who were likely to react adversely to the vaccine. He further argued in favor of a policy of TV for small-scale attacks and a policy of MV for large-scale attacks [75]. Kaplan estimated the potential number of total deaths and cases resulting from the use of MV and TV strategies. He concluded that MV was better. Kemper and colleagues reacted to Kaplan's conclusions with concern because of their own assessment of the potential complication rates that would be generated from the massive use of the smallpox vaccine [69]. Immediate responses expressing serious doubts about the figures used on adverse reactions and deaths on Kemper's paper followed (see [69]).

The use of the basic reproductive number to evaluate the effectiveness of MV and TV strategies was at the heart of the analyses. The assumption was made that the basic reproductive number was approximately 3, a number consistent with prior published estimates [3]. In [53], it was reported that estimates for reproductive number during the 1960s and 1970s was as large as 10 or even 20 [53]. Gani and Leach argued that the basic reproduction number range should be between 3.5 and 6 [46]. These ranges were used to support the initial decision by the CDC and the Working Group on Civilian Biodefense in 1999 to store 40 million doses [53]. The U.S. government stockpiled 286 million doses of which 155 million were bought from a British firm after 9/11 [34].

5.4 Model for the Deliberate Release of Communicable Diseases

Why is smallpox such a threat? Smallpox, a highly contagious deadly agent, is capable of generating high case fatality rates and lacks *specific* forms of treatment. Smallpox has access to an immense pool of susceptibles worldwide. Further, we live in a highly mobile world where infected individuals have the ability to spread smallpox over short- and long-term regions. Subways, airport hubs, and city buses provide instant access to rapid and highly effective transmission networks. New York City, for example, with a population of about 8 million (just within the city) and roughly 4.3 million individuals running around each day through its subway system (higher number on weekends), provides a prototypical example of a *vulnerable target* from where pathogens would spread quickly and efficiently to most corners of the world [56].

Daniel Bernoulli [9], one of the first mathematicians to publish a smallpox model, used New York City to reestimate, under the assumption that smallpox could be eliminated as a cause of death, smallpox-free adjusted life tables [43]. After 9/11 smallpox and anthrax were reidentified as portable dangerous biological agents that aerosolized easily and generate high case fatality rates [88]. The results of pre- and post-9/11 studies involving mathematical models used to assess potential outcomes from the deliberate release of smallpox can be found in the literature (see [31, 38, 50, 52, 67, 82] and the references therein).

In this section, we reintroduce a model that was first put forward in the context of tuberculosis transmission in urban centers [28]. The model was used, in a corrected version, in a study of the potential consequences of the deliberate smallpox release in a city like New York City [31]. The discussion in the rest of this section follows closely the formulation and results found in [31] and shown schematically in Figure 5.1.

The urban center modeled is divided into N neighborhoods. The population within each neighborhood is further subdivided into two groups: subway (or mass-transportation) users (SU) and nonsubway (non-mass-transportation) users (NSU). Individuals, in the version presented, are not assumed to change mass-transportation status, an assumption that naturally determines the time-scale of model "validity" or applicability (an assumption that

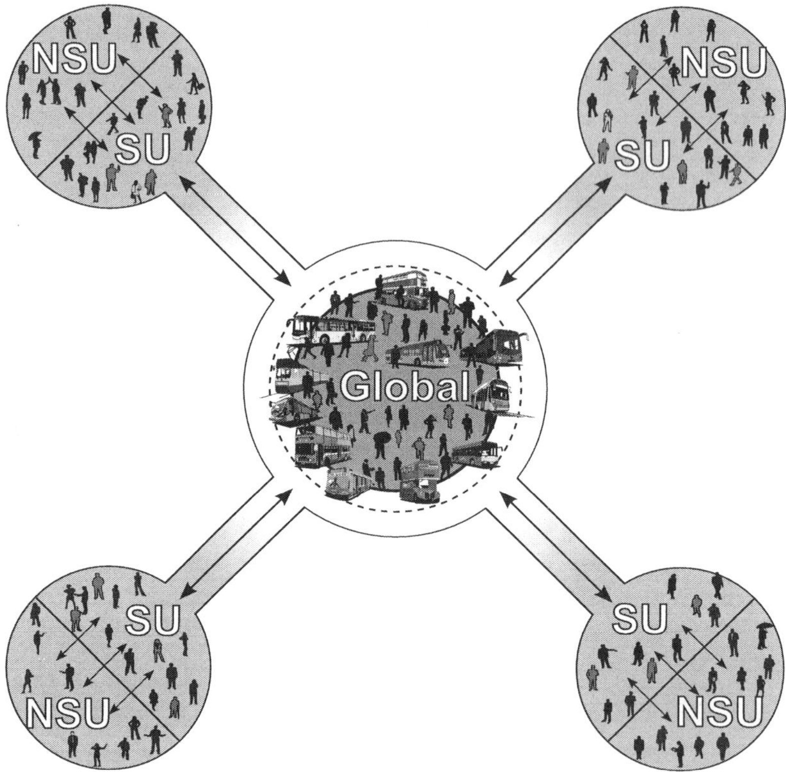

Figure 5.1. *A schematic diagram of the transportation model.*

is easily weakened). The contact structure is driven by mass-transit status: SU individuals are assumed to have contacts with *both* SU individuals *everywhere in the city* and NSU individuals but *only* within their own (home) neighborhood. In other words, SU individuals are the link connecting neighborhoods with the mass-transit system playing the role of a "mixing bowl" since SU multineighborhood connections are only active while mass-transportation, that is, SU users *share a subway–mass-transportation ride*. Hence, it is assumed that contacts between SU individuals living in distinct home neighborhoods are negligible *outside the subway–mass-transportation network*. On the other hand, NSU individuals have, by assumption, all of their contacts with individuals living in the same neighborhood while they are off the subway. The last assumptions could be easily relaxed within the same modeling framework, but as we shall soon observe the mixing makes the generation of analytical results tough (at least for us).

In the event of an epidemic outbreak, here the result of a smallpox attack, the epidemiological status of individuals would shift. Individuals in this population (SU and NSU) are therefore assumed to belong to one of the following neighborhood specific epidemiological classes: S_i, E_i, I_i, R_i, classes used to denote the number of NSU individuals with home neighborhood i that are susceptible, exposed, infectious, and recovered, respectively. Similarly, W_i, X_i, Y_i, Z_i denote the subpopulation of SU individuals with home neighborhood i

who are susceptible, exposed, infectious, and recovered, respectively. Hence total SU and NSU population sizes are $Q_i = S_i + E_i + I_i + R_i$ and $T_i = W_i + X_i + Y_i + Z_i$, respectively. In order to introduce the contact structure describing the mixing between and within individuals of these subpopulations, we let a_i and b_i denote the average per-capita contact rates for NSU and the SU neighborhood i subpopulations, respectively. Further, if we now let ρ_i and σ_i denote the per-capita rates at which SU individuals get on and off the subway, respectively, then $\omega_i = \rho_i/(\sigma_i + \rho_i)$ and $\tau_i = \sigma_i/(\sigma_i + \rho_i)$ would represent the fractions of time that SU individual spend on and off the subway, respectively ($\omega_i + \tau_i = 1$). Finally, it is assumed in the rest of this lecture that group interactions are modeled under proportional mixing model (see [18, 7, 84, 65]), an assumption that could be relaxed [10, 18].

The mixing probabilities between the SU and NSU subpopulations within and outside the subway (mass-transportation system) are therefore modeled by the following functions of the state variables (see [31]):

(1) $P_{a_i a_i} = \tilde{P}_{a_i} = \frac{a_i Q_i}{a_i Q_i + b_i \tau_i T_i}$ is the mixing probability between SU individuals from the same neighborhood i.

(2) $P_{a_i b_i} = \tilde{P}_{b_i} = \frac{b_i \tau_i T_i}{a_i Q_i + b_i \tau_i T_i}$ the mixing probability of NSU and SU individuals from the same neighborhood i.

(3) $P_{b_i a_i} = \bar{P}_{a_i} = \frac{a_i Q_i}{a_i Q_i + b_i \tau_i T_i} \tau_i$ is the mixing probability of SU and NSU individuals from the same neighborhood i.

(4) $P_{b_i b_i} = \bar{P}_{b_i} = \frac{b_i \tau_i T_i}{a_i Q_i + b_i \tau_i T_i} \tau_i$ is the mixing probability between SU individuals from the same neighborhood i.

(5) $P_{b_i b_j} = \bar{P}_{b_j^i} = \frac{b_j \omega_j T_j}{\sum_{k=1}^{N} b_k \omega_k T_k} \omega_i$ is the mixing probability between SU individuals from neighborhoods i and j.

(6) $P_{a_i a_j} = 0$ means NSU individuals from neighborhoods i and j do not have contacts assuming $i \neq j$.

(7) $P_{a_i b_j} = 0$ means NSU individuals from neighborhood i and SU individuals from neighborhood j have no contacts a ssuming $i \neq j$.

The following neighborhood identities must hold (see [31]):

$$\begin{aligned} \tilde{P}_{a_i} + \tilde{P}_{b_i} &= 1, \quad i = 1,2,\ldots,N, \\ \bar{P}_{a_i} + \bar{P}_{b_i} + \sum_{j=1}^{N} \bar{P}_{b_j} &= \tau_i + \omega_i = 1, \quad i = 1,2,\ldots,N. \end{aligned} \tag{5.4}$$

The dynamics of transmission within and between neighborhoods is therefore modeled as a nonlinear system of differential equations (parameters definitions are collected in Table 5.1). The model equations are therefore given by the following system (as in [31]):

$$\frac{dW_i}{dt} = \Lambda_i - V_i(t) - (\mu + q_i l_1) W_i, \tag{5.5}$$

$$\frac{dX_i}{dt} = V_i(t) - (\mu + \phi + q_i l_2) X_i, \tag{5.6}$$

Table 5.1. *Definitions of parameters; i is used to index the neighborhoods (modified from* [31]*).*

Parameters	Definitions
Λ_i	recruitment rate of subway users
A_i	recruitment rate of nonsubway users
μ	per-capita natural mortality rate
d	per-capita mortality rate due to smallpox
q_i	per capital vaccination rate
l_1, l_2	vaccination efficacy rates for susceptible and exposed populations
ϕ	per-capita progression rate from latent to infectious
α	per-capita recovery rate
σ_i	per-capita the rate at which subway user leaves the subway
ρ_i	per-capita the rate at which subway user takes the subway
a_i	per-capita average number of contacts of nonsubway users per unit of time
b_i	per-capita average number of contacts of subway users per unit of time
β_i	transmission rate per contact
$\frac{1}{\rho_i}$	average time spent in the subway
$\frac{\sigma_i}{\sigma_i+\rho_i}$	proportion of time spent off the subway; subway users
$\frac{\rho_i}{\sigma_i+\rho_i}$	proportion of time spent in the subway; subway users

$$\frac{dY_i}{dt} = \phi X_i - (\mu+\alpha+d)Y_i, \tag{5.7}$$

$$\frac{dZ_i}{dt} = \alpha Y_i - \mu Z_i + q_i l_1 W_i + q_i l_2 X_i, \tag{5.8}$$

$$\frac{dS_i}{dt} = A_i - B_i(t) - (\mu + q l_1) S_i, \tag{5.9}$$

$$\frac{dE_i}{dt} = B_i(t) - (\mu+\phi+q_i l_2) E_i, \tag{5.10}$$

$$\frac{dI_i}{dt} = \phi E_i - (\mu+\alpha+d) I_i, \tag{5.11}$$

$$\frac{dR_i}{dt} = \alpha I_i - \mu R_i + q_i l_1 S_i + q_i l_2 E_i, \quad i = 1,\dots,N, \tag{5.12}$$

where the infection rate for NSU individuals is

$$B_i(t) = \beta_i a_i S_i \left[\tilde{P}_{a_i} \frac{I_i}{T_i \tau_i + Q_i} + \tilde{P}_{b_i} \frac{Y_i \tau_i}{T_i \tau_i + Q_i} \right], \tag{5.13}$$

and the infection rate for SU individuals is

$$V_i(t) = \beta_i b_i W_i \left[\bar{P}_{a_i} \frac{I_i}{T_i \tau_i + Q_i} + \bar{P}_{b_i} \frac{Y_i \tau_i}{T_i \tau_i + Q_i} + \sum_{j=1}^{N} \bar{P}_{b^i_j} \frac{Y_j \omega_j}{T_j \omega_j} \right], \tag{5.14}$$

with

$$Q_i(t) = S_i(t) + E_i(t) + I_i(t) + R_i(t),$$
$$T_i(t) = W_i(t) + X_i(t) + Y_i(t) + Z_i(t).$$

The proportionate mixing model [7, 18, 65, 84] has been *slightly modified* to take into account that individuals do not always share the same mixing environments. Proportionate mixing means that the probability that a "type 1" individual has a contact with "type 2" individuals, given that he/she had contacts, is modeled by a ratio that is independent of "type 1" individuals, the ratio with numerator given by the weighted-by-activity level size of the type 2 subpopulation and denominator given by the sum of the weighted-by-activity level sizes of all population types (here only types 1 and 2). The proportionate mixing model has to be modified because SU individuals do not spend their entire unit of time (the contact rate must therefore be budgeted) *within their home neighborhood.* We budget, a crude modeling assumption, SU contacts in proportion to the time SU individuals spend on or off (assumed to be at their home neighborhood) the subway; that is, we take $b_i \times \omega_i$ $(b_i \times \rho_i/(\sigma_i + \rho_i))$ and $b_i \times \tau_i$ $(b_i \times \sigma_i/(\sigma_i + \rho_i))$ as SU individuals' effective per-capita contact rates with SU and NSU individuals, respectively. Hence, for example, $P_{a_i a_i} = \tilde{P}_{a_i} = \frac{a_i Q_i}{a_i Q_i + b_i \tau_i T_i}$ denotes the mixing "probability" (abuse of language) involving NSU individuals living in (the same) neighborhood i. The numerator $a_i Q_i$ is the total average activity level of the NSU neighborhood i population while the denominator is $a_i Q_i + b_i \tau_i T_i$, that is, the sum of the total activity of neighborhood i individuals (while in neighborhood i).

Typically, one would proceed in the standard way, that is, one would compute equilibria, compute the basic reproduction number, and study invasion conditions and stability conditions. The analyses turned out to be quite cumbersome even for the case of two neighborhoods (see [31]), and so we focused instead on discussing the results of a few simulations in the context of a simplified version of a city the size of New York (see [31]).

Finally, as noted in the prior section, although proportionate mixing is quite useful, it is not the only form of mixing available, and sometimes, for example, in the case of STDs, it may not lead to a reasonable approximate model. Several generalizations, avoiding this pitfall, can be found in [10, 11, 13, 17, 18, 22, 49] and the references therein.

5.4.1 The basic reproductive number

We calculate the basic reproductive number for the case of two neighborhoods, that is, when $N = 2$ (all the formulae come from [31]). The disease-free equilibrium of system (5.5)–(5.12) is $(w_i, 0, 0, z_i, s_i, 0, 0, r_i)$, where

$$w_i = \frac{\Lambda_i}{\mu} \frac{\mu}{\mu + q_i l_1}, \qquad z_i = \frac{\Lambda_i}{\mu} \frac{q_i l_1}{\mu + q_i l_1},$$
$$s_i = \frac{A_i}{\mu} \frac{\mu}{\mu + q_i l_1}, \qquad r_i = \frac{A_i}{\mu} \frac{q_i l_1}{\mu + q_i l_1},$$

with the local asymptotic stability (LAS) of this equilibrium determined by the basic reproductive number. The mixing probabilities, at the disease-free equilibrium, are given below (the superscript 0 highlights the fact that the population is at a demographic steady state):

$$\bar{P}^0_{b^1_1} = \frac{b_1\omega_1\Lambda_1}{\sum_{j=1}^N b_j\omega_j\Lambda_j}\omega_1, \tag{5.15}$$

$$\bar{P}^0_{b^1_2} = \frac{b_2\omega_2\Lambda_2}{\sum_{j=1}^N b_j\omega_j\Lambda_j}\omega_1, \tag{5.16}$$

$$\bar{P}^0_{b^2_1} = \frac{b_1\omega_1\Lambda_1}{\sum_{j=1}^N b_j\omega_j\Lambda_j}\omega_2, \tag{5.17}$$

$$P^0_{b^2_2} = \frac{b_2\omega_2\Lambda_2}{\sum_{j=1}^N b_j\omega_j\Lambda_j}\omega_2, \tag{5.18}$$

$$\tilde{P}^0_{a_i} = \frac{a_i A_i}{a_i A_i + b_i\tau_i\Lambda_i}, \tag{5.19}$$

$$\tilde{P}^0_{b_i} = \frac{b_i\tau_i\Lambda_i}{a_i A_i + b_i\tau_i\Lambda_i}, \tag{5.20}$$

$$\bar{P}^0_{a_i} = \tilde{P}_{a_i}\tau_i, \tag{5.21}$$

$$\bar{P}^0_{b_i} = \tilde{P}_{b_i}\tau_i. \tag{5.22}$$

The application of the next generation operator approach [30, 39, 40] is followed. Hence, we linearize the equations of X_1, Y_1, E_1, I_1, X_2, Y_2, E_2, I_2 around the disease-free equilibrium. The Jacobian matrix, 8×8, denoted by J has the nonzero entries listed in Table 5.2. J has the form

$$\begin{pmatrix} A & B \\ C & D \end{pmatrix},$$

where

$$A = \begin{pmatrix} J_{11} & J_{12} & 0 & J_{14} \\ J_{21} & J_{22} & 0 & 0 \\ 0 & J_{32} & J_{33} & J_{34} \\ 0 & 0 & J_{43} & J_{44} \end{pmatrix}, \qquad B = \begin{pmatrix} 0 & J_{16} & 0 & 0 \\ 0 & 0 & 0 & 0 \\ 0 & 0 & 0 & 0 \\ 0 & 0 & 0 & 0 \end{pmatrix},$$

$$C = \begin{pmatrix} 0 & J_{52} & 0 & 0 \\ 0 & 0 & 0 & 0 \\ 0 & 0 & 0 & 0 \\ 0 & 0 & 0 & 0 \end{pmatrix}, \qquad D = \begin{pmatrix} J_{55} & J_{56} & 0 & J_{58} \\ J_{65} & J_{66} & 0 & 0 \\ 0 & J_{76} & J_{77} & J_{78} \\ 0 & 0 & J_{87} & J_{88} \end{pmatrix}.$$

The dominant eigenvalue of MM_d^{-1}, where J is the difference $J = M - M_d$ with $M_d = \text{diag}\{J_{ii}\}$ and $M = J - M_d$, corresponds to the basic reproductive number. We use

Table 5.2. *Nonzero entries in the Jacobian matrix J (taken from* [31]*).*

$J_{11} = -(\mu+\phi+q_1l_2)$	$J_{12} = \beta_1 b_1 w_1\left(\bar{P}^0_{b_1}\frac{\tau_1}{A_1+\tau_1\Lambda_1} + \bar{P}^0_{b_1^1}\frac{1}{\Lambda_1}\right)$
$J_{14} = \beta_1 b_1 w_1 \bar{P}^0_{a_1}\frac{1}{A_1+\tau_1\Lambda_1}$	$J_{21} = J_{43} = J_{65} = J_{87} = \phi$
$J_{16} = \beta_1 b_1 w_1 \bar{P}^0_{b_2^1}\frac{1}{\Lambda_2}$	$J_{22} = J_{44} = J_{66} = J_{88} = -(\mu+d+\alpha)$
$J_{32} = \beta_1 a_1 s_1 \tilde{P}^0_{b_1}\frac{\tau_1}{A_1+\tau_1\Lambda_1}$	$J_{33} = -(\mu+\phi+q_1l_2)$
$J_{34} = \beta_1 a_1 s_1 \tilde{P}^0_{a_1}\frac{1}{A_1+\tau_1\Lambda_1}$	$J_{52} = \beta_2 b_2 w_2 \bar{P}^0_{b_1^2}\frac{1}{\Lambda_1}$
$J_{55} = -(\mu+\phi+q_2l_2)$	$J_{56} = \beta_2 b_2 w_2\left(\bar{P}^0_{b_2}\frac{\tau_2}{A_2+\tau_2\Lambda_2} + \bar{P}^0_{b_2^2}\frac{1}{\Lambda_2}\right)$
$J_{58} = \beta_2 b_2 w_2 \bar{P}^0_{a_2}\frac{1}{A_2+\tau_2\Lambda_2}$	$J_{76} = \beta_2 a_2 s_2 \tilde{P}^0_{b_2}\frac{\tau_2}{A_2+\tau_2\Lambda_2}$
$J_{77} = -(\mu+\phi+q_2l_2)$	$J_{78} = \beta_2 a_2 s_2 \tilde{P}^0_{a_2}\frac{1}{A_2+\tau_2\Lambda_2}$

Laplace's formula to expand the characteristic equation $\det(MM_d^{-1} - \lambda I) = 0$ using the fact that the matrix product MM_d^{-1} has the same form as matrix J. Hence, if we let $f(\lambda)$ denote the characteristic equation, then $f(\lambda) = f_A(\lambda)f_D(\lambda) + f_B(\lambda)f_C(\lambda)$, where

$$f_A(\lambda) = \begin{vmatrix} -\lambda & -\frac{J_{12}}{J_{22}} & 0 & -\frac{J_{14}}{J_{44}} \\ -\frac{J_{21}}{J_{11}} & -\lambda & 0 & 0 \\ 0 & -\frac{J_{32}}{J_{22}} & -\lambda & -\frac{J_{34}}{J_{44}} \\ 0 & 0 & -\frac{J_{43}}{J_{33}} & -\lambda \end{vmatrix}, \quad f_D(\lambda) = \begin{vmatrix} -\lambda & -\frac{J_{56}}{J_{66}} & 0 & \frac{J_{58}}{J_{88}} \\ -\frac{J_{65}}{J_{55}} & -\lambda & 0 & 0 \\ 0 & -\frac{J_{76}}{J_{66}} & -\lambda & -\frac{J_{78}}{J_{88}} \\ 0 & 0 & -\frac{J_{87}}{J_{77}} & -\lambda \end{vmatrix},$$

$$f_C(\lambda) = \begin{vmatrix} -\frac{J_{21}}{J_{11}} & -\lambda & 0 & 0 \\ 0 & -\frac{J_{32}}{J_{22}} & -\lambda & -\frac{J_{34}}{J_{44}} \\ 0 & 0 & -\frac{J_{43}}{J_{33}} & -\lambda \\ 0 & -\frac{J_{52}}{J_{22}} & 0 & 0 \end{vmatrix}, \quad f_B(\lambda) = \begin{vmatrix} 0 & -\frac{J_{16}}{J_{66}} & 0 & 0 \\ -\frac{J_{65}}{J_{55}} & -\lambda & 0 & 0 \\ 0 & -\frac{J_{76}}{J_{66}} & -\lambda & -\frac{J_{78}}{J_{88}} \\ 0 & 0 & -\frac{J_{87}}{J_{77}} & -\lambda \end{vmatrix}.$$

We proceed to rewrite $f_A(\lambda)$ as follows:

$$f_A(\lambda) = \lambda^2(\lambda^2 - R^{n,n,L_1}_{1,1}) - (R^{u,u,L_1}_{1,1} + R^{u,u,L_2}_{1,1})(\lambda^2 - R^{n,n,L_1}_{1,1}) - R^{n,u,L_1}_{1,1}R^{u,n,L_1}_{1,1},$$

where

$$R^{n,n,L_1}_{1,1} = \beta_1 a_1 \frac{s_1}{A_1+\tau_1\Lambda_1}\frac{1}{\mu+d+\alpha}\frac{\phi}{\mu+\phi+q_1l_2}\tilde{P}^0_{a_1}.$$

We observe that $R_{1,1}^{n,n,L_1}$, or

$$R_{1,1}^{u,u,L_1} = \frac{1}{\mu+d+\alpha}\frac{\phi}{\mu+\phi+q_1 l_2}\beta_1 b_1 \frac{w_1\tau_1}{A_1+\tau_1\Lambda_1}\bar{P}_{b_1}^0,$$

denotes the new cases of infections generated from NSUs by NSUs within the first neighborhoods; $R_{1,1}^{u,u,L_2}$, or

$$R_{1,1}^{u,u,L_2} = \frac{1}{\mu+d+\alpha}\frac{\phi}{\mu+\phi+q_1 l_2}\beta_1 b_1 \frac{w_1}{\Lambda_1}\bar{P}_{b_1^1}^0,$$

denotes the new cases of infections generated from SUs by SUs within the first neighborhood; and $R_{1,1}^{n,u,L_1}$ and $R_{1,1}^{u,n,L_1}$, given by

$$R_{1,1}^{n,u,L_1} = \left(\frac{\phi}{\mu+\phi+q_1 l_2}\right)\left(\frac{\beta_1 a_1 s_1 \tilde{P}_{b_1}^0 \frac{\tau_1}{A_1+\tau_1\Lambda_1}}{\mu+d+\alpha}\right)$$

and

$$R_{1,1}^{u,n,L_1} = \left(\frac{\phi}{\mu+\phi+q_1 l_2}\right)\left(\frac{\beta_1 b_1 w_1 \bar{P}_{a_1}^0 \frac{1}{A_1+\tau_1\Lambda_1}}{\mu+d+\alpha}\right),$$

do not have clear interpretations. However, they will eventually disappear from the equations given by (5.36)–(5.38). The superscript L_1 means that contacts take place off of the subway, while L_2 means that contacts take place on the subway.

Now, let $R_{i,j}^{\alpha,\beta,\gamma}$ describe the expected number of new distinct type cases at specific locations, with α and β denoting the type of susceptible and infectious individuals involved, respectively; i denoting the susceptible-individual neighborhood index; j denoting the infectious-individual neighborhood index; and γ denoting the place where α-individuals contact β-individuals. Hence, with this notation, we have, for example, that $R_{1,1}^{n,n,L_1}$ is the expected average number of new NSU cases of infection generated by a "typical" NSU individual within the first neighborhood; $R_{2,2}^{n,u,L_1}$ denotes the expected average number of new NSU cases generated by a "typical" SU individual within the second neighborhood; $R_{2,2}^{u,n,L_1}$ denotes the expected average number of new SU cases generated by "typical" NSU individual within the second neighborhood; and $R_{1,2}^{u,u,L_2}$ denotes the expected average number of new SU cases in neighborhood 1 generated by a "typical" SU individual from neighborhood 2 *on the subway*. The explicit relevant expressions $R_{i,j}^{\alpha,\beta,\gamma}$ are (see [31])

$$R_{1,1}^{n,n,L_1} = \frac{1}{\mu+d+\alpha}\frac{\phi}{\mu+\phi+q_1 l_2}\beta_1 a_1 \frac{s_1}{A_1+\tau_1\Lambda_1}\tilde{P}_{a_1}^0, \tag{5.23}$$

$$R_{1,1}^{u,u,L_1} = \frac{1}{\mu+d+\alpha}\frac{\phi}{\mu+\phi+q_1 l_2}\beta_1 b_1 \frac{w_1\tau_1}{A_1+\tau_1\Lambda_1}\bar{P}_{b_1}^0, \tag{5.24}$$

$$R_{1,1}^{u,u,L_2} = \frac{1}{\mu+d+\alpha}\frac{\phi}{\mu+\phi+q_1 l_2}\beta_1 b_1 \frac{w_1}{\Lambda_1}\bar{P}_{b_1^1}^0, \tag{5.25}$$

$$R_{1,1}^{n,u,L_1} = \frac{1}{\mu+d+\alpha}\frac{\phi}{\mu+\phi+q_1l_2}\beta_1 a_1 \frac{\tau_1 s_1}{A_1+\tau_1\Lambda_1}\tilde{P}^0_{b_1}, \tag{5.26}$$

$$R_{1,1}^{u,n,L_1} = \frac{1}{\mu+d+\alpha}\frac{\phi}{\mu+\phi+q_1l_2}\beta_1 b_1 \frac{w_1}{A_1+\tau_1\Lambda_1}\bar{P}^0_{a_1}, \tag{5.27}$$

$$R_{2,2}^{n,n,L_1} = \frac{1}{\mu+d+\alpha}\frac{\phi}{\mu+\phi+q_2l_2}\beta_2 a_2 \frac{s_2}{A_2+\tau_2\Lambda_2}\tilde{P}^0_{a_2}, \tag{5.28}$$

$$R_{2,2}^{u,u,L_1} = \frac{1}{\mu+d+\alpha}\frac{\phi}{\mu+\phi+q_2l_2}\beta_2 b_2 \frac{w_2\tau_2}{A_2+\tau_2\Lambda_2}\bar{P}^0_{b_2}, \tag{5.29}$$

$$R_{2,2}^{u,u,L_2} = \frac{1}{\mu+d+\alpha}\frac{\phi}{\mu+\phi+q_2l_2}\beta_2 b_2 \frac{w_2}{\Lambda_2}\bar{P}^0_{b_2^2}, \tag{5.30}$$

$$R_{2,2}^{n,u,L_1} = \frac{1}{\mu+d+\alpha}\frac{\phi}{\mu+\phi+q_2l_2}\beta_2 a_2 \frac{\tau_2 s_2}{A_2+\tau_2\Lambda_2}\tilde{P}^0_{b_2}, \tag{5.31}$$

$$R_{2,2}^{u,n,L_1} = \frac{1}{\mu+d+\alpha}\frac{\phi}{\mu+\phi+q_2l_2}\beta_2 b_2 \frac{w_2}{A_2+\tau_2\Lambda_2}\bar{P}^0_{a_2}, \tag{5.32}$$

$$R_{2,1,}^{u,u,L_2} = \frac{1}{\mu+d+\alpha}\frac{\phi}{\mu+\phi+q_2l_2}\beta_2 b_2 \frac{w_2}{\Lambda_2}\bar{P}^0_{b_2^1}, \tag{5.33}$$

$$R_{1,2}^{u,u,L_2} = \frac{1}{\mu+d+\alpha}\frac{\phi}{\mu+\phi+q_1l_2}\beta_1 b_1 \frac{w_1}{\Lambda_1}\bar{P}^0_{b_1^2}. \tag{5.34}$$

The above definitions can now be used to rewrite $f_D(\lambda)$, $f_B(\lambda)$, and $f_C(\lambda)$ as follows:

$$\begin{aligned}
f_D(\lambda) &= \lambda^2(\lambda^2 - R_{2,2}^{n,n,L_1}) - (R_{2,2}^{u,u,L_1} + R_{2,2}^{u,u,L_2})(\lambda^2 - R_{2,2}^{n,n,L_1}) - R_{2,2}^{n,u,L_1}R_{2,2}^{u,n,L_1},\\
f_B(\lambda) &= -\frac{\beta_1 b_1 w_1}{\beta_2 b_2 w_2}R_{2,1}^{u,u,L_2}(\lambda^2 - R_{2,2}^{n,n,L_1}),\\
f_C(\lambda) &= \frac{\beta_2 b_2 w_2}{\beta_1 b_1 w_1}R_{1,2}^{u,u,L_2}(\lambda^2 - R_{1,1}^{n,n,L_1}).
\end{aligned}$$

Therefore we have that

$$\begin{aligned}
f(\lambda) &= f_A(\lambda)f_D(\lambda) + f_B(\lambda)f_C(\lambda)\\
&= \left(\lambda^2(\lambda^2 - R_{1,1}^{n,n,L_1}) - (R_{1,1}^{u,u,L_1} + R_{1,1}^{u,u,L_2})(\lambda^2 - R_{1,1}^{n,n,L_1}) - R_{1,1}^{n,u,L_1}R_{1,1}^{u,n,L_2}\right)\\
&\left(\lambda^2(\lambda^2 - R_{2,2}^{n,n,L_1}) - (R_{2,2}^{u,u,L_1} + R_{2,2}^{u,u,L_2})(\lambda^2 - R_{2,2}^{n,n,L_1}) - R_{2,2}^{n,u,L_1}R_{2,2}^{u,n,L_2}\right)\\
&- \left(R_{1,2}^{u,u,L_2}(\lambda^2 - R_{1,1}^{n,n,L_1})\right)\left(R_{2,1}^{u,u,L_2}(\lambda^2 - R_{2,2}^{n,n,L_1})\right).
\end{aligned} \tag{5.35}$$

Further, the following identities hold:

$$R_{1,1}^{u,u,L_1}R_{1,1}^{n,n,L_1} - R_{1,1}^{n,u,L_1}R_{1,1}^{u,n,L_1} = 0, \tag{5.36}$$

$$R_{2,2}^{u,u,L_1}R_{2,2}^{n,n,L_1} - R_{2,2}^{n,u,L_1}R_{2,2}^{u,n,L_1} = 0, \tag{5.37}$$

$$R_{1,1}^{u,u,L_2}R_{2,2}^{u,u,L_2} - R_{1,2}^{u,u,L_2}R_{2,1}^{u,u,L_2} = 0. \tag{5.38}$$

The substitution of (5.23), (5.25), (5.26), and (5.27) into (5.36) leads to

$$R_{1,1}^{u,u,L_1} R_{1,1}^{n,n,L_1} - R_{1,1}^{n,u,L_1} R_{1,1}^{u,n,L_1} = \frac{1}{(\mu+d+\alpha)^2} \frac{\beta_1 a_1 \phi}{\mu+\phi+q_1 l_2} \frac{\beta_1 b_1 \phi}{\mu+\phi+q_1 l_2} \frac{w_1 s_1}{(A_1+\tau_1\Lambda_1)^2} \left(\tilde{P}_{a_1}^0 \tau_1 \bar{P}_{b_1}^0 - \tilde{P}_{b_1}^0 \tau_1 \bar{P}_{a_1}^0 \right).$$

Finally, (5.21) and (5.22) imply $\tilde{P}_{a_1}^0 \tau_1 \bar{P}_{b_1}^0 - \tilde{P}_{b_1}^0 \tau_1 \bar{P}_{a_1}^0 = 0$.

The same argument was used to verify that $R_{2,2}^{u,u,L_1} R_{2,2}^{n,n,L_1} - R_{2,2}^{n,u,L_1} R_{2,2}^{u,n,L_1} = 0$. The substitutions of (5.25), (5.30), (5.34), and (5.33) into (5.38) finally lead to

$$R_{1,1}^{u,u,L_2} R_{2,2}^{u,u,L_2} - R_{1,2}^{u,u,L_2} R_{2,1}^{u,u,L_2} = \frac{\beta_1 b_1 \beta_2 b_2}{(\mu+d+\alpha)^2} \frac{\phi}{\mu+\phi+q_1 l_2} \frac{\phi}{\mu+\phi+q_2 l_2} \left(\bar{P}_{b_1^1}^0 \bar{P}_{b_2^2}^0 - \bar{P}_{b_2^1}^0 \bar{P}_{b_1^2}^0 \right),$$

and, consequently, it follows from (5.15), (5.16), (5.17), and (5.18) that (5.38) holds. We observe that (5.38) is equivalent to the fact that the constant term in (5.35) vanishes (where the constant term is $R_{1,1}^{n,n,L_1} R_{2,2}^{n,n,L_1} (R_{1,1}^{u,u,L_2} R_{2,2}^{u,u,L_2} - R_{1,2}^{u,u,L_2} R_{2,1}^{u,u,L_2})$). Hence, $\lambda = 0$ is a root of the characteristic equation. The use of (5.36)–(5.37) and that 0 is a root of the characteristic equation leads finally to the following cubic equation in terms of $x = \lambda^2$:

$$x^3 - A_2 x^2 + A_1 x + A_0 = 0, \tag{5.39}$$

where

$$\begin{aligned} A_2 &= \sum_{i=1}^{2} (R_{i,i}^{n,n,L_1} + R_{i,i}^{u,u,L_1} + R_{i,i}^{u,u,L_2}), \\ A_1 &= \sum_{i=1}^{2} (R_{i,i}^{n,n,L_1} R_{i,i}^{u,u,L_2}) + \Pi_{i=1}^2 (R_{i,i}^{n,n,L_1} + R_{i,i}^{u,u,L_1} + R_{i,i}^{u,u,L_2}) - R_{1,2}^{u,u,L2} R_{2,1}^{u,u,L2}, \\ A_0 &= R_{1,2}^{u,u,L_2} R_{2,1}^{u,u,L_2} (R_{1,1}^{n,n,L_1} + R_{2,2}^{n,n,L_1}) - R_{2,2}^{n,n,L_1} R_{2,2}^{u,u,L_2} (R_{1,1}^{n,n,L_1} + R_{1,1}^{u,u,L_1} + R_{1,1}^{u,u,L_2}) \\ &\quad - R_{1,1}^{n,n,L_1} R_{1,1}^{u,u,L_2} (R_{2,2}^{n,n,L_1} + R_{2,2}^{u,u,L_1} + R_{2,2}^{u,u,L_2}). \end{aligned}$$

Therefore, the dominant root of the cubic equation (5.39), found using [93], gives the basic reproductive number [93]. That is,

$$\begin{aligned} \mathcal{R}_0 = \frac{A_2}{3} &+ \sqrt[3]{\frac{2A_2^3 - 9A_2A_1 - 27A_0}{54} + \sqrt{\left(\frac{3A_1 - A_2^2}{9}\right)^3 + \left(\frac{2A_2^3 - 9A_2A_1 - 27A_0}{54}\right)^2}} \\ &+ \sqrt[3]{\frac{2A_2^3 - 9A_2A_1 - 27A_0}{54} - \sqrt{\left(\frac{3A_1 - A_2^2}{9}\right)^3 + \left(\frac{2A_2^3 - 9A_2A_1 - 27A_0}{54}\right)^2}}. \end{aligned} \tag{5.40}$$

The average number of secondary cases generated by a "typical" infectious individual in a population of susceptible individuals at a demographic steady state must factor in the contributions across all neighborhoods of the SU and NSU susceptible and the infectious individuals. Since the contacts are not independent, hence (5.41) is not, as it is often the case, given by the arithmetic or geometric mean, but as expected by a rather convoluted expression. In [31] we discussed the following special cases of formula (5.41). Here we recollect what we had written in [31].

Case 1. If $\omega_2 = 0$, then $R_{1,2}^{u,u,L_2} = R_{2,2}^{u,u,L_2} = 0$. This reduces (5.39) to

$$\left(x - (R_{2,2}^{n,n,L_1} + R_{2,2}^{u,u,L_1})\right)$$
$$\left(x^2 - (R_{1,1}^{n,n,L_1} + R_{1,1}^{u,u,L_1} + R_{1,1}^{u,u,L_2})x + R_{1,1}^{n,n,L_1} R_{1,1}^{u,u,L_2}\right) = 0.$$

The two positive roots are given by

$$\lambda_1 = \frac{1}{2}\left(R_{1,1}^{n,n,L_1} + R_{1,1}^{u,u,L_1} + R_{1,1}^{u,u,L_2}\right)$$
$$+\frac{1}{2}\sqrt{(R_{1,1}^{n,n,L_1} + R_{1,1}^{u,u,L_1} + R_{1,1}^{u,u,L_2})^2 - 4R_{1,1}^{n,n,L_1} R_{1,1}^{u,u,L_2}},$$
$$\lambda_2 = R_{2,2}^{n,n,L_1} + R_{2,2}^{u,u,L_1}.$$

Therefore, we have that $\mathcal{R}_0 = \max\,\{\lambda_1, \lambda_2\}$. If $\omega_1 = \omega_2 = 0$, then

$$\mathcal{R}_0 = \max\,\{R_{1,1}^{n,n,L_1} + R_{1,1}^{u,u,L_1}, R_{2,2}^{n,n,L_1} + R_{2,2}^{u,u,L_1}\}.$$

Case 2. The basic reproductive number, when only one neighborhood is included ($N = 1$), reduces to the dominant root of $f_A(\lambda) = 0$, that is, to

$$\mathcal{R}_0 = \frac{R_{1,1}^{n,n,L_1} + R_{1,1}^{u,u,L_1} + R_{1,1}^{u,u,L_2}}{2}$$
$$+\frac{1}{2}\sqrt{(R_{1,1}^{n,n,L_1} + R_{1,1}^{u,u,L_1} + R_{1,1}^{u,u,L_2})^2 - 4R_{1,1}^{n,n,L_1} R_{1,1}^{u,u,L_2}}.$$

Case 3. The extreme case involving $N = 1$ and $\omega_1 = 0$ leads to the known basic reproductive number given by the simple algebraic expression $\mathcal{R}_0 = \frac{1}{2}(R_{1,1}^{n,n,L_1} + R_{1,1}^{u,u,L_1})$.

5.5 A Two-Neighborhood Example

We divide the population of our theoretical city into two neighborhoods: the resident population (neighborhood 1) and the transient or tourist population (neighborhood 2). The resident population (inspired by New York City data) is assumed to be 8 million. It should be clear from the prior section that our illustration will be based on numerical simulations, and so we need to use reasonable "data." So, since the example is taken from [31], we build a city that has some of the characteristics of New York City. Hence, since the tourist population of New York City, using 1999 data (see [4]), was roughly 36.7 million, this is the number

Table 5.3. *Parameters (taken from* [31]*).*

μ	d	l_1	l_2	ϕ	α	β	a_1	a_2	b_1	b_2
0.033	0.0116	0.97	0.3	0.086	0.086	0.5	5	10	15	30

that we use. The tourist population was estimated to include 30.1 million domestic and 6.6 million international visitors. In addition, 18.4 million of the visitors stayed overnight, while 18.3 million visited for just a day. It is therefore assumed here that international visitors stayed in the city an average of 5 days, while domestic visitors stayed overnight for 2 days. Therefore, the average number of visits per day was $(18.3+11.8\times 2+6.6\times 5)/365=0.2$ million. That is, here, it is assumed that 0.2 million tourists visited New York City per day (numerical simulation uses a day as the unit of time).

What about the rest of the parameters needed to run simulations of the two-neighborhood model? Data suggest that 30% of those infected with smallpox die during the second week following infection, and that a vaccinated person may escape death if infected with smallpox again even if the vaccine had been applied 30 years before. In 2003 when the simulations were carried out, roughly half of the population of the United States had been vaccinated 30 years prior. Therefore, we used the average case-fatality rate of 0.15. Hence, under the assumption of an exponential survivorship distribution it was estimated that the per-capita disease-induced mortality $d\approx -\log(0.85)/14=0.0116$. Table 5.3 collects the rest of the parameters; most of the values were taken from [44, 67, 46, 82] (Table 5.3 was taken from [31]). In [44] it was claimed that the effective total contact number over the entire period of infection was about 50, and so it was assumed that the daily contact rate for NSU individuals is 5. For SU individuals it was assumed (no data) that the contact rate was twice that of NSU individuals. Further the average daily contact rates for the tourist/transient subpopulation (neighborhood 2) was assumed to be triple that of the residents. The demographic parameters Λ_i, A_i, and μ were chosen so that residents and tourists would support a population of 8 and 0.2 million, respectively. The values $\tau_1=0.6$ and $\tau_2=0.1$ reflect our view then that second neighborhood SU individuals spend more time on the subway than those from the first neighborhood. These *arbitrarily* selected parameters gave a basic reproductive number of 5.8, a value computed using the expression in [31], namely, the dominant root of the cubic equation (5.39), restated here:

$$\mathcal{R}_0=\frac{A_2}{3}+\sqrt[3]{\frac{2A_2^3-9A_2A_1-27A_0}{54}+\sqrt{\left(\frac{3A_1-A_2^2}{9}\right)^3+\left(\frac{2A_2^3-9A_2A_1-27A_0}{54}\right)^2}}$$
$$+\sqrt[3]{\frac{2A_2^3-9A_2A_1-27A_0}{54}-\sqrt{\left(\frac{3A_1-A_2^2}{9}\right)^3+\left(\frac{2A_2^3-9A_2A_1-27A_0}{54}\right)^2}}. \tag{5.41}$$

Efforts to ameliorate or stop the impact of a deliberate release were modeled using the vaccination proportions for the resident and tourist, q_1 and q_2, respectively. What would be the values that minimize the prevalence of the disease and total number of deaths?

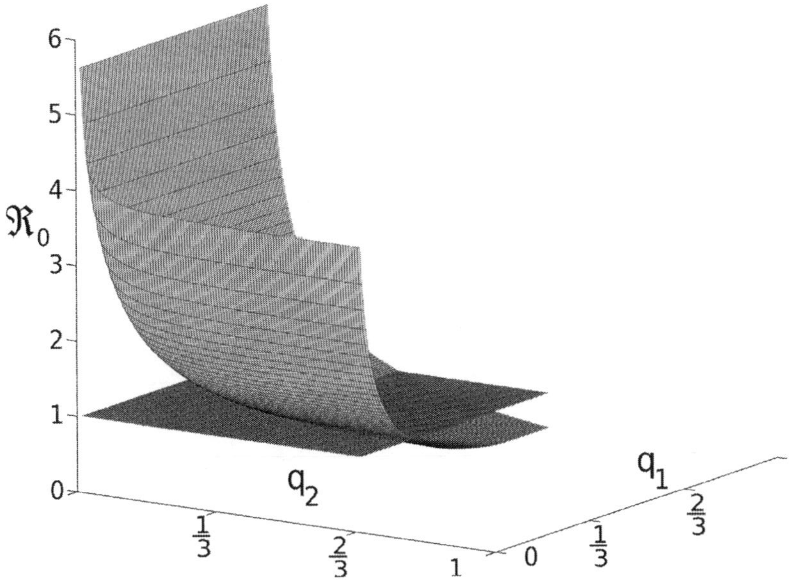

Figure 5.2. *Plot $\mathcal{R}_0$ versus q_1 and q_2. Taken from* [31].

The initial conditions for the simulations were set as follows: $Y_1(0) = 70$ and $Y_2(0) = 30$, that is, 100 infected on the subway. The initial values of W_1, S_1, W_2, and S_2 are chosen so that $W_1(0) + S_1(0) = 8{,}000{,}000$ and $W_2(0) + S_2(0) = 200{,}000$. The rest of initial conditions are set to zero ($I_1(0) = I_2(0) = X_1(0) = X_2(0) = Z_1(0) = Z_2(0) = \mathcal{R}_1(0) = \mathcal{R}_2(0) = 0$).

The last smallpox outbreak in New York City took place in 1947 with only 8 cases initially reported in a population with 6 million individuals vaccinated [44]. Simulations turned out to strongly support mass vaccination (MV) within this two-neighborhood, transient-resident population model. We used an initial population of 100 cases, which would be classified as a large-scale attack (see [37]), thus requiring MV.

What would the impact be of varying q_1 and q_2 on the basic reproductive number $\mathcal{R}_0$? Simulations using (5.41) were carried out to explore just this. The plot of $\mathcal{R}_0(q_1, q_2)$ versus q_1 and q_2 (Figure 5.2) collects these simulations. The region where $\mathcal{R}_0(q_1, q_2) < 1$ is shown in Figure 5.3.

These two graphs (taken from [31]), show that if the vaccination rate for the residence population (over 97.56% of the total population) is greater than 0.46, then the tourist population is less important than the resident population (vaccination rate as low as 0.26 would work). However, the key observation is that one *cannot ignore the tourist population.*

5.6 Review and Discussion

In this lecture, we revisited the concepts of pair formation, marriage functions, and mixing as one of the most challenging aspects associated with modeling heterogeneity. We revisited continuous and discrete modeling frameworks and briefly reviewed some of the literature

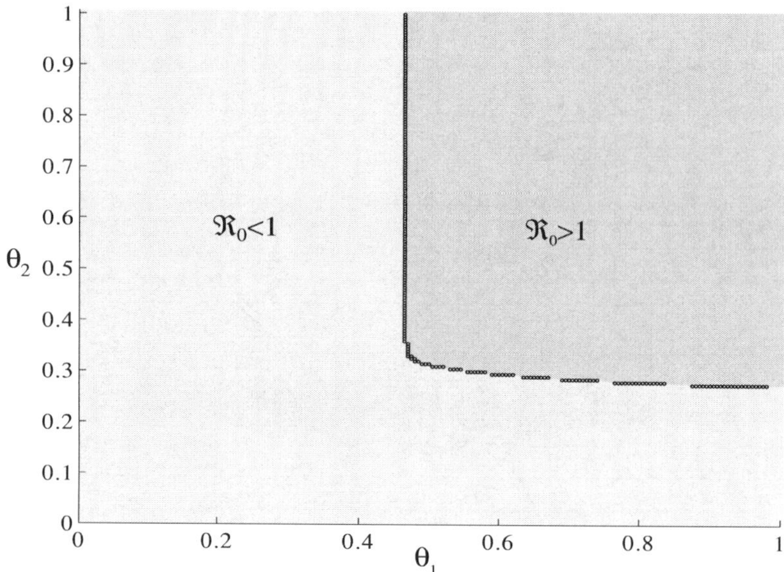

Figure 5.3. *Boundary curve of $\mathcal{R}_0(q_1,q_2) = 1$ on the (q_1q_2) plane. Taken from* [31].

[2, 3, 8, 19, 20, 48, 55, 59, 60, 62, 63, 65, 73]. We particularly relied on our own past collaborative work [10, 11, 12, 13, 17, 18, 19, 20, 21, 22, 23, 25, 26, 27, 35, 49, 58, 62, 63, 64, 83, 89]. We focused primarily on the modeling aspects, particularly multilayered mixing. The budgeting of environment-dependent contact rates was used to account for the fact that individuals spend different amounts of time as temporary residents of multiple environments as first introduced in [28, 31]. The application of this framework, in the context of an artificial city that borrows some of the statistics from New York City, was carried out via numerical simulations, and was briefly described following the presentation in [31] .

The simulations involving a deliberate release of smallpox show that an outbreak could not be controlled unless the program deployed to vaccinate the population included a fraction of the tourist population even though, in our setup, it accounts for less than 2.5% of the entire population (see Figure 5.4). It was observed that vaccinating 90% of residents and no visitors would still leave a basic reproductive number of 5.624 (under the selected parameters).

The special homogeneous artificial case of $q_1 = q_2$, a vaccination campaign that does not distinguish between residents and tourists, leads to the identification of a single critical value of $q_c = 0.4635$, the value where $\mathcal{R}_0(q_c) = 1$ when $q < q_c$, $\mathcal{R}_0(q) > 1$ and $q > q_c$ when $\mathcal{R}_0(q) < 1$ (Figure 5.5).

The number of logistical issues associated with addressing the impact of a deliberate release are immense, and the recent Hollywood production *Contagion* actually has provided the general public with a somewhat realistic perspective of the challenges posed when a new deadly pathogen emerges. Challenges arise from many factors, including the availability of responding personnel, delays, information and misinformation, and fear. Some of these issues are discussed and illustrated in [31].

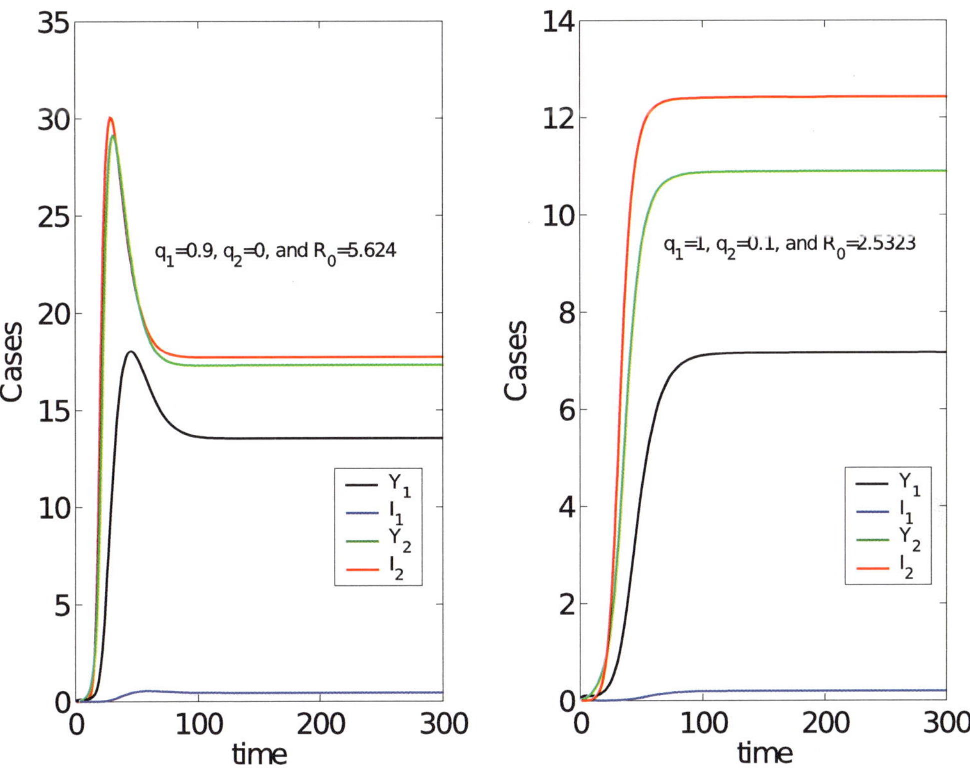

Figure 5.4. *The left graph shows the number of cases for* $q_1 = 0.9$ *and* $q_2 = 0$ *and the right* $q_1 = 0.9$ *and* $q_2 = 0.1$. *The disease becomes endemic. The units for the y-axis are* 1,000. *Taken from* [31].

Bibliography

[1] Anderson, R.M., ed. (1982) *Population Dynamics of Infectious Diseases: Theory and Applications*, Chapman and Hall, London.

[2] Anderson, R.M. (1988) *The epidemiology of HIV infection: Variable incubation plus infectious periods and heterogeneity in sexual activity*, J. Roy. Stat. Soc. A **151**: 66–93.

[3] Anderson, R. and R. May (1991) *Infectious Disease of Humans*, Oxford University Press, Oxford, New York, Toronto.

[4] Archives of the Mayor's Press Office (2000) Release 291-00, August 7, http://home.nyc.gov/html/om/html/2000b/pr291-00.html.

[5] Arino, J. and P. van den Driessche (2003) *A multi-city epidemic model*, Mathematical Population Studies **10**: 175–193.

[6] Bailey, N.T.J. (1975) *The Mathematical Theory of Infectious Diseases and Its Applications*, Griffin, London.

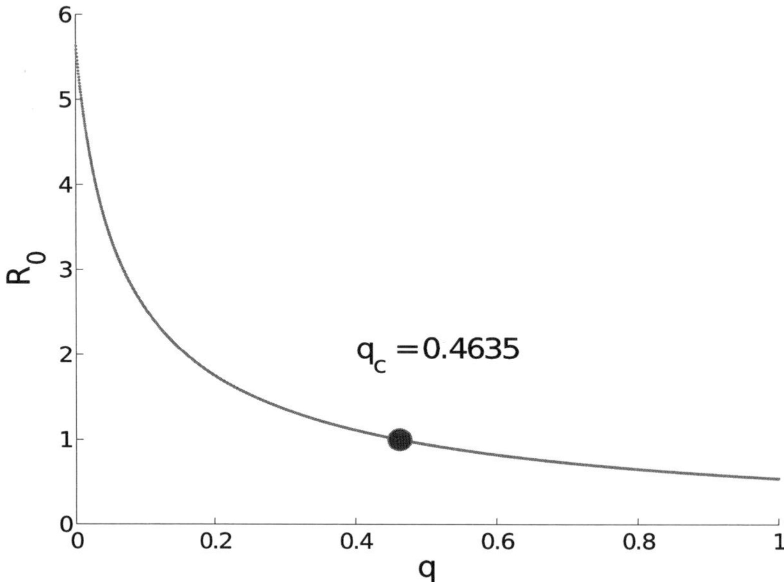

Figure 5.5. *Critical vaccination rate is* $q_c = 0.4635$. *Taken from* [31].

[7] Barbour, A.D. (1978) *Macdonald's model and the transmission of bilharzia*, Trans. Roy. Trop. Med. Hyg. **72**: 6–15.

[8] Baroyan, O.V. and L.A. Rvachev (1967) *Deterministic models of epidemics for a territory with a transport network*, Cybernetics and Systems Analysis **3**(3): 55–61.

[9] Bernoulli, D. (1971). *Essai d'une nouvelle analyse de la mortalité causée par la petite verole*, Mem. Math. Phys. Acad. R. Sci. Paris, 1–45, 1766; English translation and translation and critical commentary by L. Bradley in Smallpox Inoculation: An Eighteenth Century Mathematical Controversy (Adult Education Department, Nottingham).

[10] Blythe, S.P. and C. Castillo-Chavez (1989) *Like with like preference and sexual mixing models*, Math. Biosc. **96**: 221–238.

[11] Blythe, S.P., C. Castillo-Chavez, J. Palmer, and M. Cheng (1991) *Towards a unified theory of mixing and pair formation*, Math. Biosc. **107**: 379–405.

[12] Blythe, S.P., C. Castillo-Chavez, and G. Casella (1992) *Empirical Methods for the Estimation of the Mixing Probabilities for Socially Structured Populations from a Single Survey Sample*, Mathematical Population Studies **3**: 199–225.

[13] Blythe, S.P., S. Busenberg, and C. Castillo-Chavez (1995) *Affinity and paired-event probability*, Math. Biosci. **128**: 265–84.

[14] Brauer, F. and C. Castillo-Chavez (2001) *Mathematical Models in Population Biology and Epidemiology*, Texts in Applied Mathematics **40**, Springer-Verlag, New York.

[15] Brauer, F. and C. Castillo-Chavez (2012) *Mathematical Models in Population Biology and Epidemiology*, 2nd ed., Texts in Applied Mathematics **40**, Springer-Verlag, New York.

[16] Broad, W.J. and J. Miller (2002) *Report provides new details of Soviet smallpox accident*, The New York Times, June 15, sect. A: 1.

[17] Busenberg, S. and C. Castillo-Chavez (1989) *Interaction, pair formation and force of infection terms in sexually transmitted diseases*, in Mathematical and Statistical Approaches to AIDS Epidemiology, C. Castillo-Chavez, ed., Lect. Notes in Biomath. **83**, Springer-Verlag, Berlin, Heidelberg, New York: 289–300.

[18] Busenberg, S. and C. Castillo-Chavez (1991) *A general solution of the problem of mixing sub-populations, and its application to risk-and age-structured epidemic models for the spread of AIDS*, IMA J. of Mathematics Applied in Med. and Biol. **8**: 1–29.

[19] Castillo-Chavez, C., ed. (1989) *Mathematical and statistical approaches to AIDS epidemiology*, Lect. Notes in Biomath. **83**, Springer-Verlag, Berlin.

[20] Castillo-Chavez, C., K. Cooke, W. Huang, and S.A. Levin (1989) *Results on the dynamics for models for the sexual transmission of the human immunodeficiency virus*, Appl. Math. Letters **2**: 327–331.

[21] Castillo-Chavez, C. and S. Busenberg (1990) *On the Solution of the Two-Sex Mixing Problem*, in Proceedings of the International Conference on Differential Equations and Applications to Biology and Population Dynamics, S. Busenberg and M. Martelli, eds., Lect. Notes in Biomath. **92**, Springer-Verlag, Berlin, Heidelberg, New York: 80–98.

[22] Castillo-Chavez, C., S. Busenberg, and K. Gerow (1991) *Pair formation in structured populations*, in Differential Equations with Applications in Biology, Physics and Engineering, J. Goldstein, F. Kappel, and W. Schappacher, eds., Marcel Dekker, New York: 47–65.

[23] Castillo-Chavez, C., S.-F. Shyu, G. Rubin, and D. Umbauch (1992) *On the estimation problem of mixing/pair formation matrices with applications to models for sexually-transmitted diseases*, in AIDS Epidemiology: Methodology Issues, N.P. Jewell, K. Dietz, and V.T. Farewell, eds., Birkhäuser, Boston: 384–402.

[24] Castillo-Chavez, C., J.X. Velasco-Hernandez, and S. Fridman (1994) *Modeling contact structures in biology*, in Frontiers of Theoretical Biology, S.A. Levin, ed., Lect. Notes in Biomath. **100**, Springer-Verlag, Berlin, Heidelberg, New York: 454–491.

[25] Castillo-Chavez, C., and W. Huang (1995) *The logistic equation revisited: The two-sex case*, Math. Biosc. **128**: 299–316.

[26] Castillo-Chavez, C., W. Huang, and J. Li (1996) *On the existence of stable pairing distributions*, J. Math. Biol. **34**: 413–441.

[27] Castillo-Chavez, C. and S.-F. Hsu Schmitz (1997) *The evolution of age-structured marriage functions: It takes two to tango*, in Structured-Population Models Marine, Terrestrial, and Freshwater Systems. S. Tuljapurkar and H. Caswell, eds., Chapman and Hall, New York: 533–550.

[28] Castillo-Chavez, C., A.F. Capurro, M. Zellner, and J.X. Velasco-Hernandez (1998) *El transporte publico y la dinamica de la tuberculosis a nivel poblacional*, Aportaciones Matematicas, Serie Comunicaciones **22**: 209–225.

[29] Castillo-Chavez, C. and F.S. Roberts (2002) *Report on Dimacs Working Group Meeting: Mathematical Sciences Methods for the Study of Deliberate Releases of Biological Agents and Their Consequences*, DIMACS, Rutgers University.

[30] Castillo-Chavez, C., Z. Feng, and W. Huang (2002) *On the computation of $\mathcal{R}_0$ and its role on global stability*, in Mathematical Approaches for Emerging and Reemerging Infectious Diseases: An introduction, C. Castillo-Chavez, S. Blower, P. van den Driessche, D. Kirschner, and A.A. Yakubu, eds., IMA Vol. Math. Appl. **125**, Springer-Verlag, New York: 229–250.

[31] Castillo-Chavez, C., B. Song, and J. Zhang (2003) *An epidemic model with virtual mass transportation: The case of smallpox in a large city*, in Bioterrorism: Mathematical Modeling Applications in Homeland Security, H.T. Banks and C. Castillo-Chavez, eds., SIAM, Philadelphia: 173–197.

[32] Castillo-Chavez, C. and B. Song (2004) *Dynamical models of tuberculosis and their applications*, Math. Biosc. & Eng. **1**: 361–404.

[33] Castillo-Chavez, C. and B. Li (2008) *Spatial Spread of Sexually-Transmitted Diseases within Susceptible Populations at a Demographic Steady State*, Math. Biosc. Eng. **5**: 713–727.

[34] Check, E. (2001) *Need for vaccine stocks questioned*, Nature **414**: 677.

[35] Crawford, C.M., S.J. Schwager, and C. Castillo-Chavez (1990) *A Methodology for Asking Sensitive Questions among College Undergraduates*, Technical Report BU-1105-M in the Biometrics Unit series, Cornell University, Ithaca, NY.

[36] CSIS News (2002) http://www.homelandsecurity.org/darkwinter/index.cfm.

[37] CSIS News (2002) *Dark Winter*, http://www.csis.org/hill/darkwinter.htm#top.

[38] Del Valle, S., H. Hethcote, J.M. Hyman, and C. Castillo-Chavez (2005) *The effects of behavioral changes in a smallpox attack model*, Math. Biosc., **195**: 228–251.

[39] Diekmann, O., J.A.P. Heesterbeek, and J.A.J. Metz (1990) *On the definition and computation of the basic reproductive ratio in models for infectious diseases in heterogeneous population*, J. Math. Biol. **28**: 365–382.

[40] Diekmann, O. and J.A.P. Heesterbeek (2000) *Mathematical Epidemiology of Infectious Diseases: Model Building, Analysis and Interpretation*, John Wiley, Chichester, New York, Weinheim, Brisbane, Singapore, Toronto.

[41] Dietz, K. (1988) *Mathematical models for transmission and control of malaria*, in Malaria: Principles and Practice of Malariology, W.H. Wernsdorfer and I. McGregor, eds., Churchill Livingstone, Edinburgh.

[42] Dietz, K. and K.P. Hadeler (1988) *Epidemiological models for sexually transmitted diseases*, J. Math. Biol. **26**: 1–25.

[43] Dietz, K. and J.P.A. Heesterbeek (2000) *Bernoulli was ahead of modern epidemiology*, Nature **408**: 513–514.

[44] Fenner, F., D.A. Henderson, I. Arita, Z. Jezek, and I.D. Ladnyi (1988) *Smallpox and Its Eradication*, World Health Organization, Geneva.

[45] Fredrickson, A.G. (1971) *A mathematical theory of age structure in sexual populations: Random mating and monogamous marriage models*, Math. Biosc. **20**: 117–143.

[46] Gani, R. and S. Leach (2001) *Transmission potential of smallpox in contemporary populations*, Nature **415**: 748–751.

[47] Glasser, J., Z. Feng, A Moylan, S. Del Valle, and C. Castillo-Chavez (2012) *Mixing in age-structured population models of infectious disease*, Math. Biosc. **235**: 1–7.

[48] Hadeler, K.P. (1989) *Modeling AIDS in structured populations*, in Proceedings of the 47th Session of the International Statistical Institute, Paris, **C1-2**: 83–99.

[49] Hadeler, K.P. (2012) *Pair formation*, J. Math. Biol. **64**: 613–645.

[50] Henderson, D.A. (1999) *About the first national symposium on medical and public health response to bioterrorism*, Emerg. Infect. Dis. **5**: 491.

[51] Henderson, D.A. (1999) *Smallpox: Clinical and epidemiologic features*, Emerg. Infect. Dis. **5**: 537–539.

[52] Henderson, D.A. (1999). *The looming threat of bioterrorism*, Science **283**: 1279–1282.

[53] Henderson, D.A., T.V. Inglesby, J.G. Bartlett, M.S. Ascher, E. Eitzen, P.B. Jahrling, J. Hauer, M. Layton, J. McDade, M.T. Osterholm, T. O'Toole, G. Parker, T. Perl, P.K. Russell, and K. Tonat (1999) *Smallpox as a biological weapon*, JAMA **281**: 2127–2137.

[54] Herrera-Valdez, M.A., M. Cruz-Aponte, and C. Castillo-Chavez (2011) *Multiple outbreaks for the same pandemic: Local transportation and social distancing explain the different "wave" of A-H1N1pdm cases observed in México during* 2009, Math. Biosc. & Eng. **8**: 21–48.

[55] Hethcote, H.W. and J.W. Van Ark (1992). *Modeling HIV Transmission and AIDS in the United States*, Lect. Notes in Biomath. **95**, Springer-Verlag, Berlin, Heidelberg, New York.

[56] http://www.ore.princeton.edu/, updated on 2012, Operations Research and Financial Engineering Department, Princeton University, December 2000.

[57] Huang, W., K.L. Cook, and C. Castillo-Chavez (1992) *Stability and bifurcation for a multiple-group model for the dynamics of HIV/AIDS transmission*, SIAM J. Appl. Math. **52**: 835–854.

[58] Huang W. and C. Castillo-Chavez (2002) *Age-structured core groups and their impact on HIV dynamics*, in Mathematical Approaches for Emerging and Reemerging Infectious Diseases: Models, Methods and Theory, C. Castillo-Chavez with P. van den Driessche, D. Kirschner, and A.A. Yakubu, eds., IMA Vol. Math. Appl. **126**, Springer-Verlag, New York: 261–273.

[59] Hyman, J. M. and E.A. Stanley (1988) *A risk base model for the spread of the AIDS virus*, Math. Biosc. **90**: 415–473.

[60] Hyman, J. M. and E.A. Stanley (1989) *The effects of social mixing patterns on the spread of AIDS*, in Mathematical Approaches to Problems in Resource Management and Epidemiology, C. Castillo-Chavez, S.A. Levin, and C.A. Shoemaker, eds., Lect. Notes in Biomath. **81**, Springer-Verlag, Berlin: 190–219.

[61] Hyman, J.M. and T. Laforce (2003) *Modeling the spread of influenza among cities*, in Bioterrorism: Mathematical Modeling Applications for Homeland Security. H.T. Banks and C. Castillo-Chavez, eds., SIAM, Philadelphia: 211–236.

[62] Hsu Schmitz, S.-F. (1993). *Some Theories, Estimation Methods and Applications of Marriage Functions and Two-Sex Mixing Functions in Demography and Epidemiology*, unpublished doctoral dissertation, Cornell University, Ithaca, NY.

[63] Hsu Schmitz, S.-F. and C. Castillo-Chavez (1994) *Parameter estimation in non-closed social networks related to dynamics of sexually transmitted diseases*, in Modelling the AIDS Epidemic: Planning, Policy, and Prediction, E.H. Kaplan and M.L. Brandeau, eds., Raven Press, New York: 533–559.

[64] Hsu Schmitz, S.-F. and C. Castillo-Chavez (2000) *A note on pair-formation functions*, Math. Comput. Modeling **31**: 83–91.

[65] Jacquez, J.A., C.P. Simon, J. Koopman, L. Sattenpiel, and T. Perry (1988) *Modeling and analyzing HIV transmission: Effect of contact patterns*, Math. Biosc. **92**: 119–199.

[66] Kahn, L.H. (2002) *Smallpox transmission risks: How bad?*, Science **297**: 50.

[67] Kaplan, E.H., D.L. Craft, and L.M. Wein (2002) *Emergency response to a smallpox attack: The case for mass vaccination*, Proc. Natl. Acad. Sci. USA **99**: 10935–10940.

[68] Kasseem, G.T., S. Roudenko, S. Tennenbaum, and C. Castillo-Chavez (2006) *The role of transactional sex in spreading HIV/AIDS in Nigeria: A modeling perspective*, in Mathematical Studies on Human Disease Dynamics: Emerging Paradigms and Challenges. A. Gumel, C. Castillo-Chavez, D.P. Clemence, and R.E. Mickens, eds., American Mathematical Society, Providence, RI: 367–389.

[69] Kemper, A.R., M.M. Davis, and G.L. Freed (2002) *Expected adverse events in a mass smallpox vaccination campaign*, Eff. Clin. Pract. **5**: 84–90.

[70] Kendall, D.G. (1949) *Stochastic processes and population growth*, Roy. Stat. Soc. Ser. B **2**: 230–264.

[71] Keyfitz, N. (1949) *The mathematics of sex and marriage*, in Proceedings of the Sixth Berkeley Symposium on Mathematical Statistics and Probability, Vol. IV: Biology and Health: 89–108.

[72] Khan, K., J. Arino, W. Hu, P. Raposo, J. Sears, F. Calderon, C. Heidebrecht, M. Macdonald, J. Liauw, A. Chan et al. (2009) *Spread of a novel influenza A (H1N1) virus via global airline transportation*, New England J. Medicine **361**: 212.

[73] Koopman, J., C.P. Simon, J.A. Jacquez, J. Joseph, L. Sattenspiel, and T. Park (1988) *Sexual partner selectiveness effects on homosexual HIV transmission dynamics*, Journal of AIDS **1**: 486–504.

[74] Kribs-Zaleta, C., M. Lee, C. Román, S. Wiley, and C.M. Hernández-Suárez (2005) *The effect of the HIV/AIDS epidemic on Africa's truck drivers*, Math. Biosc. & Eng. **2**: 771–778.

[75] Larsen, R. (2003) *Smallpox: Right Topic, Wrong Debate*, Journal of Homeland Security, http://www.homelandsecurity.org/HLSCommentary/20020725.htm.

[76] Leslie, P.H. (1945) *On the use of matrices in certain population mathematics*, Biometrika **33**: 183–212.

[77] Lotka, A.J. (1922) *The stability of the normal age distribution*, Proc. Natl. Acad. Sci. USA **8**: 339–345.

[78] Lotka, A.J. (1923) *Contributions to the analysis of malaria epidemiology*, Amer. J. Hygiene **3** (Suppl.).

[79] Luo, X. and C. Castillo-Chavez (1993) *Limit behavior of pair-formation for a large dissolution rate*, J. Math. Systems, Estimation, and Control **3**: 247–264.

[80] McKendrick, A.G. (1926) *Applications of mathematics to medical problems*, Proc. Edinburgh Math. Soc. **44**: 98–130.

[81] McFarland, D.D. (1972) *Comparison of alternative marriage models*, in Population Dynamics, T.N.E. Greville, ed., Academic Press, New York: 89–106.

[82] Meltzer, M.I., I. Damon, J.W. LeDuc, and J.D. Millar (2001) *Modeling potential responses to smallpox as a bioterrorist weapon*, Emerg. Infect. Dis. **7**: 959–968.

[83] Morin, B., C. Castillo-Chavez, S.-F. Hsu Schmitz, A. Mubayi, and X. Wang (2010) *Notes from the heterogeneous: A few observations on the implications and necessity of affinity*, J. Biol. Dynamics **4**: 456–477.

[84] Nold, A. (1980) *Heterogeneity in disease-transmission modeling*, Math. Biosc. **52**: 227–240.

[85] Parlett, B. (1972) *Can there be a marriage function?*, in Population Dynamics, T.N.E. Greville, ed., Academic Press, New York: 107–135.

[86] Pollard, J.H. (1973) *The two-sex problem*, in Mathematical Models for the Growth of Human Populations, Cambridge University Press, Cambridge.

[87] Ross, R. (1911) *The Prevention of Malaria*, 2nd ed. (with Addendum), John Murray, London.

[88] Rotz, L.D., A.S. Khan, S.R. Lillibridge, S.M. Ostroff, and J.M. Hughes (2002) *Public health assessment of potential biological terrorism agents*, Emerg. Infect. Dis. **8**: 225–229.

[89] Rubin, G., D. Umbauch, S.-F. Shyu, and C. Castillo-Chavez (1992) *Application of capture-recapture methodology to estimation of size of population at risk of AIDS and/or other sexually-transmitted diseases*, Statistics in Medicine **11**: 1533–1549.

[90] Rvachev, L.A. and I.M. Longini, Jr. (1985) *A mathematical model for the global spread of influenza*, Math. Biosc. **75**: 3–22.

[91] Stearn, E.W. and A.E. Stearn (1945) *The Effect of Smallpox on the Destiny of the Amerindian*, Bruce Humphries, Boston, MA.

[92] Wehrle, P.F., J. Posch, K.H. Richter, and D.A. Henderson (1970) *An airborne outbreak of smallpox in a German hospital and its significance with respect to other recent outbreaks in Europe*, Bull. World Health Org. **43**: 669–679.

[93] Weisstein, E.W. (1999) *CRC Concise Encyclopedia of Mathematics*, CRC Press, Boca Raton, London, New York, Washington, D.C.: 362–364.

[94] *What is Smallpox*, http://www.vaccinationnews.com/DailyNews/May2002/WhatSmallpox.htm © 2001 WebMD Corporation, accessed July 2002.

Lecture 6

Modeling Influenza

6.1 Introduction to Influenza Models

Influenza causes more morbidity and mortality than all other respiratory diseases combined. There are annual seasonal epidemics that cause about 500,000 deaths worldwide each year. During the twentieth century there were three influenza pandemics. The WHO estimates that there were 40,000,000–50,000,000 deaths worldwide in the 1918 pandemic, 2,000,000 deaths worldwide in the 1957 pandemic, and 1,000,000 deaths worldwide in the 1968 pandemic. There has been concern since 2005 that the H5N1 strain of avian influenza could develop into a strain that could be transmitted readily from human to human and develop into another pandemic, and it is widely believed that even if this does not occur, there is likely to be an influenza pandemic in the near future. More recently, the H1N1 strain of influenza did develop into a pandemic in 2009, but fortunately its case mortality rate was low, and this pandemic turned out to be much less serious than had been feared. This history has aroused considerable interest in both modeling the spread of influenza and comparing the results of possible management strategies.

Vaccines are available for annual seasonal epidemics. Influenza strains mutate rapidly, and each year a judgment is made of which strains of influenza are most likely to invade. A vaccine is distributed that protects against the three strains considered most dangerous. However, if a strain radically different from previously known strains arrives, the vaccine provides little or no protection and there is danger of a pandemic. As it would take at least six months to develop a vaccine to protect against such a new strain, it would not be possible to have a vaccine ready to protect against the initial onslaught of a new pandemic strain. Antiviral drugs are available to treat pandemic influenza, and they may have some preventive benefits as well, but such benefits are present only while antiviral treatment is continued.

Various kinds of models have been used to describe influenza outbreaks. Many public health policy decisions on coping with a possible influenza pandemic are based on construction of a contact network for a population and analysis of disease spread through this network. This analysis consists of multiple stochastic simulations requiring a substantial amount of computer time. In advance of an epidemic it is not possible to know its severity, and it would be necessary to make estimates for a range of reproduction numbers. Also, model parameters for the H1N1 influenza pandemic of 2009, especially the susceptibility to infection for different age groups, were significantly different from those for seasonal epidemics. In advance of an anticipated pandemic it may be more appropriate to use simpler models until enough data are acquired to facilitate parameter estimation. Early estimation of model parameters is extremely important for coping with a serious epidemic, and one of the outcomes of the H1N1 influenza pandemic of 2009 was development of new methods, mainly based on network models, to achieve this.

Our approach is to begin with simple models and to add more structure later as more information is obtained. When an epidemic does begin, plans for management strategies need to be very detailed, and use of the simple models we describe in this lecture should be restricted to advance planning and broad understanding.

We begin this lecture by developing a simple compartmental influenza transmission model and then augmenting it to include both pre-epidemic vaccination and treatment during an epidemic. We will then develop a compartmental model with more structure and compare its predictions with those of the simpler model. We will also describe some ways in which the model can be modified to be more realistic, though more complicated. The development follows the treatment in [3, 4]. We will describe the models and the results of their analyses but omit proofs in order to focus attention on the applications of the models. Many of the results may be found in earlier lectures.

6.2 A Basic Influenza Model

Since influenza epidemics usually come and go in a time period of several months, we do not include demographic effects (births and natural deaths) in our model. Our starting point is the SIR model of Section 1.2. Two aspects of influenza that are easily added are (i) there is an incubation period between infection and the appearance of symptoms, and (ii) a significant fraction of people who are infected never develop symptoms but go through an asymptomatic period, during which they have some infectivity, and then recover and go to the removed compartment [17]. Thus a model should contain the compartments S (susceptible), L (latent), I (infective), A (asymptomatic), and R (removed). Specifically, we make the following assumptions:

- There is a small number I_0 of initial infectives in a population of constant total size N.
- The number of contacts in unit time per individual is a constant multiple β of total population size N.
- Latent members (L) are not infective.
- A fraction p of latent members proceed to the infective compartment at rate κ, while the remainder goes directly to an asymptomatic infective compartment (A), also at rate κ.
- There are no disease deaths. Infectives (I) recover and leave the infective compartment at rate α, and go to the removed compartment (R).
- Asymptomatics have infectivity reduced by a factor δ and go to the removed compartment at rate η.

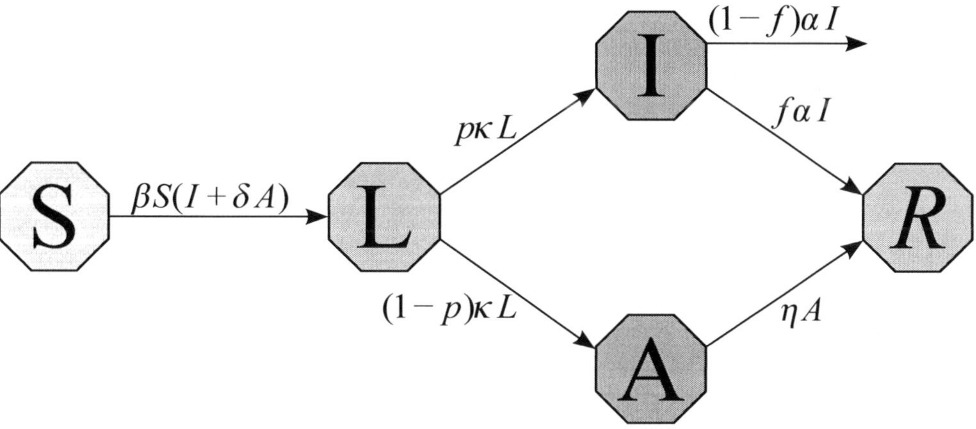

Figure 6.1. *Basic influenza model.*

These assumptions lead to the model

$$\begin{aligned} S' &= -S\beta(I+\delta A), \\ L' &= S\beta(I+\delta A) - \kappa L, \\ I' &= p\kappa L - \alpha I, \\ A' &= (1-p)\kappa L - \eta A, \\ R' &= \alpha I + \eta A, \end{aligned} \tag{6.1}$$

with initial conditions

$$S(0) = S_0, \quad L(0) = 0, \quad I(0) = I_0, \quad A(0) = 0, \quad R(0) = 0, \quad N = S_0 + I_0.$$

In analyzing this model we may remove one variable since $N = S + L + I + A + R$ is constant. It is usually convenient to remove the variable R. Our language is ambiguous in that we use S, L, I, A, R, N to denote both the names of the classes and the number of members of the classes, but this should cause no confusion. It is possible to show that the model (6.1) is properly posed in the sense that all variables remain nonnegative for $0 \le t < \infty$. A flow diagram for the model (6.1) is shown in Figure 6.1. The model is the simplest possible description for influenza having the property that there are asymptomatic infections. The question that should be in the back of our minds is whether it is a sufficiently accurate description for its predictions to be useful.

The model (6.1), like the other models that we will introduce later, consists of a system of ordinary differential equations, and the number of susceptibles in the population tends to a limit S_∞ as $t \to \infty$. There is a *final size relation*, as introduced in Section 1.2, that we may use to find this limit without the need to solve the system of differential equations. If the contact rate β is constant, the final size relation is an equality. It is more realistic to assume saturation of contacts and that β is a function of the total population size N. In general, the final size relation is an inequality. If there are no disease deaths, N is constant and β is constant even with saturation of contacts. If the disease death rate is small, it appears that the final size relation is very close to an equality and it is reasonable to assume that β is constant and use the final size relation as an equation to solve for S_∞.

We may use the next generation matrix approach of [25], described in Section 3.3, to calculate the basic reproduction number

$$\mathcal{R}_0 = \beta N \left[\frac{p}{\alpha} + \frac{\delta(1-p)}{\eta} \right]. \tag{6.2}$$

A biological interpretation of this basic reproduction number is that a latent member introduced into a population of S_0 susceptibles becomes infective with probability p, in which case he or she causes $\beta N/\alpha$ infections during an infective period of length $1/\alpha$, or becomes asymptomatic with probability $1-p$, in which case he or she causes $\delta\beta N/\eta$ infections during an asymptomatic period of length η.

The *final size relation* is given by

$$\log \frac{S_0}{S_\infty} = \mathcal{R}_0 \left[1 - \frac{S_0}{N} \right]. \tag{6.3}$$

A very general form of the final size relation that is applicable to each of the models in this lecture is derived in [4]. The final size relation shows that $S_\infty > 0$. This means that some members of the population are not infected during the epidemic. The size of the epidemic, the number of (clinical) cases of influenza during the epidemic, is

$$I_0 + S_0 - S_\infty = N - S_\infty,$$

and the number of symptomatic cases is

$$I_0 + p(S_0 - S_\infty).$$

If there are disease deaths, with a disease survival rate f and a disease death rate $(1-f)$ among infectives (assuming no disease deaths of asymptomatics), the number of disease deaths is

$$I_0 + (1-f)p(S_0 - S_\infty).$$

While mathematicians view the basic reproduction number as central in studying epidemiological models, epidemiologists may be more concerned with the *attack rate*, as this may be measured directly. For influenza, where there are asymptomatic cases, there are two attack rates. One is the clinical attack rate, which is the fraction of the population that becomes infected, defined as

$$1 - \frac{S_\infty}{N}.$$

There is also the symptomatic attack rate, the fraction of the population that develops disease symptoms, defined as

$$p\left[1 - \frac{S_\infty}{N(0)} \right].$$

The attack rates and the basic reproduction number are connected through the final size relation (6.3). If we know the parameters of the model, we can calculate $\mathcal{R}_0$ from (6.2) and then solve for S_∞ from (6.3).

We apply the model (6.1) using parameters appropriate for the 1957 influenza pandemic as suggested by [17]. The latent period is approximately 1.9 days and the infective period is approximately 4.1 days, so that

$$\kappa = \frac{1}{1.9} = 0.526, \quad \alpha = \eta = \frac{1}{4.1} = 0.244.$$

We also take

$$p = 2/3, \quad \delta = 0.5, \quad f = 0.98.$$

As in [17] we consider a population of 2,000 members, of whom 12 are infective initially. In [17] a symptomatic attack rate was assumed for each of four age groups, and the average symptomatic attack rate for the entire population was 0.326. This implies $S_\infty = 1022$. Then we obtain

$$\mathcal{R}_0 = 1.37$$

from (6.3). Now, we use this in (6.2) to calculate

$$\beta N = 0.402.$$

We will use these data as baseline values to estimate the effect that control measures might have had. The number of clinical cases is 978 (including the initial 12), the number of symptomatic cases is 664, again including the original 12, and the number of disease deaths is approximately 13.

The model (6.1) can be adapted to describe management strategies for both annual seasonal epidemics and pandemics.

6.3 Vaccination

To cope with annual seasonal influenza epidemics there is a program of vaccination before the "flu" season begins. Each year a vaccine is produced aimed at protecting against the three influenza strains considered most dangerous for the coming season. We formulate a model to add vaccination to the model described by (6.1) under the assumption that vaccination reduces susceptibility (the probability of infection if a contact with an infected member of the population is made). In addition we assume that vaccinated members who develop infection are less likely to transmit infection, more likely not to develop symptoms, and likely to recover more rapidly than unvaccinated members.

These assumptions require us to introduce additional compartments into the model to follow treated members of the population through the stages of infection. We use the classes S, L, I, A, R as before and introduce S_T, the class of treated susceptibles, L_T, the class of treated latent members, I_T, the class of treated infectives, and A_T, the class of treated asymptomatics. In addition to the assumptions made in formulating the model (6.1) we also assume the following:

- A fraction γ of the population is vaccinated before a disease outbreak, and vaccinated members have susceptibility to infection reduced by a factor σ_S.
- There are decreases σ_I and σ_A, respectively, in infectivity in I_T and A_T; it is reasonable to assume

$$\sigma_I < 1, \quad \sigma_A < 1.$$

- The rates of departure from L_T, I_T, and A_T are κ_T, α_T, and η_T, respectively. It is reasonable to assume
$$\kappa \le \kappa_T, \quad \alpha \le \alpha_T, \quad \eta \le \eta_T.$$
- The fractions of members recovering from disease when they leave I and I_T are f and f_T, respectively. It is reasonable to assume $f \le f_T$. In our analysis we will take $f = f_T = 1$.
- Vaccination decreases the fraction of latent members who will develop symptoms by a factor τ, with $0 \le \tau \le 1$.

For convenience we introduce the notation

$$Q = I + \delta A + \sigma_I I_T + \delta \sigma_A A_T. \tag{6.4}$$

The resulting model is

$$\begin{aligned}
S' &= -S\beta Q,\\
S_T' &= -\sigma_S S_T \beta Q,\\
L' &= S\beta Q - \kappa L,\\
L_T' &= \sigma_S S_T \beta Q - \kappa_T L_T,\\
I' &= p\kappa L - \alpha I,\\
I_T' &= \tau p \kappa_T L_T - \alpha_T I_T,\\
A' &= (1-p)\kappa L - \eta A,\\
A_T' &= (1-p\tau)\kappa_T L_T - \eta_T A_T,\\
R' &= \alpha I + \alpha_T I_T + \eta A + \eta_T A_T.
\end{aligned} \tag{6.5}$$

The initial conditions are

$$\begin{aligned}
S(0) = (1-\gamma)S_0, \quad S_T(0) = \gamma S_0, \quad I(0) = I_0, \quad N = S_0 + I_0,\\
L(0) = L_T(0) = I_T(0) = A(0) = A_T(0) = 0,
\end{aligned}$$

corresponding to pre-epidemic treatment of a fraction γ of the population. A flow diagram for the model (6.5) is shown in Figure 6.2.

Since the infection now is beginning in a population which is not fully susceptible, we speak of the *control reproduction number* $\mathcal{R}_c$ rather than the basic reproduction number. A computation using the next generation matrix leads to the control reproduction number

$$\mathcal{R}_c = (1-\gamma)\mathcal{R}_u + \gamma \mathcal{R}_v,$$

with

$$\begin{aligned}
\mathcal{R}_u &= N\beta\left[\frac{p}{\alpha} + \frac{\delta(1-p)}{\eta}\right] = \mathcal{R}_0, \qquad (6.6)\\
\mathcal{R}_v &= \sigma_S N\beta\left[\frac{p\tau\sigma_I}{\alpha_T} + \frac{\delta(1-p\tau)\sigma_A}{\eta_T}\right].
\end{aligned}$$

Then $\mathcal{R}_u$ is a reproduction number for unvaccinated people and $\mathcal{R}_v$ is a reproduction number for vaccinated people. There is a pair of final size relations (Section 3.6) for the two final

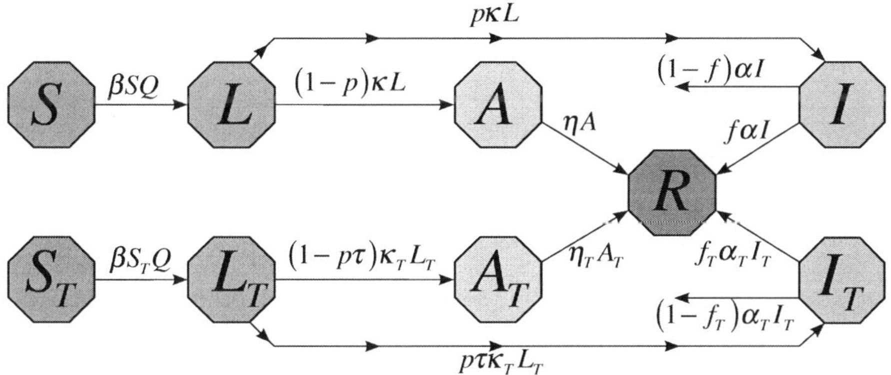

Figure 6.2. *Vaccination model.*

sizes $S(\infty)$ and $S_T(\infty)$ in terms of the group sizes $N_u = (1-\gamma)N, N_v = \gamma N$, namely,

$$\begin{aligned}\log\frac{(1-\gamma)S_0}{S_\infty} &= \mathcal{R}_u\left[1-\frac{S_\infty}{N_u}\right]+\mathcal{R}_v\left[1-\frac{S_T(\infty)}{N_v}\right],\\ \log\frac{\gamma S_0}{S_T(\infty)} &= \sigma_S\mathcal{R}_u\left[1-\frac{S_\infty}{N_u}\right]+\mathcal{R}_v\left[1-\frac{S_T(\infty)}{N_v}\right].\end{aligned} \tag{6.7}$$

The number of symptomatic disease cases is

$$I_0 + p[(1-\gamma)S_0 - S(\infty)] + p\tau[\gamma S_0 - S_T(\infty)],$$

and the number of disease deaths is

$$(1-f)[I_0 + p(1-\gamma)S_0 - S(\infty)] + (1-f_T)p\tau[\gamma S_0 - S_T(\infty)].$$

These may be calculated with the aid of (6.7). By control of the epidemic we mean vaccinating enough people (i.e., taking γ large enough) to make $\mathcal{R}_c < 1$. We use the parameters of Section 6.2, with vaccination parameters as suggested in [17], using estimates of vaccine efficacy based on those reported in [10],

$$\sigma_S = 0.3, \quad \sigma_I = \sigma_A = 0.2, \quad \kappa_T = 0.526, \quad \alpha_T = \eta_T = 0.323, \quad \tau = 0.4.$$

With these parameter values,

$$\mathcal{R}_u = 1.373, \quad \mathcal{R}_v = 0.047.$$

In order to make $\mathcal{R}_c = 1$, we need to take $\gamma = 0.28$. This is the fraction of the population that needs to be vaccinated to head off an epidemic.

We may solve the pair of final size equations with $S(0) = (1-\gamma)S_0, S_T(0) = \gamma S_0$ for $S(\infty), S_T(\infty)$ for different values of γ. We do this for the parameter values suggested above and obtain the results shown in Table 6.1, giving the treatment fraction γ, the number of untreated susceptibles $S(\infty)$ at the end of the epidemic, the number of treated susceptibles $S_T(\infty)$ at the end of the epidemic, the number of treated cases of influenza $I_0 + p[(1-\gamma)S_0 - S(\infty)]$, and the number of untreated cases $(\gamma S_0 - S_T(\infty)]$. The results indicate the

Table 6.1. *Effect of vaccination.*

Fraction treated	S_∞	$S_T\infty$	Untreated cases	Treated cases
0	1015	0	660	0
0.05	1079	84	552	4
0.1	1149	174	439	7
0.15	1224	271	323	7
0.2	1305	375	201	6
0.25	1395	487	76	3
0.3	1391	596	13	0

benefits of pre-epidemic vaccination of even a small fraction of the population in reducing the number of influenza cases. They also demonstrate the advantage of vaccination to an individual. The attack rate in the vaccinated portion of the population is much less than the attack rate in the unvaccinated portion of the population.

6.4 Antiviral Treatment

If no vaccine is available for a strain of influenza, it would be possible to use an antiviral treatment. However, antiviral treatment is more expensive and affords protection only while the treatment is continued. In addition, antivirals are in short supply and treatment of enough of the population to control an anticipated epidemic may not be feasible. A policy of treatment aimed particularly at people who have been infected or who have been in contact with infectives once a disease outbreak has begun may be a more appropriate approach. This requires a model with treatment rates for latent, infective, and asymptomatically infected members of the population that we construct building on the structure used for vaccination in (6.5).

Antiviral drugs have effects similar to vaccines in decreasing susceptibility to infection and decreasing infectivity, the likelihood of developing symptoms, and the length of infective period in case of infection. However, they are likely to be less effective than a well-matched vaccine, especially in the reduction of susceptibility.

Treatment may be given to diagnosed infectives. In addition, one may treat contacts of infectives who are thought to have been infected. This is modeled by treating latent members. In practice, some of those identified by contact tracing and treated would actually be susceptibles, but we neglect this in the model. Although we have allowed treatment of asymptomatics in the model, this is unlikely to be done, and we will describe the results of the model under the assumption $\varphi_A = \theta_A = 0$. However, for generality we retain the possibility of antiviral treatment of asymptomatics in the model. If treatment is given only to infectives, the compartments L_T, A_T are empty and may be omitted from the model.

We add to the model (6.5) antiviral treatment of latent, infective, and asymptomatically infected members of the population, but we do not assume an initial treated class. In addition to the assumptions made earlier we also assume the following:

- There is a treatment rate φ_L in L and a rate θ_L of relapse from L_T to L, a treatment rate φ_I in I and a rate θ_I of relapse from I_T to I, and a treatment rate φ_A in A and a rate θ_A of relapse from A_T to A.

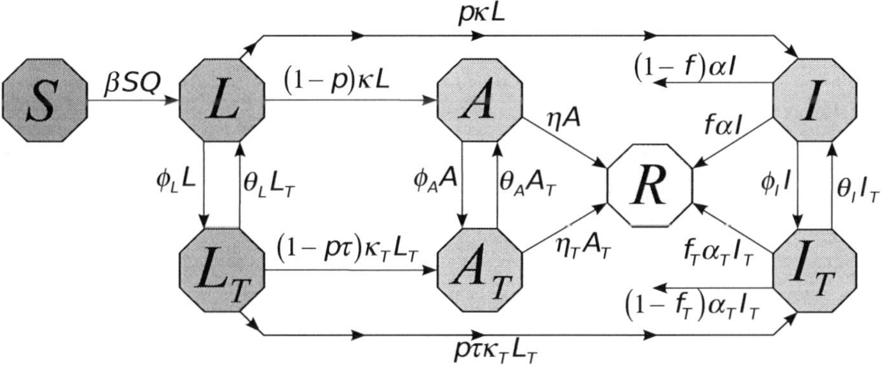

Figure 6.3. *Treatment model.*

The resulting model is

$$
\begin{aligned}
S' &= -\beta S Q, \\
L' &= \beta S Q - \kappa L - \varphi_L L + \theta_L L_T, \\
L_T' &= -\kappa_T L_T + \varphi_L L - \theta_L L_T, \\
I' &= p\kappa L - \alpha I - \varphi_I I + \theta_I I_T, \\
I_T' &= p\tau\kappa_T L_T - \alpha_T I_T + \varphi_I I - \theta_I I_T, \\
A' &= (1-p)\kappa L - \eta A - \varphi_A A + \theta_A A_T, \\
A_T' &= (1-p\tau)\kappa_T L_T - \eta_T A_T + \varphi_A A - \theta_A A_T, \\
N' &= -(1-f)\alpha I - (1-f_T)\alpha_T I_T,
\end{aligned}
\tag{6.8}
$$

with Q as in (6.4). The initial conditions are

$$S(0) = S_0, \quad I(0) = I_0, \quad L(0) = L_T(0) = I_T(0) = A(0) = A_T(0) = 0, \quad N = S_0 + I_0.$$

A flow diagram for the model (6.8) is shown in Figure 6.3.

The calculation of $\mathcal{R}_c$ for the antiviral treatment model (6.8) is more complicated than for models considered previously, but it is possible to show that $\mathcal{R}_c = \mathcal{R}_I + \mathcal{R}_A$ with

$$
\begin{aligned}
\mathcal{R}_I &= \frac{N\beta}{\Delta_I \Delta_L}\left[(\alpha_T + \theta_I + \sigma_I\varphi_I)p\kappa(\kappa_T + \theta_L) + (\theta_I + \sigma_I(\alpha + \varphi_I))p\tau\kappa_T\phi_L\right], \\
\mathcal{R}_A &= \frac{\delta N\beta}{\Delta_L}\left[\frac{(1-p)\kappa(\kappa_T + \theta_L)}{\eta} + \frac{\sigma_A(1-p\tau)\kappa_T\varphi_L}{\eta_T}\right],
\end{aligned}
\tag{6.9}
$$

where

$$
\begin{aligned}
\Delta_I &= (\alpha + \varphi_I)(\alpha_T + \theta_I) - \theta_I\varphi_I, \\
\Delta_L &= (\kappa + \varphi_L)(\kappa_T + \theta_L) - \theta_L\varphi_L.
\end{aligned}
$$

The final size equation is

$$\log \frac{S_0}{S_\infty} = \mathcal{R}_c\left[1 - \frac{S_\infty}{S_0}\right] + \frac{\beta I_0(\alpha_T + \theta_I + \sigma_I \varphi_I)}{\Delta_I}. \tag{6.10}$$

The number of people treated is

$$\int_0^\infty [\varphi_L L(t) + \varphi_I I(t)]dt,$$

and the number of disease cases is

$$I_0 + \int_0^\infty [p\kappa L(t) + p\tau\kappa_T L_T]dt,$$

which can be evaluated in terms of the parameters of the model. The number of people treated and the number of disease cases are constant multiples of $S_0 - S_\infty$ plus constant multiples of the (presumably small) number of initial infectives. Since the expressions in terms of $S_0 - S_\infty$ and I_0 are more complicated than in the cases of no treatment or vaccination, we have chosen to give these numbers in terms of integrals.

There is an important consequence of the calculation of the number of disease cases and treatments that is not at all obvious. If $\mathcal{R}_c$ is close to 1 or ≤ 1, $S_0 - S_\infty$ depends very sensitively on changes in I_0. For example, in a population of 2,000 with $\mathcal{R}_0 = 1.5$, a change in I_0 from 1 to 2 multiplies $S_0 - S_\infty$ and therefore treatments and cases by 1.4, and a change in I_0 from 1 to 5 multiplies $S_0 - S_\infty$ and therefore treatments and cases by 3. Thus, numerical predictions in themselves are of little value. However, comparison of different strategies is valid, and the model indicates the importance of early action while the number of infectives is small.

In the special case that treatment is applied only to infectives, $\mathcal{R}_c$ is given by the simpler expression

$$\mathcal{R}_c = N\beta\left[\frac{p(\alpha_T + \theta_I + \sigma_I\varphi_I)}{\Delta_I} + \frac{\delta(1-p)}{\eta}\right].$$

The number of disease cases is $I_0 + p(S_0 - S_\infty)$, and the number of people treated is

$$\frac{\varphi_I(\alpha_T + \theta_I)}{\Delta_I}[I_0 + p(S_0 - S_\infty)].$$

Since the infective period is short, antiviral treatment would normally be applied as long as the patient remains infective. Thus we assume $\theta_I = 0$, and these relations become even simpler. The control reproduction number is

$$\mathcal{R}_c = N\beta\left[\frac{p(\alpha_T + \sigma_I\varphi_I)}{\alpha_T(\alpha + \varphi_I)} + \frac{\delta(1-p)}{\eta}\right], \tag{6.11}$$

and the number of people treated is

$$\frac{\varphi_I}{\alpha + \varphi_I}[I_0 + p(S_0 - S_\infty)]. \tag{6.12}$$

Since the basic reproduction number of a future pandemic cannot be known in advance, it is necessary to take a range of contact rates in order to make predictions.

In particular, we could compare the effectiveness in controlling the number of infections or the number of disease deaths of different strategies such as treating only infectives, treating only latent members, or treating a combination of both infective and latent members. In making such comparisons, it is important to take into account that treatment of latent members must be supplied for a longer period than for infectives. In case of a pandemic, there are also questions of whether the supply of antiviral drugs will be sufficient to carry out a given strategy. For this reason we must calculate the number of treatments corresponding to a given treatment rate. It is possible to do this from the model; the result is a constant multiple of I_0 plus a multiple of $S_0 - S_\infty$.

The results of such calculations appear to indicate that treatment of diagnosed infectives is the most effective strategy [3, 4]. However, there are other considerations that would go into any policy decision. For example, a pandemic would threaten to disrupt essential services, and it could be decided to use antiviral drugs prophylactically in an attempt to protect health care workers and public safety personnel. A study including this aspect based on the antiviral treatment model given here is reported in [14].

For simulations, we use the initial values

$$S_0 = 1988, \quad I_0 = 12,$$

the parameters of Section 6.2, and for antiviral efficacy we assume

$$\sigma_S = 0.7, \quad \sigma_I = \sigma_A = 0.2,$$

based on data reported in [26].

We simulate the model (6.8) with $\theta_I = 0$, assuming that treatment continues for the duration of the infection. We assume that 80% of diagnosed infectives are treated within 1 day. Since the assumption of treatment at a constant rate φ_I implies treatment of a fraction $1 - \exp(-\varphi_I t)$ after a time t, we take φ_I to satisfy

$$1 - e^{-\varphi_I} = 0.8,$$

or $\varphi_I = 1.61$. We use different values of βN, corresponding to different values of $\mathcal{R}_0$, and use (6.10) and (6.11), obtaining the results shown in Table 6.2.

Table 6.2. *Control by antiviral treatment.*

βN	$\mathcal{R}_0$	$\mathcal{R}_c$	Disease cases	Treatments
0.402	1.37	0.92	64	56
0.435	1.49	1.00	130	113
0.5	1.71	1.15	373	314
0.7	2.39	1.61	865	751

We calculate from (6.11) that $\mathcal{R}_c = 1$ if $N\beta = 0.435$ and $\mathcal{R}_0 = 1.49$, corresponding to a symptomatic attack rate of 39%. This is the critical attack rate beyond which treatment at the rate specified cannot control the pandemic.

In the next section, we will formulate and analyze a compartmental model that describes influenza more precisely. Then we will choose parameters so that the behavior agrees with the behavior of the model (6.1) without treatment as simulated in Section 6.2 and compare simulation of a corresponding model with the simulation of Section 6.4.

6.5 A More Detailed Model

Recent re-examination of data from past influenza epidemics [1, 6, 12, 14, 23] has indicated a more complicated compartmental structure than that of (6.1). It is suggested that susceptibles go first to a noninfectious first latent stage, then either to an asymptomatic stage and removal, or to a second latent stage with some infectivity, followed by two infective stages with different infectivity. Treatment is applied only during the first infective stage. This leads to the following model, taken from [1]:

$$
\begin{aligned}
S' &= -\beta S Q, \\
L_1' &= \beta S Q - \kappa_1 L_1, \\
L_2' &= p\kappa_1 L_1 - \kappa_2 L_2, \\
I_1' &= \kappa_2 L_2 - (\alpha_1 + \varphi) I_1, \\
I_2' &= \alpha_1 I_1 - \alpha_2 I_2, \\
I_T' &= \varphi I_1 - \alpha_T I_T, \\
A' &= (1-p)\kappa_1 L_1 - \eta A, \\
N' &= -(1-f)\alpha_2 I_2 - (1-f_T)\alpha_T I_T,
\end{aligned}
\tag{6.13}
$$

with

$$Q = \sigma_L L_2 + I_1 + \sigma_I I_2 + \sigma_T I_T + \sigma_A A.$$

The parameters $\sigma_L, \sigma_I, \sigma_T, \sigma_A$ are the relative infectivities in the compartments L_2, I_2, I_T, A, respectively. The initial conditions are

$$S(0) = S_0, \quad I_1(0) = I_0, \quad L_1(0) = L_2(0) = I_2(0) = I_T(0) = A(0) = 0, \quad N(0) = S_0 + I_0.$$

A flow diagram for the model (6.13) is shown in Figure 6.4.

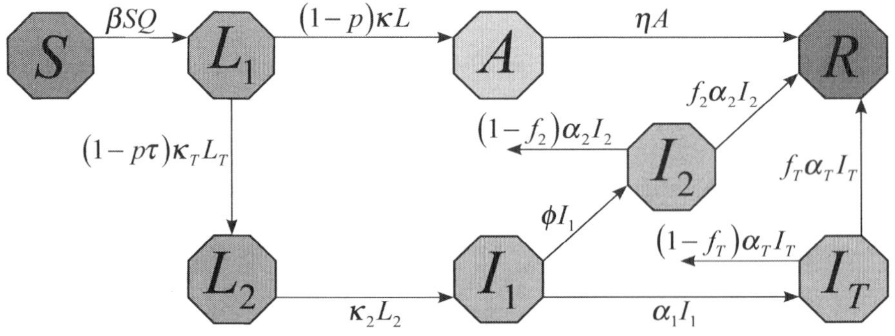

Figure 6.4. *Refined model.*

Then we calculate

$$\mathcal{R}_c = \beta N\left[\frac{p\sigma_L}{\kappa_2} + \frac{p}{\alpha_1+\varphi} + \frac{p\sigma_I\alpha_1}{\alpha_2(\alpha_1+\varphi)} + \frac{p\sigma_T\varphi}{\alpha_T(\alpha_1+\varphi)} + \frac{(1-p)\sigma_A}{\eta}\right]. \tag{6.14}$$

The basic reproduction number is given by (6.14) with $\varphi = 0$,

$$\mathcal{R}_0 = \beta N\left[\frac{p\sigma_L}{\kappa_2} + \frac{p}{\alpha_1} + \frac{p\sigma_I}{\alpha_2} + \frac{(1-p)\sigma_A}{\eta}\right]. \tag{6.15}$$

The final size relation is

$$\log\frac{S_0}{S_\infty} = \mathcal{R}_c\left[1 - \frac{S_\infty}{S_0}\right] + \beta I_0 \rho, \tag{6.16}$$

with

$$\rho = \frac{1}{\alpha_1+\varphi} + \frac{\sigma_I\alpha_1}{\alpha_2(\alpha_1+\varphi)} + \frac{\sigma_T\varphi}{\alpha_T(\alpha_1+\varphi)}.$$

The number of disease cases is $I_0 + p(S_0 - S_\infty)$, and the number of people treated is

$$\frac{\varphi}{\alpha_1+\varphi}[I_0 + p(S_0 - S_\infty)].$$

In [14], suggested parameter values are

$$\kappa_1 = 0.8, \quad \kappa_2 = 4.0, \quad \alpha_1 = 1.0, \quad \alpha_2 = \frac{1}{2.85}, \quad \alpha_T = \frac{1}{1.35},$$
$$\eta = \frac{1}{4.1}, \quad \delta_L = 0.286, \quad \delta_I = 0.143,$$

and we take

$$\delta_T = 0.2, \quad \delta_A = 0.5$$

as in [3, 4, 17]. With these parameter values,

$$\mathcal{R}_0 = 1.669\beta N.$$

In order to obtain $\mathcal{R}_0 = 1.37$ as in the simulation of Section 6.2 using (6.15), we take $N\beta = 0.823$ (note that this is not the same value as in Section 6.2). Next, we take a treatment rate $\varphi = 1.61$, as in the simulation of Section 6.4. Using (6.14) we obtain $\mathcal{R}_c = 0.74$, compared with the value $\mathcal{R}_c = 0.50$ obtained in Section 6.4. From (6.16) we obtain $S_\infty = 1962$, corresponding to 29 cases of disease compared with 19 cases found in Section 6.4. The number of people receiving antiviral treatment is 12.

There are significant differences between the predictions of the models (6.8) and (6.13), with the number of disease cases and disease deaths higher for (6.13). Presumably, the model (6.13) is closer to the truth than (6.8). However, use of (6.13) requires more knowledge of the course of the epidemic period and more information about parameter values. Also, it should be noted that the model (6.13), having treatment only during one infective stage, is not suitable for modeling pre-epidemic vaccination.

There are other, probably more serious, omissions in the model. In many past influenza epidemics it has been observed that much of the transmission of infection can be traced to school children, while many of the disease fatalities are in elderly or immune-compromised people who make many fewer contacts. This suggests that in order to give a more accurate description of influenza transmission it is important to separate the population into subgroups with different contact rates and different disease mortality rates, as in Section 3.5. This is also essential for choosing a vaccination or treatment strategy that targets particular age groups.

6.6 The Influenza Pandemic of 2009

In the spring of 2009 a new strain (H1N1) of influenza A developed, apparently first in Mexico, and spread rapidly through much of the world. Initially, it was thought that there was no resistance to this strain, although it developed later that people who were old enough to have been exposed to similar strains in the 1950s appeared to be less susceptible than younger people. It also appeared initially that this strain had a high case fatality rate, but it was later learned that since many cases were mild enough not to be reported, the early data were weighted towards severe cases, and the case fatality rate was actually lower than for most seasonal influenza strains.

Management of the H1N1 influenza pandemic of 2009 made use of mathematical models and the experience gained from previous epidemics, but it also exposed some gaps between a well-developed mathematical theory of epidemics and real-life epidemics, notably in the acquisition of reliable data early in the pandemic, understanding of spatial spread of a pandemic, and the development of multiple epidemic waves.

There are important differences in the kinds of models that are of value to different types of scientists. There are *strategic* disease transmission models aimed at the understanding of broad general principles, and *tactical* models with the goal of helping make decisions in specific and detailed situations on short-term policies. A model that predicts how many people will become ill in an anticipated epidemic is quite different from a model that helps to identify which subgroups of a population should have highest priority for preventive vaccination with an uncertain prediction of how much vaccine will be available in a given time frame.

6.6.1 A tactical influenza model

There was a second wave of infections in the 2009 H1N1 influenza pandemic, just as in several previous influenza pandemics. As soon as possible during the first wave, work began on the development of a vaccine matched to the virus to be used to combat the expected second wave [20]. Since a vaccine requires at least six months for development, and the second wave could begin within six months of the first wave, there was an urgent need to prepare a vaccine distribution strategy.

In this section we describe the model of [9] as an example of a tactical model. This model was used by the British Columbia Centre for Disease Control in making planning decisions for vaccination distribution during the second wave of the 2009 H1N1 influenza pandemic. Because of the need to make such decisions rapidly, the development and application of the model was more urgent than the writing of the paper that described the work, and use of the results preceded the write-up. In a pandemic, there is still much to be done after the model has been developed and applied, and frequently there is not time to explore basic theoretical questions that may arise in the study. Ideally, these questions can be studied in more depth after the urgency of coping with a pandemic has passed, and this is an opportunity to return to more general strategic models.

Infection rates in an influenza epidemic depend strongly on the (demographic) age of the individuals in contact. This dependence of transmission and infection rates on age (the age profile) may vary significantly between locations and from year to year for seasonal epidemics. Also, the age profile in a pandemic is probably unlike that for seasonal epidemics. For this reason, real-time planning during an epidemic must make use of surveillance data obtained as soon as possible after the epidemic has begun. The data gathered during the first wave in the spring of 2009 were used to project the age profile to be expected in the second wave. A compartmental model with 6 compartments in each of 40 population subgroups, covering 8 age classes and 5 activity levels using this age profile and existing estimates of the Vancouver contact network structure, was developed to project the results of different vaccination strategies.

The analysis of the model was carried out using numerical simulations, because comparisons of different strategies, including numerical estimates of disease cases and vaccine quantities required, were needed quickly and because general theoretical analysis of this high-dimensional system would have been too complicated. The numerical simulations indicated that a good estimate of the epidemic peak would be essential for making policy decisions on vaccination strategies. In a pandemic situation, delays in vaccine production may mean that vaccination cannot be started until an epidemic is already underway, and the model suggested that an early start to vaccine distribution makes a big difference in the effectiveness of the vaccination program. This raises a general theoretical question of the relation between the starting time of vaccination and the effectiveness of the vaccination program. Future theoretical study of models of this type would be very useful for planning vaccination strategies for epidemics in the future.

During the 1918 Spanish flu pandemic, North America and much of Western Europe experienced two waves of infection, with the second wave more severe than the first [7, 8]. Unlike seasonal influenza epidemics, which occur at predictable times each year, influenza pandemics are often shifted slightly from the usual "influenza season" and have multiple waves of varying severity. This suggests a modeling question that does not arise with seasonal influenza. During a first wave of a pandemic it should be possible to isolate virus samples and begin development of a vaccine matched to the virus in time to allow vaccination against the virus that could help to manage a second wave. One question that arises concerns prediction of the timing of a second wave. This is not yet possible because there is not yet a satisfactory explanation of the causes of a second wave. One suggestion that has been made is that transmissibility of virus varies seasonally, and this has been used to try to predict whether an endemic disease will exhibit seasonal outbreaks [19, 24]. The same approach can be used to formulate an SIR epidemic model with a periodic contact rate that can exhibit two epidemic waves. However, the behavior of such a model depends strongly on the timing of the epidemic. If we assume that the contact rate is highest in the winter, lowest in the summer, and varies sinusoidally with a period of one year, we could use a simple SIR model with a variable contact rate. With N as the (constant) total population size, this suggests a model

$$\begin{aligned} S' &= -\beta(t)\frac{SI}{N}, \qquad (6.17) \\ I' &= \beta(t)\frac{SI}{N} - \alpha I, \end{aligned}$$

where

$$\beta(t) = \beta\left[1 + c\cos\left(\frac{\pi(t+t_0)}{180}\right)\right],$$

with parameter values

$$\alpha = 0.25, \quad \beta = 0.45, \quad c = 0.45,$$
$$N = 1000, \quad S_0 = 999, \quad I_0 = 1, \quad t_0 = 85, 90, 95.$$

The choice of t_0 determines where in the oscillation of $\beta(t)$ the epidemic begins, because at the start of the epidemic ($t = 0$)

$$\beta(0) = \beta\left[1 + c\cos\left(\frac{\pi t_0}{180}\right)\right].$$

Thus t_0 is the number of days after the maximum transmissibility that the epidemic begins. By numerical integration of (6.17), we obtain the following three epidemic curves (giving the number of infectious individuals as a function of time), with the same parameters except that by varying t_0 the starting date of the epidemic is moved five days later from one curve to the next.

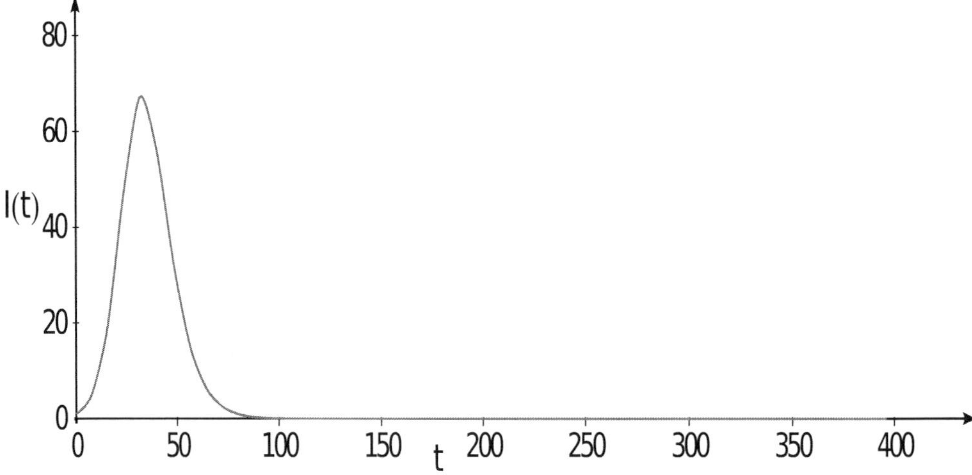

Figure 6.5. *A one-wave epidemic curve,* $t_0 = 85$.

An interpretation of these curves is that if the epidemic begins when the contact rate is decreasing and is close to its minimum value and the contact rate is relatively small over the course of the epidemic, the wave may end while there are still enough susceptibles to support a second wave when the contact rate increases, as in Figures 6.6 and 6.7. However, if the epidemic begins earlier, it may continue until enough individuals are infected that a second wave cannot be supported, even when the contact rate becomes large, as in Figure 6.5.

Simulations indicate that for the model (6.17) with the parameter values used here there is a small window of starting times corresponding to the interval $90 \le t_0 \le 110$ for

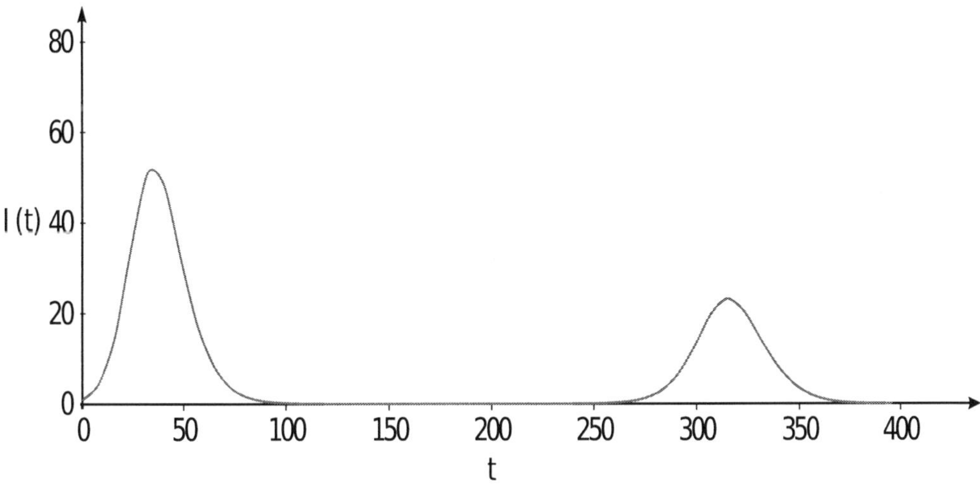

Figure 6.6. *A two-wave epidemic curve, first wave more severe,* $t_0 = 90$.

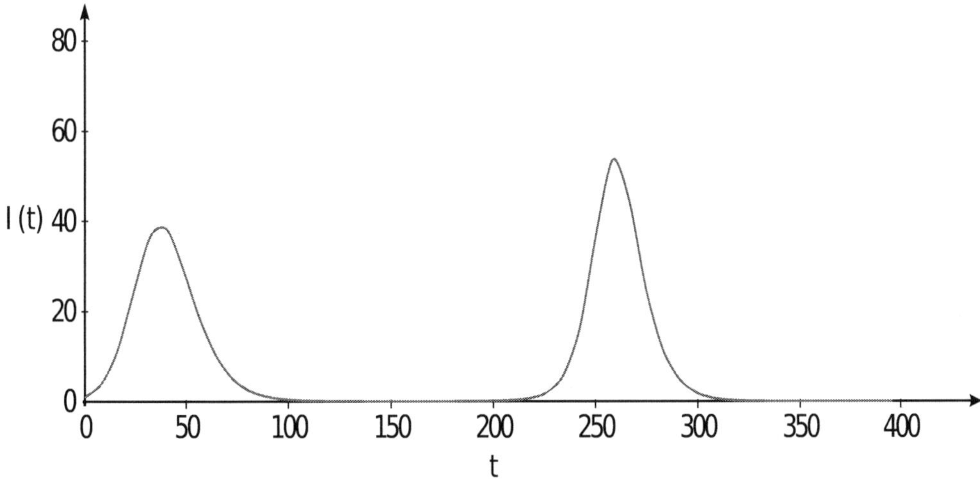

Figure 6.7. *A two-wave epidemic curve, second wave more severe,* $t_0 = 95$.

which a second wave is possible (Figures 6.6 and 6.7). The nature of the epidemic curves indicates that the behavior depends critically on timing, and this means that such a model is not suitable for precise predictions. Note that there may be a single wave or two waves, and if there are two waves, either one may be more severe. Not only does the prediction depend on the timing of the introduction of infection, but this timing is also stochastic and by its very nature unpredictable. It depends on mutations of the virus and importations of new cases.

We have here a strategic model that predicts the possibility of a second wave, but this is not sufficient to inspire confidence in using it to advise policy, because we do not have enough evidence to be sure about the cause of a second wave. Before we can make predictions we need more evidence about factors that could cause a second wave, as well as more detailed tactical models, including sensitivity analysis. Another factor that has been suggested as a possible explanation for a second epidemic wave is coinfection with other respiratory infections that might increase susceptibility, and some experimental data would be needed that might confirm or deny that either seasonal variation in transmission or coinfection, or both, could explain multiple pandemic waves.

In the H1N1 influenza pandemic of 2009, there were some concerns about the development of drug resistance as a consequence of antiviral treatment. While this did not appear to have widespread consequences, in a more severe disease outbreak in which more patients receive antiviral treatment there could be major effects. The modeling of drug resistance effects in an influenza pandemic has begun [1, 2, 16, 21, 22, 23], but much more needs to be understood. A full analysis of the development of drug resistance will require nested models, including immunological in-host aspects as well as effects on the population level.

Data from the 1918 pandemic indicate clearly that behavioral response, including both individual and public health measures, had significant effects on the outcome of the epidemic [5]. Incorporating behavioral responses is a new aspect of epidemic modeling, and there is much to be learned about the factors that influence behavioral responses when a disease outbreak begins.

6.7 Extensions and Other Types of Model

We have considered only compartmental models for influenza in this lecture, but there are other useful approaches. Many of the estimates being made for use in policy-making decisions for coping with an influenza pandemic are based on network models [11, 12, 15, 16, 17, 18]. These are based on a detailed study of mixing patterns in populations and assume a great deal of knowledge of the contact structure. They divide a population into subgroups having different contact patterns and are able to give very detailed predictions, including the effects of management strategies that treat different segments of the population differently. Their analyses involve large-scale stochastic simulations; while they give a great deal of information it is difficult to estimate their sensitivity to uncertainties in the parameter values. In addition to their current use in pandemic influenza preparation, they would also be useful in coping with seasonal influenza epidemics.

In Section 3.5 we have introduced heterogeneous mixing as an aspect of a model. Another heterogeneity arises from considering a population as a collection of separate units or patches with travel between them rather than as a single entity.

We have assumed mass-action incidence, but it is probably more realistic to assume some density dependence in the contact rates. In this case, the final size relations are inequalities rather than equations. If there are no disease deaths, the total population remains constant and mass action is equivalent to general incidence. It appears that if the disease death rate is small, mass-action incidence is a good approximation, and the use of final size equations in place of actually solving the systems of differential equations is a valid approximation.

We have not built into our models any assumptions of behavioral change by the population during an epidemic. It would be reasonable to expect infectives to withdraw from contact, either because of weakness caused by infection or because of public health encouragement to infectives to reduce contacts in order to avoid spreading infection. This could be modeled by the addition of an isolated compartment with reduced contacts. Another response to be expected is that at least part of the population would try to reduce contacts and take hygienic measures to decrease risk of infection. These factors have not been built into models here but are obvious candidates for consideration.

We have assumed rates of transition between compartments to be proportional to compartment sizes, which is equivalent to assuming negative exponential distributions of times in compartments. The assumption of more realistic distributions would lead to more complicated models, formulated as integral or integro-differential equations. An important question is whether such realistic assumptions—and therefore models that are much more difficult to analyze—would yield a worthwhile return in more accurate information.

A new and important question that is beginning to be studied is the possibility of development of resistance to antiviral drugs [1, 22, 23]. Models currently being developed build on compartmental models of the type studied in this lecture, and there are many questions coming under study.

In studying epidemic models in general there is a trade-off between the ease of analyzing a model and the amount of detail and accuracy provided by the model. The appropriate model for a given situation depends on the nature of the information sought and the amount and reliability of the data.

Bibliography

[1] Alexander, M.E., C.S. Bowman, Z. Feng, M. Gardam, S.M. Moghadas, G. Röst, J. Wu, and P. Yan (2007) *Emergence of drug resistance: Implications for antiviral control of pandemic influenza*, Proc. Roy. Soc. B **274**: 1675–1684.

[2] Arino, J., C.S. Bowman, and S.M. Moghadas (2009) *Antiviral resistance during pandemic influenza: Implications for stockpiling and drug use*, BMC Infectious Diseases **9**: 1–12.

[3] Arino, J., F. Brauer, P. van den Driessche, J. Watmough, and J. Wu (2006) *Simple models for containment of a pandemic*, J. Roy. Soc. Interface **3**: 453–457.

[4] Arino, J., F. Brauer, P. van den Driessche, J. Watmough, and J. Wu (2008) *A model for influenza with vaccination and antiviral treatment*, Theor. Pop. Biol. **253**: 118–130.

[5] Bootsma, M.C.J. and N.M. Ferguson (2007) *The effect of public health measures on the 1918 influenza pandemic in U.S. cities*, Proc. Natl. Acad. Sci. USA **104**: 7588–7593.

[6] Cauchemez, S., F. Carrat, C. Viboud, A.J. Valleron, and P.Y. Boëlle (2004) *A Bayesian MCMC approach to study transmission of influenza: Application to household longitudinal data*, Stat. in Med. **232**: 3469–3487.

[7] Chowell, G., C.E. Ammon, N.W. Hengartner, and J.M. Hyman (2006) *Transmission dynamics of the great influenza pandemic of* 1918 *in Geneva, Switzerland: Assessing the effects of hypothetical interventions*, J. Theor. Biol. **241**: 193–204.

[8] Chowell, G., C.E. Ammon, N.W. Hengartner, and J.M. Hyman (2007) *Estimating the reproduction number from the initial phase of the Spanish flu pandemic waves in Geneva, Switzerland*, Math. Biosc. & Eng. **4**: 457–479.

[9] Conway, J.M., A.R. Tuite, D.N. Fisman, N. Hupert, R. Meza, B. Davoudi, K. English, P. van den Driessche, F. Brauer, J. Ma, L.A. Meyers, M. Smieja, A. Greer, D.M. Skowronski, D.L. Buckeeridge, J. Kwong, J. Wu, S.M. Moghadas, D. Coombs, R.C. Brunham, and B. Pourbohloul (2010) *Vaccination against* 2009 *pandemic H1N1 in a population dynamic model of Vancouver, Canada: timing is everything*, submitted for publication.

[10] Elveback, L.R., J.P. Fox, E. Ackerman, A. Langworthy, M. Boyd, and L. Gatewood (1976) *An influenza simulation model for immunization studies*, Am. J. Epidem. **103**: 152–165.

[11] Ferguson, N.M., D.A.T. Cummings, S. Cauchemez, C. Fraser, S. Riley, A. Meeyai, S. Iamsirithaworn, and D.S. Burke (2005) *Strategies for containing an emerging influenza pandemic in Southeast Asia*, Nature **437**: 209–214.

[12] Ferguson, N.M., D.A.T. Cummings, C. Fraser, J.C. Cajka, P.C. Cooley, and D.S. Burke (2006) *Strategies for mitigating an influenza pandemic*, Nature **442**: 448–452.

[13] Gani, R., H. Hughes, T. Griffin, J. Medlock, and S. Leach (2005) *Potential impact of antiviral use on hospitalizations during influenza pandemic*, Emerg. Infect. Dis. **11**: 1355–1362.

[14] Gardam, M., D. Liang, S.M. Moghadas, J. Wu, Q. Zeng, and H. Zhu (2007) *The impact of prophylaxis of healthcare workers on influenza pandemic burden*, J. Roy. Soc. Interface **4**: 727–734.

[15] Germann, T.C., K. Kadau, I.M. Longini, and C.A. Macken (2006) *Mitigation strategies for pandemic influenza in the United States*, Proc. Natl. Acad. Sci. USA **103**: 5935–5940.

[16] Lipsitch, M., T. Cohen, M. Murray, and B.R. Levin (2007) *Antiviral resistance and the control of pandemic influenza*, PLoS Med. **4**: e15.

[17] Longini, I.M., M.E. Halloran, A. Nizam, and Y. Yang (2004) *Containing pandemic influenza with antiviral agents*, Am. J. Epidem. **159**: 623–633.

[18] Longini, I.M., A. Nizam, S. Xu, K. Ungchusak, W. Hanshaoworakul, D.A.T. Cummings, and M.E. Halloran (2005) *Containing pandemic influenza at the source*, Science **309**: 1083–1087.

[19] Olinsky, R., A. Huppert, and L. Stone (2008) *Seasonal dynamics and threshold governing recurrent epidemics*, J. Math. Biol. **56**: 827–839.

[20] Public Health Agency of Canada, *Vaccine Development Process*, http://www.phac-aspc.gc.ca/influenza/pandemic-eng.php.

[21] Qiu, Z. and Z. Feng (2010) *Transmission dynamics of an influenza model with vaccination and antiviral treatment*, Bull. Math. Biol. **72**: 1–33.

[22] Regoes, R.R. and S. Bonhoeffer (2006) *Emergence of drug-resistant influenza virus: Population dynamical considerations*, Science **312**: 389–391.

[23] Stillianakis, N.I., A.S. Perelson, and F.G. Hayden (1998) *Emergence of drug resistance during an influenza epidemic: Insights from a mathematical model*, J. Inf. Diseases **177**: 863–873.

[24] Stone, L., R. Olinsky, and A. Huppert (2007) *Seasonal dynamics of recurrent epidemics*, Nature **446**: 533–536.

[25] Van den Driessche, P. and J. Watmough (2002) *Reproduction numbers and subthreshold endemic equilibria for compartmental models of disease transmission*, Math. Biosc. **180**: 29–48.

[26] Welliver, R., A.S. Monto, O. Carewicz, E. Schatteman, M. Hassman, J. Hedrick, H.C. Jackson, L. Huson, P. Ward, and J.S. Oxford (2001) *Effectiveness of Oseltamivir in preventing influenza in household contacts: A randomized controlled trial*, JAMA **285**: 748–754.

Lecture 7

Models for the Dynamics of Influenza

7.1 Influenza Modeling and Cross-Immunity

The global dynamics of influenza at the population level provides an important example of an *epidemiological* complex adaptive systems. The results in this chapter have been published in a series of studies on the transmission dynamics of *influenza A* in human populations for the past two and a half decades [3, 9, 10, 28, 34, 35, 39, 40, 41, 42, 43, 44]. It is difficult (if not impossible) to discuss the dynamics of influenza without at least superficially addressing its evolutionary dynamics. The evolution of influenza type A, the only one specifically considered here, is intimately tied in to the dynamics of recurrent influenza outbreaks including infrequent pandemics. The dynamics of influenza type A involves strains (variants) of three subtypes, A/H1N1, A/H2N2, and A/H3N2. The interest in this complex adaptive system reached new heights after the emergence of a novel strain of A/H1N1 influenza in Mexico on April 13, 2009 (see [49, 57]). The World Health Organization (WHO) declared a pandemic alert (WHO level-5 warning) a couple of weeks after the new virus was identified. Governments and worldwide media provided minute-by-minute accounts of the number of cases, morbidity, age-specific mortality, and interventions (professional soccer games being played in empty stadiums, school closings, surveillance at airports, traveler quarantine or isolation, and more) while identifying possible outcomes, including worst-case scenarios. The lightening speed of spread of A/H1N (in May 16, 2009, Japan reported its first incidence peak [39, 54]), when combined with the unavailability of a vaccine and the lack of facilities capable of producing massive vaccine amounts over a short time scale, put the pandemic at the forefront of health policy challenges worldwide during 2009–2010. The challenges posed by the short- and long-term dynamics of influenza naturally raised questions concerning our inability to determine, for example, what generates strain-variability and severity; the kinds of scenarios that we have faced year after year are a natural outcome of the genetic changes continuously generated by existing influenza A subtypes.

While the generation of new subtypes is (so far) infrequent possibly because it requires dramatic genetic shifts, this has not been the case for novel strains (new subtype-specific variants). Novel strains typically emerge from the accumulation of point mutations within specific regions of the influenza HA molecule. The frequent emergence of new strains and the rare emergence or re-emergence of new subtypes has played a fundamental role in the short-term and long-term global transmission dynamics of influenza A. Perhaps, the most important consequence associated with influenza mutations is tied to its ability, after invasion, to reduce the effectiveness of new strains as a result of the strain-specific gradients of cross-immunity, *the ability of an individual's immune system to use his/her history of prior infections in reducing the likelihood of infection or severity from novel but related strains*, generated in human populations by prior subtype-specific strains. The aggregated dynamic effect of cross-immunity and intervention measures (including social distancing) have played and continue to play a key role in the transmission dynamics of influenza at the population level [3, 9, 10, 12, 34, 35, 38, 40, 41, 42, 43, 44, 58], which is the primary focus of this chapter.

Social dynamics and population structure, factors that determine who interacts with whom, heterogeneity in the levels of susceptibility, and the intensity and duration of interactions that facilitate or limit transmission are but some of the drivers of recurrent influenza outbreaks [3, 9, 10, 12, 28, 38, 58]. The effects of social dynamics and population structure proved to be significant during the 2009 A/H1N1 influenza pandemic. The transmission patterns were *atypical* since an unusually large percentage of young adults experienced severe infections [15, 36, 56]. As a result, some researchers focused on exploring the potential similarities between the 2009 and the 1918 H1N1 influenza pandemics [16], and such comparisons identified cross-immunity as central to such discussions. It was noted that secondary 1918 A/H1N1 waves were responsible for most influenza-related deaths (over 90% according to some reports). Canada's second 2009 A/H1N1 wave was bigger than the spring wave, but the associated outbreaks were on the mild side in terms of disease severity [26], a most welcome outcome. The 2009 pandemic did not reach the levels of morbidity and mortality patterns observed during the 1918–1920 (Spanish influenza), 1957–1959 (Asian influenza), or 1968–1970 (Hong Kong influenza) pandemics. It was a "mild" pandemic, raising questions on the value of the WHO's system of ranking all pandemics as "level five" regardless of their severity. It seems clear that the WHO's future grading system must account for disease severity and not just on its ability to infect. This is an evident recommendation given the mortality levels linked to the 1918 pandemic (approximately forty million individuals [13, 52]), the roughly 69,800 deaths in the U.S. alone associated with the 1957 pandemic, and the relatively low severity of the 2009 pandemic. Marc Lipsitch and colleagues concluded after analyzing New York and Minneapolis 2009 pandemic data that "0.048% of people who developed symptoms of H1N1 died ... [with] 1.44% [requiring] hospitalization." *Seasonal influenza*, for example, is believed to be responsible for about 35,000 deaths each winter in the U.S. [53]. Lipsitch and colleagues, according to *Time*, predicted that the total number of U.S. deaths attributed to H1N1 to be most likely between 10,000 and 15,000, that is, between 30% and 45% of the deaths attributed each year to seasonal influenza in the U.S.

The collection of articles [12] on the challenges posed and lessons learned from the A/H1N1 2009 pandemic provides interesting perspectives primarily by U.S., Canadian, and Mexican researchers. This volume explores the impact of constraints faced by many communities as a result of the inability of nations to respond effectively. Questions raised, some partially addressed in this volume, include: Was the knowledge of past pandemics useful in dealing with this global outbreak? What kinds of state of preparedness limitations emerged during this pandemic? How did the world manage the limited global supply of antiviral drugs and later vaccine stockpiles? What was the impact of mass-transportation systems and human mobility on the spread or control of influenza? What were the lessons learned from international mitigating and response efforts? How should severity be factored in the definition of a pandemic? (see [12]).

The role of measures that alter the transmission patterns of communicable diseases like influenza, including quarantine and population-level immunological responses like strain-specific cross-immunity, are explored in this lecture. Emphasis is placed on discussing the impact of *naturally* reduced susceptibility (the result of recovery from *strain-specific* influenza A prior infections [22, 47, 48, 50, 51]). Further, since there are no quantitatively documented population-level measures of *subtype*-specific cross-immunity (reduced susceptibility to subtype invasion) in the case of influenza A [17, 23], the focus is on the outcomes generated by *within* subtype influenza A *strain* cross-immunity. In other words, we work under the assumption that influenza transmission and severity, within each subtype (H1N1, H2N2, or H2N3), are mediated by cross-immunity. Cross-immunity values are derived from field study data [22, 51] that estimated the levels of protection acquired from prior infections to novel emergent or re-emergent influenza strains *within the same subtype* at the population level. The impact of individuals' acquired cross-immunity on population-level transmission processes is carried out with mathematical models involving nonlinear systems of ordinary or partial differential equations (see [9, 10, 38, 40, 41, 42, 43, 58] and the references therein).

Data from field studies are used to determine simple coefficients of cross-immunity (σ). Data naturally give values $\sigma \in [0,1]$ (see [9, 10, 17, 23]). This coefficient was incorporated, for the first time, as a coupling parameter, in models for the transmission dynamics of multistrain influenza models [9, 10]. The case $\sigma = 1$ corresponds to the situation when no protection is acquired from a prior infection against an incoming new infection, while the case $\sigma = 0$ corresponds to the case of *total cross-immunity*, in which incoming strains are incapable of infecting recovered hosts. Over twenty years ago, the articles [9, 10] showed that cross-immunity mediated competition, a regulator in the "fight" for susceptible and/or partially susceptible individuals to invading *related* influenza strains variants of a given subtype, enhanced the likelihood of population-level multistrain coexistence, and as a result it increased the diversity of population-level dynamics supported (oscillations). The qualitative "discrepancies" observed as σ was varied $\in [0,1]$, not surprisingly, turned out to be intimately tied in to the time required to replenish strain-specific populations of susceptible individuals, the resource for new invasions. The closer σ was to zero, the longer it would take to replenish the critical mass of susceptible individuals needed to support an outbreak [9, 10, 38, 40, 41, 42, 43, 58].

Susceptible-infectious-recovered, or SIR, models [6], that is, nonlinear systems of differential equations where it is assumed that all infected individuals are infectious and where all individuals acquire permanent strain-specific immunity after recovery, have been used to show, under quite general conditions, that when an outbreak is possible, the long-term disease dynamics will approach a unique endemic state, with slowly damped oscillations as the dynamics trademark [9, 20, 28, 29]. The introduction of a quarantine class, called Q, required the modification of SIR transmission terms. It was assumed that the Q-class would alter the rate of secondary infections through its impact, in single-strain epidemic models, on the incidence rate [20, 28, 29]. The inclusion of the Q class supported disease (persistence) and sustained oscillations via a Hopf bifurcation, under some conditions. Models supporting recurrent epidemic outbreaks (periodic solutions) have also emerged as a result of the coupling generated by cross-immunity [9, 10, 28, 29, 38, 40, 41, 42, 43, 58], or by age-dependent variability in survivorship rates [9, 10, 28, 38], or in two-strain models coupled by cross-immunity involving quarantine classes [38, 40, 41, 42, 43, 58]. We will discuss some of these models in this chapter.

In Section 7.2 some of the results in Feng [19] and Feng and Thieme [20] are revisited in order to highlight the impact of the inclusion of quarantine and/or isolation classes in generating sustained periodic solutions ($SIQR$ epidemic models). Section 7.3 reviews a two-strain model where the competitive dynamics between related disease strains are mediated by cross-immunity. Section 7.4 sketches historical results on the role of age structure and cross-immunity on influenza dynamics. Section 7.5 brings the material together in a pedagogical effort to address future research possibilities.

7.2 Basic Model

It was during the Black Death in the 14th century in Venice that a system of quarantine was first put in operation. It demanded ships to lay at anchor for 40 days (in Italian *quaranti giorni*) before sailors and guests could come on land. Quarantine is often thought of as a policy that separates individuals who may have been exposed to a contagious agent regardless of symptoms. Isolation is, generally speaking, considered a severe form of quarantine, often put in place in response to high morbidity and mortality. Quarantine was used extensively in the treatment and control of tuberculosis first in Europe and later, at end of the 19th century, in the U.S. The emergence of SARS in 2003 reinstated the world's interests in the concepts of isolation and quarantine (I & Q), the only initial methods available of disease control [7, 14].

The concepts of I & Q have multiple working meanings and uses. Hence, selecting a definition depends on the disease, the suspected level of risk that it poses to others, the means and modes of transmission, and the system's knowledge and experience with the infectious agent. Regardless of the definition used, one of the challenges associated with I & Q strategies is that there is hardly any reliables assessments of their *population level* efficacy. There are no effective quantitative frameworks that account for direct and indirect economic losses and/or the costs associated with the implementation of I & Q strategies (but see [12, 21, 24, 25, 32, 33, 37, 45]).

Critical to any method of assessment comes from the fact that dynamic models that include the I & Q classes disease must be prepared to account for their sometimes destabilizing impact on the disease dynamics (sustained oscillations). The introduction of I & Q classes can generate the kind of dynamics where assessing the effectiveness of interventions may be difficult. Feng showed [19, 20], for example, that the incorporation of a quarantine or isolation class (Q) was enough to destabilize the unique disease endemic equilibrium in an SIR model. Feng's results were confirmed by Hethcote and collaborators [29] using alternative $SIQR$ modeling frameworks.

Tracing exposed individuals—assuming that a test exists that determines if an individual is infected or not and their contacts would make it possible to quarantine or isolate diagnosed infectives, a first step towards assessing the impact of I & Q [11]. Models are used to address questions such as the following: What impact will placing a fixed proportion of individuals living in the "neighborhood" of an index case in quarantine have on disease control? (We observe that when large numbers are involved, the costs and challenges become immense.) Should isolated individuals be kept at their homes or moved to designated quarantine facilities?

A discussion of the models and results that emerge from the incorporation of quarantine in single-strain models [19, 20, 28] will be carried out after the introduction of a

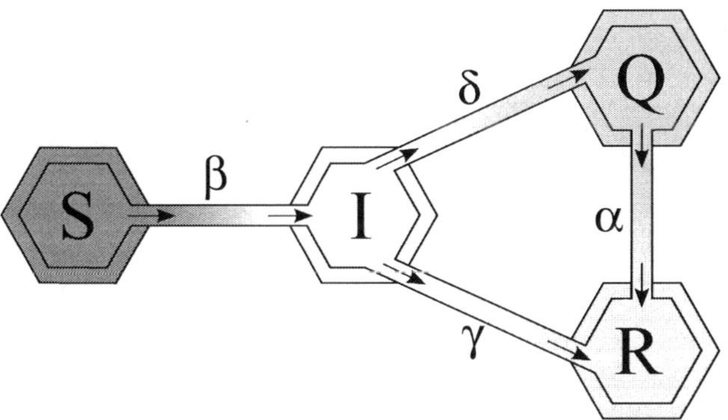

Figure 7.1. *Flow diagram for the classical $SIQR$ model (modified from Figure* 1 *of* [42, p. 5]*).*

simple model capable of capturing the impact of the Q class. Specifically, aversion of the $SIQR$ model in [19, 20] is introduced next. We let $S(t)$, $I(t)$, $Q(t)$, and $R(t)$ denote the susceptible, infective (assumed to be infectious), quarantined, and recovered classes, respectively, all members of a population of size N ($N = S + I + Q + R$). The total birth rate is μN, where μ denotes the natural per-capita death rate, assumed to be the same for all four epidemiological classes. That is, deaths due to disease are assumed to be negligible and at a demographic equilibrium; in other words, it is assumed to be constant. Further, we let γ denote the per-capita recovery rate, δ the per-capita quarantine rate, c the average per-capita contact rate, with $\beta = qc$ ($0 < q < 1$) denoting the effective per-infective transmission rate. From the flow diagram in Figure 7.1, it is easily concluded that an $SIQR$ model can be formulated in terms of the following set of nonlinear ordinary differential equations:

$$\begin{aligned} \frac{dS}{dt} &= \mu N - \beta S \frac{I}{N-Q} - \mu S, \\ \frac{dI}{dt} &= \beta S \frac{I}{N-Q} - (\mu + \gamma) I, \\ \frac{dQ}{dt} &= \gamma I - (\mu + \delta) Q, \end{aligned} \tag{7.1}$$

where $R = N - (S + I + Q)$ and the initial conditions are $S(0) = N - I_0, I(0) = I_0$, and $Q(0) = 0 = R(0)$. What makes the above model "distinct" is that the incidence rate now accounts for the possibility that a large number—those in the class Q—do not participate (by request, mandate, or personal decision) in the transmission process. Hence, the "randomly mixing" infected proportion with susceptible and recovered individuals is $\frac{I}{N-Q}$ rather than $\frac{I}{N}$. Since the total population is constant, we can assume without loss of generality that $N = 1$. We observe that the case $\delta =$ "∞" collapses model (7.1) into the classical SIR epidemic model [6, 27]. Up-to-date references on recent theoretical work on SIR models can be found in the excellent review by Hethcote [28].

The *basic reproductive number,* $\mathcal{R}_0$, a dimensionless quantity (number or ratio), discussed in every lecture in this volume, was introduced by physicians that include Nobel Laureate Sir Ronald Ross and McKendrick (with Kermack). $\mathcal{R}_0$ gives the average number of secondary infections generated by a *typical* infectious individual in a population of noninfected and nonimmune individuals, members of a population at a *demographic* steady state. The theory developed by Ross [46] and Kermack and McKendrick [31] confirms the epidemiological intuitive understanding that a *basic reproductive number* greater than one must be able to generate an epidemic outbreak, while $\mathcal{R}_0 < 1$ would not. The basic reproductive number for the above $SIQR$ model is

$$\mathcal{R}_0 = \frac{\beta}{\mu + \gamma} = \beta \times D,$$

where β is the transmission rate and $D = \frac{1}{\mu+\gamma}$ the death-adjusted infectious period [5]. The classical SIR model (no Q class) can support up to two equilibria [6, 27]: the disease-free state $E_0 = (1,0)$, and when $\mathcal{R}_0 > 1$, the unique endemic state, $E_1 = (\frac{1}{\mathcal{R}_0}, \frac{\mu}{\beta}(\mathcal{R}_0 - 1))$. It is known that E_0 is globally asymptotically stable whenever $\mathcal{R}_0 \leq 1$ and that E_1 is globally asymptotically stable whenever it exists, that is, when $\mathcal{R}_0 > 1$ (see [28]).

Model (7.1) supports at most two equilibria: the disease-free state $\mathcal{F}_0 = (1,0,0)$ and, whenever $\mathcal{R}_0 > 1$, the unique endemic state $\mathcal{F}_1 = (\frac{1}{\mathcal{R}_0}, \frac{\mu}{\beta}[\mathcal{R}_0 - 1], \frac{\delta}{\mu+\gamma}\frac{\mu}{\beta}[\mathcal{R}_0 - 1])$, where $\mathcal{R}_0 = \frac{\beta}{\mu+\gamma+\delta} = \beta D_Q$, with β is the transmission rate and D_Q the quarantine-death-adjusted infectious period. $\mathcal{F}_1$ is "globally asymptotically" stable when the quarantine period $(\frac{1}{\delta})$ is either very large or very small. It turns out that for intermediate values of the quarantine period, the endemic state becomes unstable. In fact, the existence of periodic solutions can be established via Hopf bifurcation. Reasonable value ranges for the quarantine period $(\frac{1}{\delta})$ capable of generating sustained oscillations were not found in this setting [19, 20]. The framework modifications discussed later manage to reduce the $\frac{1}{\delta}$ window, bringing it into a realistic region. In [19, 20] the following result on the possibility of periodic solutions via Hopf bifurcation was established:

Theorem 7.1. *If we let θ denote the rescaled per-capita recovery period, then there is a function, $\zeta_0(\nu)$, defined for small $\nu > 0$,*

$$\zeta_0(\nu) = \theta^2(1-\theta) + O(\nu^{1/2}),$$

with the following properties: (a) *The endemic equilibrium is locally asymptotically stable if $\zeta > \zeta_0(\nu)$ and unstable if $\zeta < \zeta_0(\nu)$, as long as ζ does not become too small.* (b) *There is a Hopf bifurcation of periodic solutions at $\zeta = \zeta_0(\nu)$ for small enough $\nu > 0$. Further, the length of periods can be approximated by the formula*

$$T = \frac{2\pi}{|\Im \omega_{\pm}|} \approx \frac{2\pi}{(1-\theta)^{1/2}\nu^{1/2}} \approx \frac{2\pi}{(\theta y^*)^{1/2}},$$

where y^* is the proportion of infectious individuals at equilibrium.

In fact, Hopf bifurcations turned out to be possible in two *separate* regions, not identified in the above theorem, specified by the average length of the quarantine period. Figure 7.2 shows bifurcations occurring for values of the average quarantine periods in two distinct ranges with only the region that includes "low" values relevant for most infectious diseases. Feng et al. [19, 20] observed that the data on the length of reported isolation periods during the 1897–1978 scarlet fever epidemics in England and Wales [2] were almost in the range of those supporting periodic solutions for model (7.1). Interesting dynamics

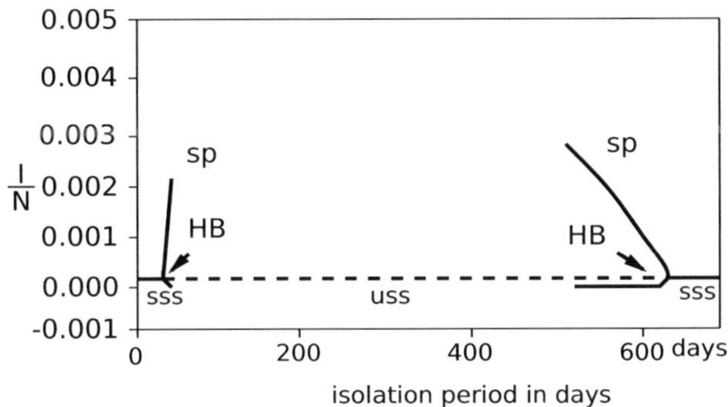

Figure 7.2. *Auto plot of the steady state solutions (fraction of infectives $\frac{I}{N}$) versus the isolation period (modified from Figure 2 of* [42]*).*

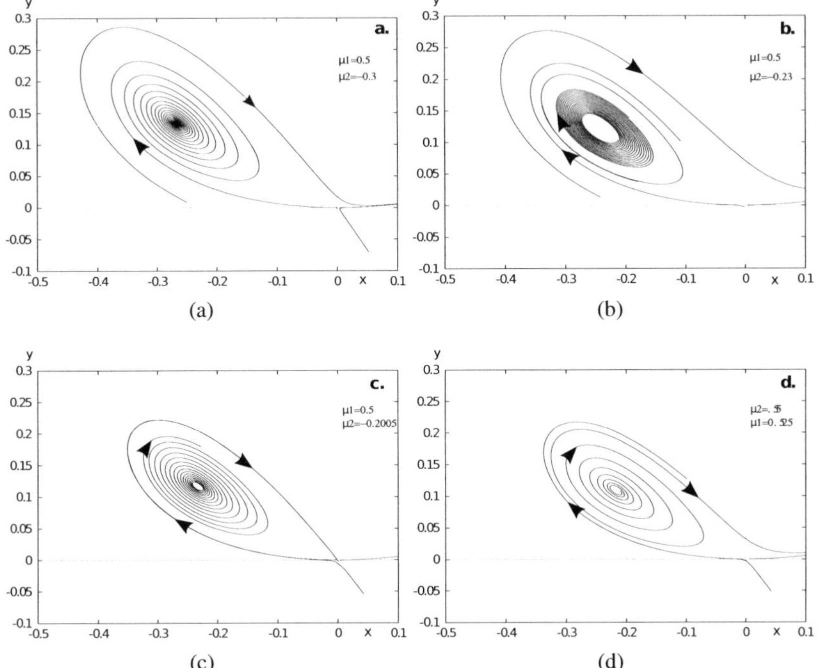

Figure 7.3. *As μ_2 (rescaled life expectation parameter) increases, the interior equilibrium changes from stable to unstable (see* (b) *and* (c)*), and Hopf bifurcation (see* (a) *and* (b)*) and homoclinic bifurcation (see* (b) *and* (c)*) may occur (modified from Figure 3 of* [42, p. 9]*).*

were also identified as quite possible. Wu and Feng [59] showed that using a perturbed system (tied in to the above model) could support a homoclinic bifurcation (see Figure 7.3).

The relevance of the work in [19, 20] arises from the fact that, under moderate periods of quarantine, an endemic state could destabilize. In a multistrain influenza model with cross-immunity, it has been shown using numerical simulations that oscillations are indeed possible under mainstream flu parameters.

7.3 Cross-Immunity and Quarantine

Initial cross-immunity studies, as reported in the literature [17, 52], gave no option but to imagine models of the immune system not only at the individual level but also at the superorganism level. These studies allowed us to consider the average immune system population-level response to influenza invasions. The historical immunological precedent (the signature) left by prior influenza outbreaks on a population *sometimes* plays a fundamental role on individuals' response to virus "invasions" since they may modify the susceptibility profile of recovered individuals by limiting the severity of subsequent new infections or by reducing the probability of success of an individual virus influenza-strain invasion. The geographical path, infectiousness, transmissibility, and time of arrival of novel strains of influenza that sweep a nation or region over a few months are quite often modified by the history of prior sweeps. Hence, the impact of a new invasion depends on initial conditions, e.g., time of the year, population density, and the immunological history of past influenza infections on local populations. The so-called epidemic waves (not the same as the traveling wave solutions that are characteristic of reaction-diffusion systems) tend to leave heterogeneous pockets of susceptible individuals, nonuniform patterns of spread, that may alter the invasion routes of the future. In other words, the distribution of cross-immunity within a population defines the regional, and possibly global, population immune responses to invasions by novel but related (to existing) influenza strains. If the relation is minimal, then whatever the population immune system learned against influenza A will be useless. On the other hand if the new strain is recognized as a minor variant of one that hit over the past couple of seasons, then we would expect the kind of outcome that results from weak invasive strains.

Cross-immunity studies [17, 22, 23, 47, 51, 52] have helped generate a crude measure of the risk that a population may expect from the invasion of related (within the same subtype) incoming strains. A novel strain may replace local strains (competitive exclusion) or it may manage to coexist with present strains [9, 10]. Simple $SIQR$ models have proved capable of supporting recurrent epidemic single-strain outbreaks, but the fact remains that recurrent behavior was shown to be possible for unrealistic parameters.

Earlier influenza mathematical research [9, 10] provided theoretical support to the view that either competition for hosts by *related* pathogens or *age structure* may be enough to support periodic epidemic outbreaks in regions of parameter space that are relevant to the flu. Recently, Nuño et al. [40, 41] extended the work in [9, 10, 18] through the inclusion quarantine class to SIR two-strain models showing that such modifications lead to oscillatory coexistence.

The system in [40, 41], which includes those in [9, 10, 18], divides the host population into 10 epidemiological classes. Susceptible (S) individuals who, if infected by strain i (at a rate β_i), move to the class I_i of infected and infectious individuals; I_i individuals are either isolated, moved into the class Q_i at the rate δ_i, or moved into the recovered (from strain i) class R_i at the rate γ_i; R_i individuals who become infected with strain j do so at the rate $\beta_j\sigma_{ij}$ (a rate reduced by cross-immunity $\sigma_{ij} \in [0,1]$) and are moved to the class V_j. Finally, individuals who have recovered from both strains are moved into the W class at the rates γ_l, $l = 1$ or 2. The model assumes that once an individual is infected

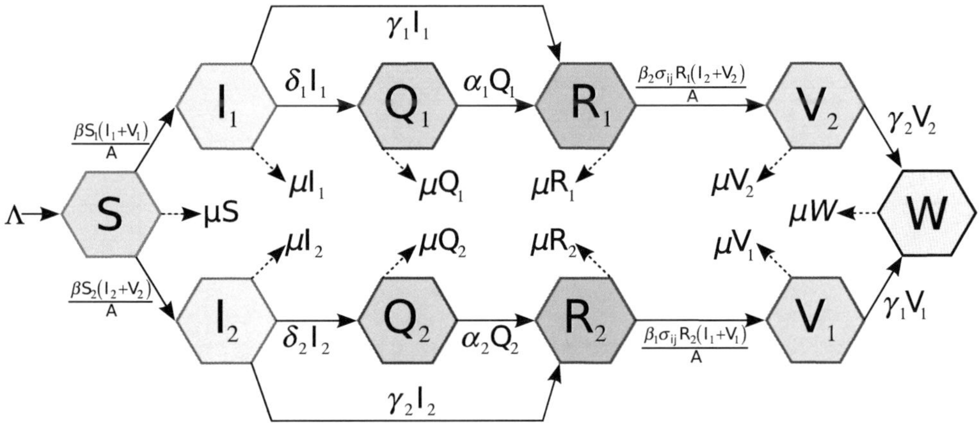

Figure 7.4. *Schematic diagram for the two-strain model with quarantine and cross-immunity (modified from Figure* 1 *of* [42, p. 10]*).*

with a particular strain, no future infections with the same strain are possible ($\sigma_{ii} \equiv 0$); no individuals can carry two infections simultaneously or "equivalently" that the number of coinfections is so small that it can be neglected; and only I_i (infected) individuals are isolated or quarantined. This last assumption is partially justified from reported studies that show that cross-immunity often reduces flu symptoms [22, 23]. The stated assumptions can be weakened, but such a decision would result in less tractable models generating (we suspect) the same qualitative results also in the regions of parameter space relevant to the flu.

The system of equations modeling the competition of two strains mediated by competition (see Figure 7.4) is given by

$$
\begin{aligned}
\frac{dS}{dt} &= \Lambda - \frac{\beta_1 S(I_1+V_1)}{A} - \frac{\beta_2 S(I_2+V_2)}{A} - \mu S, \\
\frac{dI_i}{dt} &= \beta_i S\frac{(I_i+V_i)}{A} - (\mu+\gamma_i+\delta_i)I_i, \\
\frac{dQ_i}{dt} &= \delta_i I_i - (\mu+\alpha_i)Q_i, \\
\frac{dR_i}{dt} &= \gamma_i I_i + \alpha_i Q_i - \beta_j\sigma_{ij}R_i\frac{(I_j+V_j)}{A} - \mu R_i, \qquad j \neq i \\
\frac{dV_i}{dt} &= \beta_i\sigma_{ij}R_j\frac{(I_i+V_i)}{A} - (\mu+\gamma_i)V_i, \qquad j\neq i \\
\frac{dW}{dt} &= \gamma_1 V_1 + \gamma_2 V_2 - \mu W, \\
A &= S+W+I_1+I_2+V_1+V_2+R_1+R_1 \text{ or } A = 1-Q,
\end{aligned}
\tag{7.2}
$$

where A denotes the population of nonisolated individuals.

In the study of system (7.2), it was shown that influenza may survive in three possible states or become extinct. Extinction corresponds to the case when $\mathcal{R}_i < 1, i = 1$ and 2, where

$\mathcal{R}_i$ denotes the ith strain-specific basic reproductive number; that is, no strain becomes established [40, 41]. The strain with the highest ability to invade (largest $\mathcal{R}_i$ greater than one) persists and eliminates competitors under appropriate conditions and boundary; one-strain endemic equilibria can become destabilized, giving rise to periodic solutions [40, 41]. The analysis is somewhat similar to the one carried out in [9, 10]. It uses the significant differences in epidemiological and demographic time scales, common to "fast" communicable diseases like influenza. Specifically, the difference in the life span of the host (decades) and the lifetime of an individual influenza infection (days) is used through the introduction of a small parameter that makes the analysis possible. The possibility of periodic solutions via a Hopf bifurcation was established using time scale arguments, and formulae for the approximate periods of oscillatory solutions were also computed. Numerical simulations showed that the oscillations' period was not too sensitive to the length of the isolation period and that the amplitude of the outbreaks increased as $\frac{1}{\delta}$ grew. Fixing the quarantine period and varying the levels of cross-immunity generated periodic patterns that became irregular as the coefficient of cross-immunity $\sigma \to 0^+$. Although the analyses were carried out only for the case of symmetric cross-immunity ($\sigma_{ij} = \sigma_{ji} = \sigma$), asymmetric cases were also investigated numerically when $|\sigma_{ij} - \sigma_{ji}| \approx$ small. Simulations showed that outbreaks could occur every 10–13 years with alternating strain-specific peaks (highs and lows) for both strains observed (Figure 7.5).

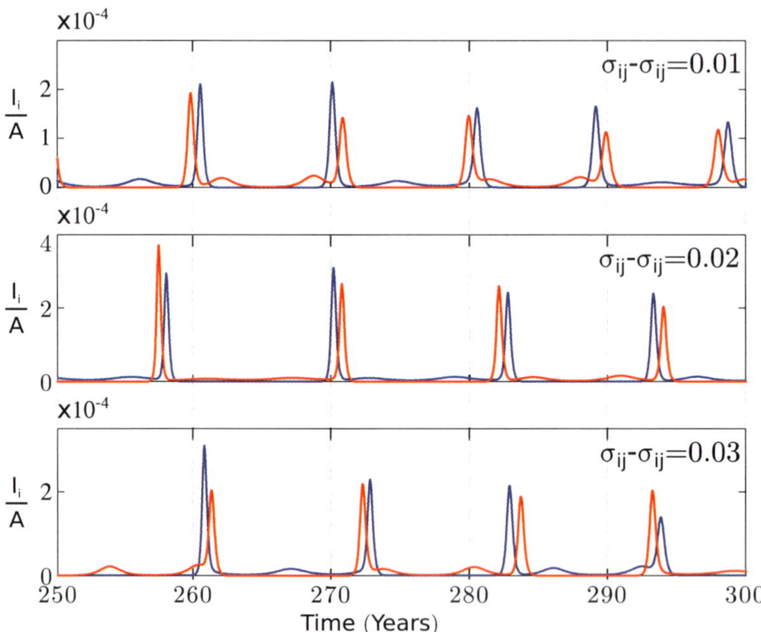

Figure 7.5. *Numerical integration of system* (7.2). *The infective fractions of individuals (nonisolated) with strain* 1 *(solid red line) and strain* 2 *(solid blue line) are shown. Differences in cross-immunity between strains* 1 *and* 2 *(*$|\sigma_{12} - \sigma_{21}|$*) are increased (from top to bottom), starting at* 0.01*, then* 0.02*, and finally* 0.03*. Cross-immunity for strains* 1 *and* 2 *are set by* $\sigma_{12} = 0.36$ *and* $\sigma_{21} = 0.33$ *(bottom panel). Taken from* [42].

Alternating peaks arise as a result of the competition for adaptive pools of susceptibles, their likelihood of becoming infected, mediated by their own history of cross-immunity relative to the invading strain. Increases and decreases in susceptible strain-specific pools are intimately tied to differences in levels of cross-immunity and the timing of the initial invasion.

The stability results were used to investigate the possibility that established strains, boundary equilibria, could be displaced by nonresident strains [40, 41]. The reproductive number $\mathcal{R}_i^j$ describing the number of secondary infections generated by strain i in a population living under a resident strain j at an endemic level. Strain i will invade (not necessarily replace) resident strain j as long as $\mathcal{R}_i^j > 1$. We observe that $\mathcal{R}_i^j$ is an increasing function of σ, a result that follows directly from expression (7.3) below:

$$\mathcal{R}_i^j = \frac{\beta_i}{\mu+\gamma_i+\delta_i}\frac{\tilde{S}_j}{\tilde{A}} + \frac{\beta_i\sigma}{\mu+\gamma_i}\frac{\tilde{R}_j}{\tilde{A}}, \tag{7.3}$$

where $\mathcal{R}_i^j$ ($i,j = 1,2$ and $i \neq j$) and $\beta_i/(\mu+\gamma_i+\delta_i)$ gives the number of secondary cases that strain-i infected individuals generate in the susceptible population $\tilde{S}_j/\tilde{A}$ (infection prior to cross-immunity). The expression $\beta_i\sigma/(\mu+\gamma_i)$ defines the number of secondary cases that a strain-i infected individual is capable of generating in the "cross-immune" susceptible fraction $\tilde{R}_i/\tilde{A}$.

We see, from (7.3), that strong cross-immunity ($\sigma \downarrow 0$) reduces the likelihood that strain i would successfully invade a population where strain j is endemic. Conversely, the likelihood of strain coexistence becomes enhanced when cross-immunity is weak ($\sigma \uparrow 1$), a result that also follows from (7.3). We conclude that the dependence of $\mathcal{R}_i^j > 1$ on cross-immunity (σ) enhances the ability of strain i to invade the resident strain j.

Numerical simulations illustrate oscillatory coexistence under reasonable quarantine periods (in the context of influenza). We observe that increasing the length of the quarantine period enhances the disease-outbreak amplitude. On the other hand, increasing cross-immunity ($\sigma \to 0^+$) while keeping the quarantine period fixed increases the distance between epidemic peaks.

In short, the dynamics of the *two-strain model* under reasonable quarantine periods support disease patterns (under parameter values acceptable for influenza) that matched reported trends. Cross-immunity facilitates strain coexistence and, consequently, strain diversity by enhancing the survival of less fit strains—a function of the ineffectiveness of a resident strain to "prevent" new infections by related strains. Cross-immunity facilitates "group" selection by enhancing the survival probability of related, possibly weaker, strains that may not have survived on their own.

7.4 Epidemic SIR Models with Age Structure and Cross-Immunity

The age structure of a population introduces the kind of heterogeneity that is considered central to the dynamics of childhood diseases like measles, rubella, and others [1]. SIR (susceptible-infected-recovered) models with age structure have been analyzed extensively [28], although only a few studies have been carried out in the context of influenza.

The complications arise from the fact that influenza changes, and, consequently, the role of age structure must be studied in the context of cross-immunity [9, 10].

The classical SIR single-strain age-structured model has been modified to include a quarantine (q) density class. In order to describe such a model, the four densities $s(a,t)$, $i(a,t)$, $q(a,t)$, and $r(a,t)$, where $\int_{a_1}^{a_2} l(a,t)da$ denotes the number of l-individuals ($l = s$, i,q, or r) with ages in $[a_1,a_2]$ at time t, must be considered.

The transition rates must now be assumed to be age-dependent. Consequently, $\mu(a)$, $\gamma(a)$, and $\delta(a)$ denote the age-specific mortality, recovery, and quarantine rates, respectively. Nonlinear effects come from the way we model the incidence rate, i.e., new cases of infection per unit time. Modeling the incidence rate requires the incorporation of age-specific interactions (or contacts) among individuals of different ages. The earlier work in "mixing" [4, 8] introduced a framework that allows for the construction of age-specific incidence rates. We let $p(a,a',t)$ denote the proportion of contacts of age-a individuals with individuals of age a' at time t under the assumption that these individuals had contact with somebody (susceptible, infected, quarantined, or recovered individuals). Letting $n(a,t) = s(a,t)+i(a,t)+q(a,t)+r(a,t)$ and $C(a)$ denote the age-structure per-capita contact rate, we observe that $p(a,a',t)$ must satisfy the following "mixing" axioms:

(i) $p(a,a',t) \geq 0$.
(ii) $\int_0^\infty p(a,a',t)da' = 1$.
(iii) $C(a)n(a,t)p(a,a',t) = C(a')n(a',t)p(a',a,t)$.

It was shown in [8] that the only separable solution, that is, a solution of the form $p(a,a',t) = g(a,t)f(a',t)$, is given by mixing the function commonly referred to as proportionate mixing or $\bar{p}(a')$, where

$$\bar{p}(a',t) = \frac{C(a')n(a',t)}{\int_0^\infty C(l)n(l,t)dl}.$$

Proportionate mixing has been used as the "prototype" for modeling age-dependent contact rates in the study of the transmission dynamics of communicable diseases [1, 28], and, consequently, here we consider only proportionate mixing, that is, we let $p(a,a',t) \equiv \bar{p}(a',t)$ in the remainder of this lecture.

Finally, we let $m(a)$ denotes the age-specific susceptibility to infection per contact and conclude that the incidence rate under proportionate mixing is given by

$$B(a,t) = \beta(a)s(a,t)\int_0^\infty \bar{p}(a',t)\frac{i(a',t)}{n(a',t)-q(a',t)}da',$$

where $\beta(a) = m(a)C(a)$. The remaining equations for our $SIQR$ model are

$$\begin{aligned}
\left(\frac{\partial}{\partial a}+\frac{\partial}{\partial t}\right)s(a,t) &= -B(a,t)-\mu(a)s(a,t),\\
\left(\frac{\partial}{\partial a}+\frac{\partial}{\partial t}\right)i(a,t) &= B(a,t)-[\mu(a)+\gamma(a)+\delta(a)]i(a,t),\\
\left(\frac{\partial}{\partial a}+\frac{\partial}{\partial t}\right)q(a,t) &= \delta(a)i(a,t)-[\mu(a)+\gamma(a)]q(a,t),\\
\left(\frac{\partial}{\partial a}+\frac{\partial}{\partial t}\right)r(a,t) &= \gamma(a)[q(a,t)+i(a,t)]-\mu(a)r(a,t),
\end{aligned} \tag{7.4}$$

where

$$
\begin{aligned}
s(a,0) &= n_0(a) - i_0(a),\\
i(a,0) &= i_0(a),\\
q(a,0) &= q_0(a),\\
s(0,t) &= n(0,t) = \int_0^\infty \lambda(a)n(a,t)\,d\bar{a},\\
i(0,t) &= q(0,t) = r(0,t) = 0.
\end{aligned}
$$

It follows that $n(a,t)$ satisfies the Kermack and McKendrick [6, 31] initial boundary problem, that is, the linear initial boundary value problem system given by

$$
\begin{aligned}
\left(\frac{\partial}{\partial a} + \frac{\partial}{\partial t}\right) n(a,t) &= -\mu(a)n(a,t),\\
n(0,t) &= \int_0^\infty \lambda(a)n(a,t)\,da,\\
n(a,0) &= n_0(a),
\end{aligned}
$$

where $\lambda(a)$ is the age-specific fertility rate.

Any solution $n(a,t)$ of the Kermack and McKendrick model approaches (uniformly) as $t \to \infty$ a separable solution $n^*(a)e^{p^*t}$, where p^* is the unique real root of Lotka's characteristic equation [30]. Further, if $z = u + iv$ is a complex root of Lotka's characteristic equation, then $p^* > u$ [30]. Here, it is assumed that $p^* = 0$ with $n_0(a) = n^*(a)$, the so-called stable age distribution [6, 30]. Ignoring the quarantine class (that is, setting $\delta(a) =$ "∞" for all a), then using the results on asymptotically autonomous systems [55], the study of (7.4) is reduced to the following equivalent system:

$$
\begin{aligned}
\left(\frac{\partial}{\partial a} + \frac{\partial}{\partial t}\right) s(a,t) &= -\hat{B}(a,t) - \mu(a)s(a,t),\\
\left(\frac{\partial}{\partial a} + \frac{\partial}{\partial t}\right) i(a,t) &= \hat{B}(a,t) - [\mu(a) + \gamma(a)]i(a,t),
\end{aligned}
\tag{7.5}
$$

and

$$
r(a,t) = n^*(a) - s(a,t) - i(a,t),
$$

with

$$
\begin{aligned}
\hat{B}(a,t) &= \beta(a)s(a,t)\int_0^\infty \bar{p}(a')\frac{i(a',t)}{p^*(a')}\,da',\\
s(a,0) &= n_0^*(a) - i_0(a),\\
i(a,0) &= i_0(a),
\end{aligned}
$$

and $n(0,t) =$ constant.

The Castillo-Chavez et al. [9, 10] version of the above model with

$$
B(a,t) = \hat{\beta}(a)s(a,t)\int_0^\infty c(a')i(a',t)\,da'
$$

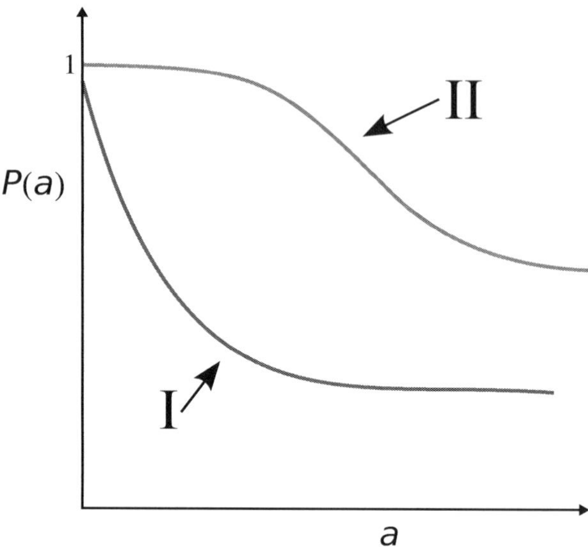

Figure 7.6. *Here $P(a)$ denotes the survivorship function as a function of age. I corresponds to the case when $P(a)$ is a negative exponential, while II models the type of survivorship that one could expect in populations with long life expectancy. The work in* [9, 10] *supports the hypothesis that as curve I is continuously deformed into curve II, the appearance of periodic solutions takes place. Taken from* [42].

was used, with the help of its analysis and simulations, to put forward two hypotheses:

(H1) Single-strain models with age-specific activity levels and constant levels of mortality (exponentially distributed survivorship) are incapable of supporting sustained oscillations.

(H2) In models with uniform activity levels, $C(a) \equiv$ constant, and age-dependent (nonexponentially distributed survivorship) mortality rates, the existence of periodic solutions is possible (see Figure 7.6).

Extensions of single-strain to two-strain models can be found in [9, 10], where strain competition is mediated by cross-immunity. The analysis and simulations of these two-strain models supported the possibility of sustained oscillations [9, 10]. Simulations using related (discrete in time and age) two-strain age-structured models supported the possibility of periodic solutions under reasonable cross-immunity values [9, 10]. Recurrent outbreaks with between-epidemic peaks in the 3–5 year range were generated under intermediate levels of cross-immunity, while outbreaks with between-epidemic peaks in the 10–20 year range could only be generated using strong levels of cross-immunity ($\sigma \downarrow 0$). The results of the simulations presented in [9, 10] seem to be in agreement with the patterns supported by the data [17, 52]. In these numerical studies a significant difference in the amplitudes was observed. These simulations seem to capture, for intermediate values of cross-immunity, high strain-specific flu peaks followed by very low disease levels, which fits (in a rather crude way) the results reported in [52]. The extremely long periods (10–20 years) supported by values of cross-immunity close to zero support the logical view that the "same" strain cannot reappear too soon, in crude agreement with the observations made in [17].

7.5 Discussion and Future Work

This chapter provides a limited perspective on the role of quarantine, age-structured, and cross-immunity on influenza dynamics. The difference associated with the role that quarantine, age structure, and cross-immunity plays on disease dynamics has been studied for some time [9, 10, 18, 19, 20, 29]. $SIQR$ nonstructured and SIR age-structured models have been shown to be capable of supporting recurrent outbreaks. It seems that cross-immunity on its own is not enough to support sustained oscillations in nonstructured populations [9, 10]. On the other hand, strain competition mediated by cross-immunity can support recurrent epidemics in the presence of quarantine (which is not surprising), but in a way that it is consistent with reasonable quarantine periods, which may not be possible in the context of single-strain models [19, 20].

Models that include a quarantine class and age structure within single- and multiple-strain systems (mediated by cross-immunity) can be found in [38, 58]. The analysis of such models exploits differences in times scales to gauge the role of the joint effects of age structure in models that include strongly or poorly isolated (quarantine) classes.

The study of multistrain systems has been the focus of intense research, more so after the 2009 A/H1N1 pandemic. Excellent places to start can be found in the studies [3, 9, 10, 28, 34, 35, 38, 39, 40, 41, 42, 43, 44, 58] and in the references therein.

Bibliography

[1] Anderson, R. and May, R. (1991) *Infectious Diseases of Humans: Dynamics and Control*, Oxford University Press, Oxford.

[2] Anderson, G.W., R.N. Arnstein, and M.R. Lester (1962) *Communicable Disease Control*, Macmillan, New York.

[3] Andreasen, V., J. Lin, and S.A. Levin (1997) *The dynamics of co-circulating influenza strains conferring partial cross-immunity*, J. Math. Biol. **35**: 825–842.

[4] Blythe, S.P. and C. Castillo-Chavez (1989) *Like with like preference and sexual mixing models*, Math. Biosc. **96**: 221–238.

[5] Brauer, F. and C. Castillo-Chavez (2001) *Mathematical Models in Populations Biology and Epidemiology*, Springer-Verlag, New York.

[6] Brauer, F. and C. Castillo-Chavez (2012) *Mathematical Models in Population Biology and Epidemiology*, 2nd ed., Texts in Applied Mathematics **40**. Springer-Verlag, New York.

[7] Brown, D. (2003) *A model of epidemic control*, The Washington Post, May 3: A 07.

[8] Busenberg, S.N. and C. Castillo-Chavez (1991) *A general solution of the problem of mixing of subpopulations and its application to risk and age-structure models for the spread of AIDS*, IMA J. Math. Appl. Med. Biol. **8**: 1–29.

[9] Castillo-Chavez, C., H.W. Hethcote, V. Andreasen, S.A. Levin, and W.M. Liu (1988) *Cross-immunity in the dynamics of homogeneous and heterogeneous populations*, in Mathematical Ecology, World Sci. Publishing: 303–316.

[10] Castillo-Chavez, C., H.W. Hethcote, V. Andreasen, S.A. Levin, and W.M. Liu (1989) *Epidemiological models with age structure, proportionate mixing, and cross-immunity*, J. Math. Biol. **27**: 233–258.

[11] Castillo-Chavez, C., C. Castillo-Garsow, and A.A. Yakubu (2003) *Mathematical models of isolation and quarantine,* JAMA **290**: 2876–2877.

[12] Castillo-Chavez, C. and G. Chowell (2011) Special Issue: *Mathematical models, challenges, and lessons learned from the* 2009 *A/H1N1 influenza pandemic*, Math. Biosc. Eng. **8**(1).

[13] CDC (Centers for Disease Control), *Recent Avian Influenza Outbreaks in Asia*, http://www.cdc.gov/flu/avian/outbreaks/asia.htm (April 26, 2005).

[14] Chowell, G., P.W. Fenimore, M.A. Castillo-Garsow, and C. Castillo-Chavez (2003) *SARS outbreaks in Ontario, Hong Kong and Singapore: The role of diagnosis and isolation as a control mechanism*, J. Theor. Biol. **24**: 1–8.

[15] Chowell G., S.M. Bertozzi, M.A. Colchero, H. Lopez-Gatell, C. Alpuche-Aranda, M. Hernandez, and M.A. Miller (2009) *Severe respiratory disease concurrent with the circulation of H1N1 influenza*, New England J. Medicine **361**: 674–679.

[16] Cohen, J. (2010) *Swine Flu Pandemic Reincarnates* 1918 *Virus,* 24 *March* 2010, http://news.sciencemag.org/sciencenow/2010/03/swine-flu-pandemic-reincarnates-.html?rss=1.

[17] Couch, R.B. and J.A. Kasel (1983) *Immunity to influenza in man*, Ann. Rev. Micro. **31**: 529–549.

[18] Dietz, K. (1979) *Epidemiological interference of virus populations*, J. Math. Biol. **8**: 291–300.

[19] Feng, Z. (1994) *Multi-annual Outbreaks of Childhood Diseases Revisited: The Impact of Isolation*, Ph.D. Thesis, Arizona State University.

[20] Feng, Z. and H. R. Thieme (1995) *Recurrent outbreaks of childhood diseases revisited: The impact of isolation*, J. Math. Biosc. **128**: 93–130.

[21] Fenichel, E.P., C. Castillo-Chavez, M.G. Ceddia, G. Chowell, P.A. Gonzalez Parra, G.J. Hickling, G. Holloway, R. Horan, B. Morin, C. Perrings, M. Springborn, L. Velazquez, and C. Villalobos (2011) *Adaptive human behavior in epidemiological models*, Proc. Natl. Acad. Sci. USA **108**: 6306–6311.

[22] Fox, J.P., C.E. Hall, M.K. Cooney, and H.M. Foy (1982) *Influenza virus infections in Seattle families*, 1975–1979, Amer. J. Epidemiology **116**: 212–227.

[23] Glezen, W.P. and R.B. Couch (1978) *Interpandemic influenza in the Houston area,* 1974–76, New England J. Medicine **298**: 587–592.

[24] Gonzalez-Parra, P., S. Lee, C. Castillo-Chavez, and L. Velazquez (2011) *A note on the use of optimal control on a discrete time model of influenza dynamics*, Math. Biosc. & Eng. **8**: 193–205.

[25] Gonzalez-Parra, P.A., L. Velazquez, M.C. Villalobos, and C. Castillo-Chavez (2010) *Optimal control applied to a discrete influenza model*, in Proceedings of the 36th International Operation Research Applied to Health Services, F. Angeli, ed.

[26] Helferty, M., J. Vachon, J. Tarasuk, R. Rodin, J. Spika, and L. Pelletier (2010) *Incidence of hospital admissions and severe outcomes during the first and second waves of pandemic (H1N1)* 2009, Canadian Medical Association Journal **182**: 1981–1987.

[27] Hethcote, H.W. (1976) *Qualitative analyses of communicable disease models*, Math. Biosc. **28**: 335–356.

[28] Hethcote, H.W. (2000) *The mathematics of infectious diseases*, SIAM Rev. **42**: 599–653.

[29] Hethcote, H.W., M. Zhien, and L. Shengbing (2002) *Effects of quarantine in six endemic models for infectious diseases*, Math. Biosc. **180**: 141–160.

[30] Hoppensteadt, F. (1974) *An age dependent epidemic model*, J. Franklin Inst. **297**: 325–333.

[31] Kermack, W.O. and A.G. McKendrick (1927) *Contributions to the mathematical theory of epidemics, part I*, Proc. Roy. Soc. Edinb. Sect. A. **115**: 700–721.

[32] Lee, S., R. Morales, and C. Castillo-Chavez (2011) *A note on the use of influenza vaccination strategies when supply is limited*, Math. Biosc. & Eng. **8**: 179–191.

[33] Lee, S., G. Chowell, and C. Castillo-Chavez (2010) *Optimal control of influenza pandemics: The role of antiviral treatment and isolation*, J. Theor. Biol. **265**: 136–150.

[34] Levin, S.A., J. Dushoff, and J.B. Plotkin (2004) *Evolution and persistence of influenza A and other diseases*, Math. Biosc. & Eng. **188**: 17–28.

[35] Lin, J., V. Andreasen, R. Casagrandi, and S.A. Levin (2003) *Traveling waves in a model of influenza a drift,* J. Theor. Biol. **222**: 437–445.

[36] Miller, M. A., C. Viboud, M. Balinska, and L. Simonsen (2009), *The signature features of influenza pandemics–implications for policy*, New England J. Medicine **360**: 2595–2598.

[37] Mubayi, A., C. Kribs-Zaleta, M. Martcheva, and C. Castillo-Chavez (2010) *A cost-based comparison of quarantine strategies for new emerging diseases*, J. Math. Biosc. Eng. **7**: 687–717.

[38] Mustafa, E. (2007) *Epidemic in Structured Populations with Isolation and Cross-immunity*, Ph.D. Thesis, Arizona State University.

[39] Nishiura, H., C. Castillo-Chavez, M. Safan, and G. Chowell (2009) *Transmission potential of the new influenza A(H1N1) virus and its age-specificity in Japan,* Eurosurveill. **14**: 19227.

[40] Nuño, M. (2005) *A Mathematical Model for the Dynamics of Influenza at the Population and Host Level*, Ph.D. Thesis, Cornell University.

[41] Nuño, M., Z. Feng, M. Martcheva, and C. Castillo-Chavez (2005) *Dynamics of two-strain influenza with isolation and partial cross-immunity*, SIAM J. Appl. Math. **65**: 964–982.

[42] Nuño, M., C. Castillo-Chavez, Z. Feng, and M. Martcheva (2008) *Mathematical model of influenza: The role of cross-immunity, quarantine and age-structure*, in Mathematical Epidemiology, P. van den Driessche, J. Wu, and F. Brauer, eds., Springer-Verlag, Berlin: 349–364.

[43] Nuño, M., M. Martcheva, and C. Castillo-Chavez (2009) *Immune level structure model for influenza strains*, J. Biol. Systems **17**(4): 713–737.

[44] Plotkin, J.B., J. Dushoff, and S.A. Levin (2002) *Hemagglutinin sequence clusters and the antigenic evolution of influenza A virus*, Proc. Natl. Acad. Sci. USA **99**: 6263–6268.

[45] Prosper, O., O. Saucedo, D. Thompson, G. Torres-Garcia, X. Wang, and C. Castillo-Chavez (2011) *Control strategies for concurrent epidemics of seasonal and H1N1 influenza*, Math. Biosc. & Eng. **8**: 147–177.

[46] Ross, R. (1911) *The Prevention of Malaria*, 2nd ed. (with Addendum), John Murray, London.

[47] Sigel, M.M., A.W. Kitts, A.B. Light, and W. Henle (1950) *The recurrence of influenza A-prime in a boarding school after two years*, J. Immunol. **64**: 33–38.

[48] Smith, A.J. and J.R. Davies (1976) *Natural infection with influenza A (H3N2). The development, persistence and effect of antibodies to the surface antigens*, J. Hyg. **77**: 271–282.

[49] Smith, G.J., D. Vijaykrishna, J. Bahl, S.J. Lycett, M. Worobey, O.G. Pybus, S.K. Ma, C.L. Cheung, J. Raghwani, S. Bhatt, J.S. Peiris, Y. Guan, and A. Rambaut (2009) *Origins and evolutionary genomics of the* 2009 *swine-origin H1N1 influenza A epidemic,* Nature **459**: 1122–1125.

[50] Stuart-Harris, C.H. (1979) *Epidemiology of influenza in man*, Br. Med. Bull. **35**: 3–8.

[51] Taber, L.H., A. Paredes, W.P. Glezen, and R.B. Couch (1981) *Infection with influenza A/Victoria virus in Houston families,* 1976, J. Hyg. Cam. **86**: 303–313.

[52] Thacker, S.B. (1986) *The persistence of influenza in human populations*, Epidemi. Rev. **8**: 129–142.

[53] Thompson, W.W., D.K. Shay, E. Weintraub, L. Brammer, N. Cox, L.J. Anderson, and K. Fukuda (2003) *Mortality associated with influenza and respiratory syncytial virus in the United States,* JAMA **289**: 179–186.

[54] Tokyo: Ministry of Health, Labor and Welfare, *Japan, Influenza A(H1N1),* Available from: (http://www.mhlw.go.jp/english/topics/influenza_a/index.html), Accessed on June 1, 2009.

[55] Thieme, H.R. (1979) *Asymptotic estimates of the solutions of nonlinear integral equations and asymptotic speeds for the spread of populations*, J. Reine Angew. Math. **306**: 94–121.

[56] Taubenberger, J. and D.M. Morens (2006) 1918 *Influenza: The Mother of All Pandemics,* Emerg. Infect. Dis. **12**: 15–22.

[57] Trifonov, V., H. Khiabanian, B. Greenbaum, and R. Rabadan (2009) *The origin of the recent swine influenza A(H1N1) virus infecting humans,* Eurosurveill. **14**: 19193.

[58] Vivas, A.L. (2011) *Dynamics of a "SAIQR" Influenza Model*, Ph.D. Thesis, New Mexico State University.

[59] Wu, L. and Z. Feng (2000) *Homoclinic bifurcation in an SIQR model for childhood disease*, J. Differential Equations **168**: 150–167.

Lecture 8

Models for the Transmission Dynamics of HIV

8.1 Introduction

The identification of HIV [9, 42, 43, 46, 91] captured the attention of theoreticians and modelers as AIDS became one of the most feared diseases nearly three decades ago. Most of the initial modeling contributions focused on the study of the transmission dynamics of HIV at the population level since little was known about the epidemiology of the virus, and, as expected, modeling was carried out first under simple settings and crude assumptions [1, 2, 3, 4, 5, 8, 11, 17, 23, 24, 25, 26, 36, 38, 39, 45, 47, 52, 54, 55, 56, 57, 58, 62, 64, 66, 68, 72, 79, 80, 81, 85, 86]. An overview of the state of the art on the transmission dynamics of HIV modeling in the 1980s is found in [21], the review papers [81, 84], and in the books [6, 21, 51].

Our first contributions [23, 24, 25, 26, 54, 85, 86] focused on the impact that changes in the pool of susceptibles, disease-induced mortality, heterogeneous mixing, vertical transmission, asymptomatic carriers, variable infectivity, and incubation and infectious periods may have on the dynamics of sexually transmitted HIV. Efforts to model the risk of infection from sexual-partner selection or from within and between group mixing became central to the research of various groups studying HIV dynamics. We focused on the role of gender, core populations, and heterogeneous mixing contact rates on HIV dynamics and therefore were naturally involved in the development of sexual-behavior surveys and data collection on sexual and dating activity as well as on the mathematical modeling and analysis of heterogeneous "mixing" frameworks (see [12, 13, 15, 16, 18, 19, 27, 28, 29, 30, 32, 37, 65, 77]). The overview in [70] highlights the potential role of sexual activity and drinking on the dynamics of STDs [37, 52, 53, 77], and while the adaptive dynamics generated by changing behaviors in response to a multitude of factors were rarely explored, some early attempts were also carried out as a result of the HIV pandemic [14, 48]. This lecture first revisits earlier models with the purpose of highlighting epidemiological factors such as variable and long periods of incubation or infectiousness on the dynamics of sexually transmitted HIV. The lecture also revisits the joint dynamics of HIV-tuberculosis coinfections [76].

The following, not quite standard, definitions are used throughout: the *latent period* is the time from the acquisition of infection to the time when the host becomes infectious; the *infectious period* is the time during which the infected individual is capable of transmitting the disease; the *incubation period* is the time interval between the point of acquisition of infection and the appearance of symptoms. As described in these historical papers [1, 2, 3] knowledge of these periods was quickly identified as critical to initial efforts to predict the dynamics of HIV. In [26] it is observed that:

> The duration of the latent period is thought to be a few days to a few weeks [1, 2, 3], and while the duration of the infectious period is not yet known, those individuals that develop full-blown AIDS have an average incubation period estimated variously at 35–47 months [72], 66 months [1], and as high as 96 months [68]. This estimate is continually being revised as information and experience accumulate. However, even the most conservative estimate suggests that it may be reasonable to approximate the infectious period by the incubation period; that is, to assume a negligible latent period. Pickering et al. [72] stress that the ability to transmit HIV is not constant, as individuals are most infectious 3–16 months following exposure, and recent studies [46, 63, 78] report the existence of two peaks of infectiousness, one taking place a few weeks after exposure and the other before the onset of "full-blown" AIDS. The models in this study have been modified to take variable infectivity into consideration, with the intention of looking at how variable infectivity affects the conclusions in this paper (see [85, 86]).

The disease's reproductive number ($\mathcal{R}_0$), as has been noted, is defined as the number of secondary infections generated by an infectious individual in a population of susceptibles at a demographic steady state. In the context of the dynamics of a homosexually active homogeneously mixing population, the reproductive number is given by $\mathcal{R}_0 = \lambda C(T)D$, where λ denotes the probability of transmission per partner, $C(T)$ the mean number of sexual partners an average individual has per unit time when the population density is T, and D the death-adjusted mean infectious period (see [26]). Since HIV is a slow disease, we have that if $\mathcal{R}_0 \leq 1$, it will die out, while if $\mathcal{R}_0 \geq 1$, it will persist in the presence of a small number of infected/infectious individuals. The mathematical analysis and numerical simulations in [26] suggest that whenever the incubation period distribution is exponential, the reproductive number $\mathcal{R}$ is a global bifurcation parameter (transcritical bifurcation); that is, as $\mathcal{R}$ crosses 1 a global transfer of stability from the infection-free state to the endemic equilibrium takes place, and vice versa. *Local* results do not depend on the distribution of times spent in the infectious categories (the survivorship functions). Keeping a suite of parameters fixed [26] allowed for the comparison of the exponential incubation period distribution versus a piecewise constant survivorship (individuals remain infectious for a fixed length of time). It was found that for "some realistic parameters we can see (at least in these cases) that the reproductive numbers corresponding to these two extreme cases do not differ by more than 18% whenever the two distributions have the same mean." [26]

The inclusion of heterogeneity via the introduction of a large number of subgroups limited the forecasting capability of these models due to factors that included increased levels of uncertainty (more parameters). The use of multigroup models raised the *expected* modeling and parameter estimation challenges [12, 13, 15, 16, 18, 19, 27, 28, 29, 32, 52, 53, 77]. In addition, the analyses of some of these models generated novel dynamic behavior, questioning, possibly for the first time in epidemiology the centrality of the role of the basic reproduction number in the identification and development of control, education, and intervention measures. For example, the natural asymmetry present in disease transmission as a result of prevalent alternative modes of sexual engagement proved to be capable of giving rise to the existence of multiple equilibria [24, 25, 54], an unexpected outcome at that time.

This lecture is organized as follows: Section 8.2 introduces an HIV model in a homosexually active population that involves constant rates of movement out of the infectious classes into the AIDS or into the sexually inactive classes, a variant of the models in [1, 2]. Section 8.2 assumes that the duration of infectiousness is given by a negative exponential distribution and studies its consequences. Section 8.3 assumes that the duration of infectiousness is given by an arbitrary distribution; criteria for the maintenance of an endemic state and its stability are also established. Section 8.4 revisits an HIV/TB model [76] that is used to study the dynamics of slow disease coinfections. Section 8.5 collects our thoughts on the consequences of modeling under different waiting time distributions and the role of coinfections on HIV dynamics.

8.2 Model with Exponential Waiting Times

A single homosexually active population is divided into five classes: S, denoting the number of susceptible individuals; I, infectious individuals (somehow we know a priori the fraction that will move to this compartment) that will go on to develop AIDS; Y, infectious individuals that will not develop full-blown AIDS (complementary fraction); Z, former Y-individuals who are no longer sexually active; and A, former I-individuals who have developed full-blown AIDS (see Figure 8.1). It is assumed that individuals in the A and Z classes no longer play a role on the transmission dynamics of HIV. We notice that a latent class (i.e., those exposed individuals that are not yet infectious) was not included because it was believed then that the time spent in that class is short. It is further assumed that individuals who develop full-blown AIDS are no longer actively infectious, that is, that they have no sexual contacts; it is also assumed that infected individuals become immediately infectious. Finally, it is assumed that individuals in this population become sexually inactive or acquire AIDS at the constant rates α_Y and α_I, respectively, per unit time. Therefore, $1/(\mu+\alpha_I)$ gives the average or mean incubation period with the fraction $1/(\mu+\alpha_Y)$ denoting the average or mean sexual-life expectancy.

The introduction of the model requires additional definitions. Λ will denote the constant recruitment rate into the susceptible class (individuals who are sexually active);

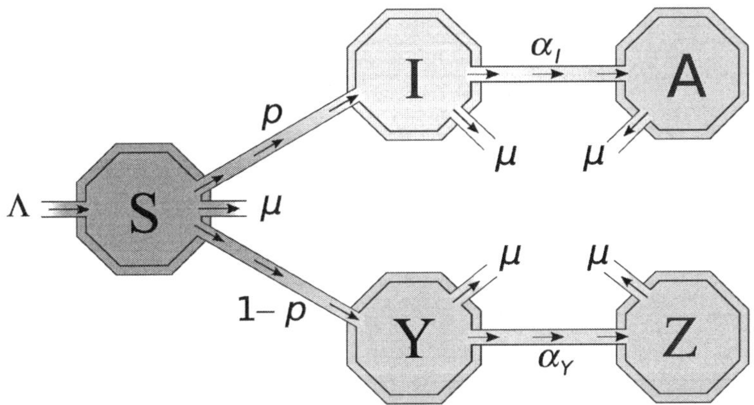

Figure 8.1. *Flow diagram: single group model with constant removal rates.*

μ the constant per-capita natural mortality rate; d the per-capita constant disease-induced mortality due to AIDS; p the constant fraction of susceptibles that become infectious and eventually go into the AIDS class; and $(1-p)$ the fraction of susceptible individuals that do not. Using the modeling framework published in [1, 2] with the help of Figure 8.1, we arrive at the following epidemiological model [26] for sexually transmitted HIV under the assumption of exponential waiting times in the infection classes:

$$\frac{dS(t)}{dt} = \Lambda - \lambda C(T(t))\frac{S(t)W(t)}{T(t)} - \mu S(t), \tag{8.1}$$

$$\frac{dI(t)}{dt} = \lambda p C(T(t))\frac{S(t)W(t)}{T(t)} - (\alpha_Y + \mu)Y(t), \tag{8.2}$$

$$\frac{dY(t)}{dt} = (\lambda - p)C(T(t))\frac{S(t)W(t)}{T(t)} - (\alpha_Y + \mu)Y(t), \tag{8.3}$$

$$\frac{dA(t)}{dt} = \alpha_I I(t) - (d+\mu)A(t), \tag{8.4}$$

$$\frac{dZ(t)}{dt} = \alpha_Y Y(t) - \mu Z(t), \tag{8.5}$$

where

$$W = I + Y \quad \text{and} \quad T = W + S. \tag{8.6}$$

In the above system, the function $C(T)$ models the mean number of sexual partners an average individual has per unit time when the population density is T; λ (a constant) denotes the average sexual risk per infected partner; and λ is often thought as the product $i\phi$ [55], where ϕ is the average number of contacts per sexual partner and i is the conditional probability of infection from a sexual contact when the latter is infected. Kingsley et al. [59] had presented (not surprising) evidence that the probability of seroconversion (infection) increases with the number of infected sexual partners. Hence, $\lambda C(T)$ models the transmission rate per unit time per infected partner when the size of the sexually active population is T.

The fraction W/T can be thought as representing the fraction of contacts that a susceptible individual has with a randomly selected infectious individual. Here $\lambda C(T)SW/T$ denotes the number of newly infected individuals per unit time since individuals in classes A and Z are sexually inactive. One may believe that a solid way of modeling $C(T)$ would be to assume that it is approximately linear for small T approaching a saturation level for large values of T [50]. Here, it is assumed that $C(T)$ is differentiable and increasing function of T (except when noted). Anderson et al. [2] observe that $C(T)$ the mean number of sexual partners per unit time underestimates the importance of highly active individuals and that, consequently, modifications should be made to this framework in order to properly account for their role.

The results associated with three cases of system (8.1)–(8.6) listed in [26] are as follows.

Case 1: $p = 1$. This, unfortunately, may be the most realistic as evidence accumulates that AIDS is a progressive disease. It now seems highly probable that most of the infected individuals will eventually develop "full-blown" AIDS (unless they die first from other causes). In this case, the Y and Z classes do not exist, and we may work only with Eqs. (8.1), (8.2), (8.4) and with $W = I$, $T = W + S$.

Case 2: $0 < p < 1$, $\alpha_I = \alpha_Y$. In this case, we may interpret I as the class of infected individuals who develop "full-blown" AIDS and Y as the class of individuals who develop ARC (AIDS-related complex). We assume that individuals with either AIDS or ARC are no longer sexually active, so that $T = W + S$ is the total number of sexually active individuals.

Case 3: $0 < p < 1$, $\alpha_i \neq \alpha_Y$. We may not interpret I as the class of individuals who spend a mean time $1/(\mu + \alpha_I)$ infected and then develop AIDS. The class Y consists of individuals who remain infective for a time $1/(\mu + \alpha_Y)$ and then withdraw from the sexually active group into a group that does not develop AIDS symptoms. In this situation presumably $\alpha_I > \alpha_Y$, so that the infection time in Y is longer than that in I. An alternative interpretation of the Z class is obtained by assuming that an individual moves into this group after testing seropositive, and then refrains from sexual intercourse. It is appropriate again to take $T = W + S$ to be the number of sexually active individuals. [26]

The analysis of system (8.1)–(8.6) found in [26] makes the following assumptions concerning $C(T)$:

$$C(T) > 0, \qquad C'(T) \geq 0, \tag{8.7}$$

with prime denoting the derivative with respect to T. The dynamics of S, Y, and I are independent of A and Z (by construction). Hence, it is enough to analyze (8.1), (8.2), (8.3) with (8.6). The system is well-posed; that is, if $S(0) \geq 0$, $I(0) \geq 0$, $Y(0) \geq 0$, then a unique solution exists with $S(t) \geq 0$, $I(t) \geq 0$, $Y(0) \geq 0$ for $t \geq 0$.

As is the case with most of the epidemiological systems addressed in this monograph, system (8.1)–(8.3) always has the disease-free equilibrium given by

$$(S, I, Y) = \left(\frac{\Lambda}{\mu}, 0, 0\right), \tag{8.8}$$

and under certain assumptions it also supports a unique endemic equilibrium.

The stability of the disease-free equilibrium (8.8) is determined by the nondimensional ratio

$$\mathcal{R}_0 = \lambda \left(\frac{p}{\sigma_I} + \frac{1-p}{\sigma_Y}\right) C\left(\frac{\Lambda}{\mu}\right), \tag{8.9}$$

that is, by the *basic reproductive number*. In the definition of $\mathcal{R}_0$, $\sigma_I = \alpha_I + \mu$, $\sigma_Y = \alpha_Y + \mu$, and $\mathcal{R}_0$ denotes the number of secondary infections generated by a single infectious individual in a population of susceptibles at a demographic steady state. $\mathcal{R}_0$ is given by the product of the following three factors (epidemiological parameters): λ (the probability of transmission per partner), $C(\Lambda/\mu)$ (the mean number of sexual partners that an average susceptible individual has per unit time when everybody in the population is susceptible), and

$$D = \left(\frac{p}{\sigma_I} + \frac{1-p}{\sigma_Y}\right). \tag{8.10}$$

The death-adjusted mean infectious period is $D = pD_I + (1-p)D_Y$, with D_I and D_Y denoting the death-adjusted mean infectious periods, $1/\sigma_I$ and $1/\sigma_Y$ of the I and Y classes, respectively. The use of the dimensionless ratio, $\mathcal{R}_0 = \lambda C(\Lambda/\mu)D$, leads to the following result [26].

Theorem 8.1. *If $\mathcal{R}_0 \leq 1$, then the equilibrium $(\Lambda/\mu, 0, 0)$ of system* (8.1)–(8.5) *is globally asymptotically stable.*

That is, any solution of (8.1)–(8.3) $(S(t), I(t), Y(t))$ with $S(0) \geq 0$, $I(0) \geq 0$, $Y(0) \geq 0$ tends to $(\Lambda/\mu, 0, 0)$ as $t \to +\infty$. That is, the condition $\mathcal{R}_0 \leq 1$ is sufficient to guarantee that the disease will eventually die out in this population.

In [26] the following result has also been established (following some of the same arguments used in other chapters).

Theorem 8.2. *If $\mathcal{R}_0 > 1$, there is a unique endemic equilibrium (S^*, I^*, Y^*), which is locally asymptotically stable, and the infection-free state $(\Lambda/\mu, 0, 0)$ is unstable.*

We can summarize the situation (full details of all proofs in [26]) as follows:

The disease-free state of system (8.1)–(8.3) is globally asymptotically stable when $\mathcal{R}_0 > 1$ and unstable if $\mathcal{R}_0 > 1$. When $\mathcal{R}_0 > 1$, this system has a unique locally asymptotically stable endemic equilibrium. There is a transfer of stability to the endemic state as $\mathcal{R}_0$ crosses one. Furthermore, when $\sigma_I = \sigma_Y$ (both death-adjusted mean infectious periods agree) and $\mathcal{R}_0 > 1$ it was shown, as one would expect, that the endemic equilibrium is also globally asymptotically stable.

The reproductive number $(\mathcal{R}_0)$ increases proportionately with the transmission probability and the average number of sexual partners; it may also increase in proportion to the rate of recruitment of individuals to the susceptible class (through $C(T)$). $\mathcal{R}_0$ is an increasing function of the mean infectious period D and may be a decreasing function of the mortality rate (depending on the functional expression for $C(T)$).

8.2.1 Outlines of some of proofs

Sketches of the proofs of Theorems 8.1 and 8.2 follow (as carried out in the appendices in [26]).

***Proof of Theorem* 8.1.** If (S_0, I_0, Y_0) is in $Q = [0, \infty]^3$, the nonnegative orthant in $\mathbf{R}^3$, then $(S(t), I(t), Y(t))$ remains in Q for $t \geq 0$ and any $p \in [0, 1]$. We have, from (8.1), that

$$\frac{dT}{dt} = \Lambda - \mu T - \alpha_I I - \alpha_Y Y,$$

which implies that $\limsup_{t\to+\infty} T(t) \leq \Lambda/\mu$.

Given our interest in the study of the asymptotic behavior of solutions as $t \to +\infty$, it is assumed, without loss of generality, that $T(t) \leq \Lambda/\mu$ for all $t \geq 0$. Since the function $C(T)$ is by assumption an increasing function of T, then $C(T) \leq C(\Lambda/\mu)$. Introducing the function

$$f(t) = \frac{I(t)}{\sigma_I} + \frac{Y(t)}{\sigma_Y}$$

and taking its derivative leads to the estimates

$$
\begin{aligned}
df(t) &= \left[\left(\frac{p}{\sigma_I}+\frac{1-p}{\sigma_Y}\right)\lambda\frac{C(T(t))S(t)}{T(t)}-1\right]W(t)\\
&\leq \left[\left(\frac{p}{\sigma_I}+\frac{1-p}{\sigma_Y}\right)\lambda C\left(\frac{\Lambda}{\mu}\right)-\lambda\left(\frac{p}{\sigma_I}+\frac{1-p}{\sigma_Y}\right)\frac{W(t)C(T(t))}{T(t)}-1\right]W(t)\\
&= (R-1)W(t)-\lambda\left(\frac{p}{\sigma_I}+\frac{1-p}{\sigma_Y}\right)\frac{C(T(t))}{T(t)}W^2(t)\\
&\leq -\Lambda\sigma^2\left(\frac{p}{\sigma_I}+\frac{1-p}{\sigma_Y}\right)\frac{C(T(t))}{T(t)}f^2(t),
\end{aligned}
$$

where $\sigma = \min \sigma_I, \sigma_Y$. Hence $f(t) \to 0$ as $t \to +\infty$ and, consequently, $I(t) \to 0, Y(t) \to 0$, and $C(T)SW/T \to 0$ as $t \to +\infty$. It follows that $S(t) \to \Lambda/\mu$ as $t \to +\infty$, and this completes the proof of Theorem 8.1. □

In order to establish that if $\mathcal{R}_0 > 1$, the disease-free equilibrium is unstable (Theorem 8.1) and there exists a unique positive *endemic* equilibrium (S^*, I^*, Y^*) we need Lemma 8.3.

Lemma 8.3. *Suppose that β_0, β_1, and H are positive numbers, and that $\beta_1 > \beta_0$, $C(\Lambda/\mu) > H$. Then there is a unique number $I^* > 0$ such that*

$$
C\left(\frac{\Lambda}{\mu}-\beta_0 I^*\right)\left(\frac{\Lambda}{\mu}-\beta_1 I^*\right) = H\left(\frac{\Lambda}{\mu}-\beta_0 I^*\right), \quad \frac{\Lambda}{\mu}-\beta_1 I^* > 0.
$$

Proof. We introduce the function $g(I) = C(\Lambda/\mu - \beta_0 I)(\Lambda/\mu - \beta_1 I)/(\Lambda/\mu - \beta_0 I)$ and note that $g(0) = C(\Lambda/\mu) > H$ and $g(\Lambda/(\mu\beta_1)) = 0$. Further, from

$$
\frac{dg}{dI} = -\beta_0\left(\frac{\Lambda}{\mu}-\beta_1 I\right)\frac{C'(u)}{u}-(\beta_1-\beta_0)\frac{\Lambda}{\mu}\frac{C(u)}{u^2}, \quad u = \frac{\Lambda}{\mu}-\beta_0 I \tag{8.11}
$$

and the observation that $I \in [0, \Lambda/(\mu\beta_1)]$, we see that

$$
u > 0, \quad C'(u) \geq 0, \quad C(u) > 0. \tag{8.12}
$$

Therefore (8.11) implies that $g(I)$ is a strictly decreasing function of I on the interval $[0, \Lambda/(\mu\beta_1)]$, and hence there is a unique I^* in the open interval $(0, \Lambda/(\mu\beta_1))$ such that $g(I^* = H)$ with $\Lambda/\mu - \beta_1 I^* > 0$. □

Corollary 8.4. *If $\Re_0 > 1$, there is a unique positive endemic equilibrium (S^*, I^*, Y^*).*

Proof. We let

$$
\beta_1 = \frac{1}{p\mu D_I}, \quad \beta_0 = \beta_1 - \frac{D}{pD_I}, \quad H = \frac{1}{\lambda D} \tag{8.13}
$$

and make use of $\beta_1 > \beta_0$ and of the lower bound estimate for β_0,

$$\begin{aligned}\beta_0 &= \frac{\sigma_I}{p\mu} - \frac{\sigma_I D}{p} = \frac{1}{p}\left[\frac{\sigma_I}{\mu} - \sigma_I\left(\frac{p}{\sigma_I} + \frac{1-p}{\sigma_Y}\right)\right] \\ &\geq \frac{1}{p}\left[\frac{\sigma_I}{\mu} - p - \frac{\sigma_I(1-p)}{\mu}\right] = \frac{1}{p}\left[\frac{\sigma_I p}{\mu} - p\right] = \frac{\alpha_I}{\mu} > 0,\end{aligned}$$

the definition of $\mathcal{R}_0 = \lambda C(\Lambda/\mu)D$, or equivalently that $C(\Lambda/\mu) = \mathcal{R}_0/(D\lambda) > H$, and we apply Lemma 8.3. Hence, there is a unique I^* in $(0, \Lambda/(\mu\beta_1))$ such that

$$C(\Lambda/\mu - \beta_0 I^*)(\Lambda/\mu - \beta_1 I^*)/(\Lambda/\mu - \beta_0 I^*) = H. \tag{8.14}$$

Further since at equilibrium we have the expressions

$$S^* = \frac{\Lambda}{\mu} - \frac{1}{\mu p D_I} I^*, \quad Y^* = \left(\frac{D}{pD_I} - 1\right) I^*, \quad W^* = I^* + Y^* = \frac{D}{pD_I} I^*, \tag{8.15}$$

then making use of $I^* < \Lambda/(\mu\beta_1) = \lambda p D_I$, $S^* > 0$, and $D/(pD_I) > 1$ we obtain $Y^* > 0$ (if $p = 1$, there is no equation for Y). Therefore using (8.15) we conclude that

$$T^* = S^* + W^* = \frac{\Lambda}{\mu} - \beta_0 I^*,$$

with which (8.14) implies that $C(T^*)S^*/T^* = H$. It can be verified that (S^*, I^*, Y^*) is a positive equilibrium of (8.1)–(8.3). Uniqueness is established by letting $(S^\wedge, I^\wedge, Y^\wedge)$ denote any positive equilibrium. Introducing $M(T) = C(T)/T$, we observe from (8.2) and (8.3) that $[(1-p)/D_I]I^\wedge = [p/D_Y]Y^\wedge$ and $\lambda D M(T^\wedge)S^\wedge W^\wedge = I^\wedge + Y^\wedge = W^\wedge$, and since

$$M(T^\wedge)S^\wedge = H = \frac{1}{\lambda D}, \quad Y^\wedge = \left(\frac{D}{pD_I} - 1\right) I^\wedge, \quad W^\wedge = \frac{D}{pD_I} I^\wedge, \tag{8.16}$$

where $W^\wedge = I^\wedge + Y^\wedge, T^\wedge = S^\wedge + W^\wedge$, and (8.1) holds, we conclude that

$$S^\wedge = \frac{\Lambda}{\mu} - \frac{1}{p\mu D_I} I^\wedge, \quad T^\wedge = S^\wedge + \frac{D}{pD_I} I^\wedge, \quad \text{and} \quad M(T^\wedge)S^\wedge = H = \frac{1}{\lambda D}.$$

Making use of Lemma 8.3, we see that $I^\wedge = I^*$ and hence that $Y^\wedge = Y^*$ and $S^\wedge = S^*$. □

The nature of the stability of the endemic equilibrium is resolved as follows.

***Proof of Theorem* 8.2.** The Jacobian matrix for (8.1)–(8.3) is

$$\begin{aligned} J &= \frac{\partial(f_1, f_2, f_3)}{\partial(S, I, Y)} \\ &= \begin{bmatrix} -\lambda W(M + SM') - \mu & -\lambda S(M + WM') & -\lambda S(M + WM') \\ p\lambda W(M + SM') & p\lambda S(M + WM') - \sigma_I & p\lambda S(M + WM') \\ (1-p)\lambda W(M + SM') & (1-p)\lambda S(M + WM') & (1-p)\lambda S(M + WM') - \sigma_Y \end{bmatrix}, \end{aligned}$$

where M' denotes $dM(T)/dt$. Evaluating the Jacobian at the disease-free equilibrium $(W = S = \Lambda/\mu)$ with $SM = (\Lambda/\mu)M(\Lambda/\mu) = c(\Lambda/\mu)$ leads to the following characteristic equation:

$$\det[zI - J] = (z+\mu)(z^2 + az + b) = 0,$$

where

$$a = \sigma_I + \sigma_Y - \lambda C\left(\frac{\Lambda}{\mu}\right), \quad b = \sigma_I \sigma_Y \left[1 - \lambda C\left(\frac{\Lambda}{\mu}\right)\left(\frac{p}{\sigma_I} + \frac{1-p}{\sigma_Y}\right)\right] = \sigma_I \sigma_Y (1 - R).$$

We observe that $b < 0$ whenever $\mathscr{R}_0 > 1$, that is, the disease-free equilibrium is unstable. The characteristic equation in the endemic case $((S^*, I^*, Y^*))$ is given by the cubic polynomial $\det(zI - J) = z^3 + a_1 z^2 + a_2 z + a_3$, where a_1, a_2, a_3 are given by

$$a_1 = \sigma_I + \sigma_Y - \frac{1}{D} + \mu + \lambda WM = \left[p\frac{\sigma_Y}{\sigma_I} + (1-p)\frac{\sigma_I}{\sigma_Y}\right]\frac{1}{D} + \mu + \lambda WM$$
$$> \left[p\frac{\sigma_Y}{\sigma_I} + (1-p)\frac{\sigma_I}{\sigma_Y}\right]\frac{1}{D} + \mu > 0,$$

$$\begin{aligned}
a_2 &= \mu(\sigma_I + \sigma_Y) + (\sigma_I + \sigma_Y)\lambda(WM + SWM') + \sigma_I\sigma_Y \\
&\quad - [\mu + \sigma_I(1-p) + \sigma_Y p]\lambda(SM + SWM') \\
&= \lambda(\sigma_I + \sigma_Y)(WM + SWM') + \mu(\sigma_I + \sigma_Y - \lambda SM) - \mu\lambda SWM' \\
&\quad - [\sigma_I(1-p) + \sigma_Y p]\lambda SWM',
\end{aligned}$$

where $W^* = I^* + Y^*$, $T^* = S^* + W^*$, $M^* = M(T^*)$, $M'^* = (dM/dt)T^*$ and where we have used the fact that

$$\sigma_I\sigma_Y - [\sigma_I(1-p) + \sigma_Y p]\lambda SM = 0.$$

Further, using the fact that

$$M'(T) = \left(\frac{C(T)}{T}\right)' = \frac{C'(T)}{T} - \frac{C(T)}{T^2}$$

and that $\sigma_1 + \sigma_2 - \lambda SM > 0$, we find that

$$\begin{aligned}
a_2 &= \lambda W\frac{C(T)}{T}\left[(\sigma_I + \sigma_Y)\left(1 - \frac{S}{T}\right) + (\sigma_I(1-p) + \sigma_Y p)\frac{S}{T}\right] \\
&\quad + \lambda[\sigma_I + \sigma_Y - \mu - \sigma_I(1-p) - \sigma_Y p]SW\frac{C'(T)}{T} \\
&\quad + \mu(\sigma_I + \sigma_Y - \lambda SM) + \lambda\mu\frac{SWC(T)}{T^2} \\
&> \lambda W\frac{C(T)}{T}\left[(\sigma_I + \sigma_Y)\left(1 - \frac{S}{T}\right) + (\sigma_I(1-p) + \sigma_Y p)\frac{S}{T}\right] \\
&\quad + \lambda[\alpha_I p + \alpha_Y(1-p)]SW\frac{C'(T)}{T} > 0,
\end{aligned}$$

as well as

$$\begin{aligned}
a_3 &= \lambda\sigma_I\sigma_Y(WM+SWM')+\mu[\sigma I\sigma_Y-((1-p)\sigma_I+p\sigma_Y)\lambda SM] \\
&\quad -\mu[(1-p)\sigma_I+p\sigma_Y]\lambda SWM' \\
&= \sigma_I\sigma_Y\lambda(WM+SWM')-\mu\lambda[\sigma_I(1-p)+p\sigma_Y]SWM' \\
&\le \lambda W\frac{C(T)}{T}\left\{\sigma_I\sigma_Y\left(1-\frac{S}{T}\right)+\mu[\sigma_I(1-p)+p\sigma_Y]\right\} \\
&\quad +\lambda SW\{\sigma_I\sigma_Y-\mu[\sigma_I(1-p)p\sigma_Y]\}\frac{C'(T)}{T} \\
&= \lambda W\frac{C(T)}{T}\left\{\sigma_I\sigma_Y\left(1-\frac{S}{T}\right)+\mu[\sigma_I(1-p)+p\sigma_Y]\right\} \\
&\quad +\lambda(\alpha_I\alpha_Y+\mu[\alpha_I p+(1-p)\alpha_Y])SW\frac{C'(T)}{T}.
\end{aligned}$$

The use of the above relations and the inequalities

$$\left[p\frac{\sigma_Y}{\sigma_I}+(1-p)\frac{\sigma_I}{\sigma_Y}\right]\frac{1}{D}(\sigma_I+\sigma_Y)>\sigma_I\sigma_Y,$$

$$\left[p\frac{\sigma_Y}{\sigma_I}+(1-p)\frac{\sigma_I}{\sigma_Y}\right]\frac{1}{D}[p\alpha_I+(1-p)\alpha_Y]\alpha_I\alpha_Y$$

can be use to show that $a_1a_2>a_3$. That is, the Routh–Hurwitz stability criteria are satisfied, completing the proof of Theorem 8.2. □

8.3 HIV Model with Arbitrary Incubation Period Distributions

The use of exponential waiting distributions in the I and Y classes corresponds to the requirement that the per-capita removal rate from the I class (by the development of full-blown AIDS symptoms) into the A class be constant. It would clearly be an improvement in the model of Section 8.2 if we were to move from constant to variable removal rates, and this is what we do in this section (the ideas follow those in [11, 26]). Hence, it is still assumed that individuals become immediately infectious (that is, we continue to neglect the latent period) and continue to divide the at-risk population into the five classes: S, I, Y, Z, and A. The parameters $\lambda=i\phi$, Λ, μ, d, and p have the same meaning as in Section 8.2; however, the removal rates are modified through the introduction of two functions, $P_I(s)$ and $P_Y(s)$ (see Figure 8.2), representing the proportion of individuals who become I- or Y-infective at time t and that, if alive, are still infectious at time $t+s$ (survive as infectious). P_I and P_Y, survivorship functions, are nonnegative and nonincreasing, and $P_I(0)=P_Y(0)=1$. It is further assumed that

$$\int_0^\infty P_I(s)ds<\infty,\qquad \int_0^\infty P_Y(s)ds<\infty,$$

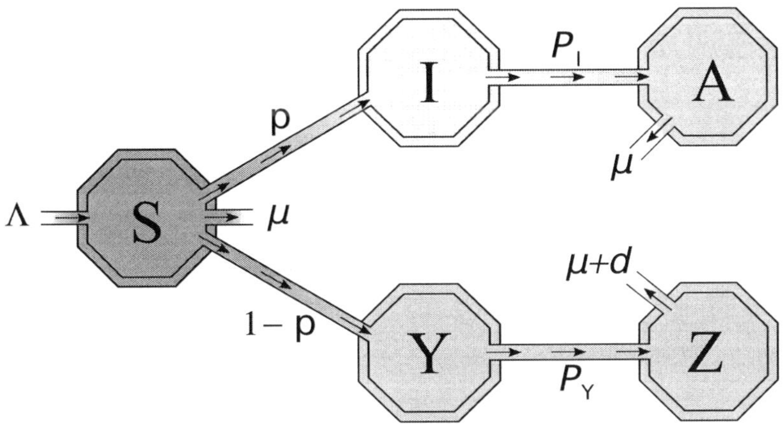

Figure 8.2. *Flow diagram for a single-group model with distributed periods of infectiousness.*

and thus $-\dot{P}(x)$ and $-\dot{P}_Y(x)$ are the rates of removal of individuals from classes I and Y into classes A and Z, x time units after infection.

The number of new infections occurring at time x is $\lambda C(T(x))S(x)W(x)/T(x)$, where we have kept the meaning of $C(T)$, W, and T as in Section 8.2. The rate of change in the susceptible class is given now by the expression

$$\frac{dS(t)}{dt} = \Lambda - \lambda C(T(t))S(t)\frac{W(t)}{T(t)} - \mu S(t), \tag{8.17}$$

with

$$p\int_0^t \lambda C(T(x))S(x)\frac{W(x)}{T(x)}e^{-\mu(t-x)}P_I(t-x)dx$$

representing the number of individuals who have been infected from times 0 to t and are still in class I (similar expression for class Y). The discount factor $\exp(-\mu(t-x))$ takes into account removals due to deaths by natural causes (not HIV). Hence, if $I_0(t)$ and $Y_0(t)$ denote individuals in either class I or Y at time $t = 0$ that are still infectious at time t, then the total numbers of I- and Y-infectives at time t are given by

$$I(t) = I_0(t) + p\int_0^t \lambda C(T(x))S(x)\frac{W(x)}{T(x)}e^{-\mu(t-x)}P_I(t-x)dx, \tag{8.18}$$

$$Y(t) = Y_0(t) + (1-p)\int_0^t \lambda C(T(x))S(x)\frac{W(x)}{T(x)}e^{-\mu(t-x)}P_Y(t-x)dx, \tag{8.19}$$

where $I_0(t)$ and $Y_0(t)$ are assumed (for biological and mathematical reasons) to have compact support (vanishing for large enough t).

The expression for $A(t)$ turns out to be the sum of three terms: $A_0e^{-(\mu+d)t}$, where $A_0 = A(0)$, representing individuals who had full-blown AIDS at time zero and are still alive; $A_0(t)$ representing individuals initially in class I who moved into class A and are still alive at time t; and those who joined the I class after time $t = 0$ (see below). We assume that

$A_0(t)$ approaches zero as t approaches infinity. The term representing I infected individuals "born" after time $t = 0$ is given by

$$\int_0^\tau \left\{ \int_0^t \lambda C(T(x))S(x)\frac{W(x)}{T(x)}e^{-\mu(\tau-x)}[-\dot{P}_I(\tau-x)e^{-(\mu+d)(t-\tau)}]dx \right\} d\tau,$$

where $-\dot{P}_I(\tau - x)$ denotes the rate of removal from the class I at time τ or $(\tau - x)$ units after infection. Therefore

$$\begin{aligned} A(t) = p \int_0^\tau \left\{ \int_0^t \lambda C(T(x))S(x)\frac{W(x)}{T(x)}e^{-\mu(t-x)}[-\dot{P}_Y(\tau-x)e^{-(t-\tau)}]dx \right\} d\tau \\ + A_0 e^{-(\mu+d)t} + A_0(t). \end{aligned} \tag{8.20}$$

The corresponding expression for the Z class is given by

$$\begin{aligned} Z(t) = (1-p) \int_0^\tau \left\{ \int_0^t \lambda C(T(x))S(x)\frac{W(x)}{T(x)}e^{-\mu(t-x)}[-\dot{P}_Y(\tau-x)e^{-(t-\tau)}]dx \right\} d\tau \\ + Z_0 e^{-\mu t} + Z_0(t). \end{aligned} \tag{8.21}$$

The model given by (8.17)–(8.21) is a system of nonlinear integral equations. The standard results on well-posedness for these systems, as found in [69], guarantee the existence and uniqueness of solutions and their continuous dependence on parameters. The proof of positivity is given in [23].

The dynamics of the S, Y, and I classes are governed autonomously, and so the analyses can be restricted to the study of system (8.17)–(8.19). The basic reproductive number ($\mathcal{R}_0$) is given by

$$\mathcal{R}_0 = \lambda C\left(\frac{\Lambda}{\mu}\right)\int_0^\infty [pP_I(x) + (1-p)P_Y(x)]e^{-\mu x}dx, \tag{8.22}$$

where

$$\int_0^\infty [pP_I(x) + (1-p)P_Y(x)]e^{-\mu x}dx$$

is the death-adjusted mean infectious period, D. If $P_I(x) = e^{-\alpha_I x}$ and $P_Y(x) = e^{-\alpha_Y x}$, then (8.22) reduces to (8.9). We also observe that as before

$$D = pD_I + (1-p)D_Y,$$

where

$$D_I = \int_0^\infty P_I(s)e^{-\mu s}ds \quad \text{and} \quad D_Y = \int_0^\infty P_Y(s)e^{-\mu s}ds$$

denote the mean infectious periods of classes I and Y, respectively.

System (8.17)–(8.19) with $I_0(t) = Y_0(t) = 0$ always has the equilibrium

$$(S, I, Y) = \left(\frac{\Lambda}{\mu}, 0, 0\right), \tag{8.23}$$

but no other constant solutions. However, since $I_0(t)$ and $Y_0(t)$ must be zero for large t, one would expected, under appropriate assumptions, that $(\Lambda/\mu, 0, 0)$ will be an attractor or "asymptotic equilibrium" as $t \to +\infty$. We have shown [23, 26] that the following results hold.

Theorem 8.5. *The infection-free state* $(\Lambda/\mu, 0, 0)$ *of the limiting system* (8.17)–(8.19) *is a global attractor; that is,* $\lim_{t\to+\infty}(S(t), I(t), Y(t)) = (\Lambda/\mu, 0, 0)$ *for any positive solution of system* (8.17)–(8.19) *as long as* $\mathcal{R}_0 \leq 1$.

Theorem 8.6. *The infection-free state of system* (8.17)–(8.19) *is unstable when* $\mathcal{R}_0 > 1$ *and there exists a constant* $W^* > 0$, *such that any positive solution* $(S(t), I(t), Y(t))$, (8.17)–(8.19), *satisfies* $\limsup_{t\to+\infty}[I(t) + Y(t)] \geq W^*$.

In other words, if $\mathcal{R}_0 > 1$, the disease-free state (8.8) cannot be an attractor of any positive solution. That is, every solution has at least approximately W^* infectives (this W^* is the same as that in the statement of Theorem 8.7 below) for a sequence of times t tending to $+\infty$. Will $S(t)$, $I(t)$, $Y(t)$ approach nonzero constants as $t \to +\infty$, when $\mathcal{R}_0 > 1$? If that were the case, then the results in [69] guarantee that these constants must satisfy the limiting system associated with (8.17)–(8.19), which is given by the following set of equations:

$$\frac{dS}{dt} = \Lambda - \lambda C(T(t))S(t)\frac{W(t)}{T(t)} - \mu S(t), \tag{8.24}$$

$$I(t) = p\int_0^t \lambda C(T(x))S(x)\frac{W(x)}{T(x)}e^{-\mu(t-x)}P_I(t-x)dx, \tag{8.25}$$

$$Y(t) = (1-p)\int_0^t \lambda C(T(x))S(x)\frac{W(x)}{T(x)}e^{-\mu(t-x)}P_Y(t-x)dx; \tag{8.26}$$

if the equations for I and Y are added, we have

$$W(t) = \int_0^t \lambda C(T(x))S(x)\frac{W(x)}{T(x)}e^{-\mu(t-x)}P(t-x)dx, \tag{8.27}$$

where

$$P(x) = pP_I(x) + (1-p)P_Y(x).$$

The limiting system (8.24)–(8.27) is an autonomous system for which we have established the following result.

Theorem 8.7. *If* $\mathcal{R}_0 > 1$, *the limiting system* (8.24)–(8.27) *has a unique positive equilibrium* (S^*, W^*). *If in addition* $(d/dT)(C(T)/T) \leq 0$, *then this endemic equilibrium is locally asymptotically stable.*

Theorem 8.7 indicates that there is a switch of stability from $(\Lambda/\mu, 0)$ to (S^*, W^*) as $\mathcal{R}_0$ crosses 1. We also conjecture but have not proved that the asymptotic dynamics of system (8.17)–(8.19) and the limiting system (8.24)–(8.27) agree. An alternative approach can be found in [49]. The proofs of these results can be found in [26].

8.4 HIV and Tuberculosis: Dynamics of Coinfections

Tuberculosis, a bacterial disease with *M. tuberculosis* as its etiological agent, is *the leading cause of death* among HIV-infected individuals [44]. TB-infected individuals remain possible latently infected for life. In 2006, it was reported that roughly one-third of the world population are infected with TB [90].

HIV, on the other hand, is not casually transmitted. It can be acquired through sexual intercourse or needle sharing with HIV-infected persons. It can also be acquired through HIV-contaminated blood transfusions or vertical transmission, that is, infants may acquire at birth or through breast feeding from HIV-positive mothers. HIV diminishes the ability of the immune system to respond to invasions by infectious agents such as *M. tuberculosis*. Furthermore, as HIV infection progresses, immunity often declines, with patients becoming more susceptible to typical or rare infections. In wealthier societies HIV and TB treatments are common; these drugs have altered significantly the joint dynamics of TB and HIV.

Health disparities mean that HIV-TB dynamics are still in high gear in poor nations. The WHO reports that about a third of the estimated 39.5 million HIV-infected individuals worldwide suffer of TB coinfections [89]. Furthermore, even after a decade HIV-infected TB carriers are 30 to 50 times more likely to develop active TB than HIV-free individuals [87]. In the 1990s roughly one-third of the observed increases in TB-active cases were attributed to HIV [87]. On the other hand, TB in HIV-infected individuals often increases the rate of HIV replication, which may result in rapid progression towards the AIDS stage.

The modeling literature on the independent dynamics of HIV or TB is quite extensive. TB efforts include, for example, [7, 10, 31, 33, 34, 35, 40, 41, 73], while HIV/AIDS include [22, 51, 67, 86] to name a few more. TB/HIV coinfection modeling efforts have also been published. Kirschner [60] developed an immunological model describing HIV-1 and TB coinfections within a host. Naresh et al. [71] introduced a model involving a population subdivided into four epidemiological classes: susceptible, TB infective, HIV infective, and those with AIDS; the model focused on the transmission dynamics of HIV and treatable TB in variable size populations. Schulzer et al. [83] looked at HIV/TB joint dynamics using actuarial methods. West and Thompson [88] introduced models for the joint dynamics of HIV and TB that were explored via numerical simulations; their main goal was to estimate parameters and use their estimates to forecast the future transmission of TB in the United States. Porco et al. [74], using a discrete event simulation model, examined the impact of HIV on the probability and expected severity of TB outbreaks. Additional efforts include those in [75, 82].

As noted in [76],

> Our approach differs from those found in the literature ... we focus on the joint dynamics of HIV and TB [at the population level] in a pseudo-competitive environment.... The model is not for a specific country or nation, and our approach does not preclude the possibility of joint infections. The model assumes that invasions are bad news for each single host and that joint invasions are worse. This model is used to explore the impact of factors associated with co-infections on the prevalence of each of the two diseases. The possibility of HIV infections is incorporated within "typical" epidemiological frameworks that have been developed for the transmission dynamics of TB. The enhanced deterministic system is used to carry out a qualitative study of the joint transmission dynamics of TB and HIV.

8.4.1 Model for the dynamics of TB/HIV co-infections

A system of differential equations is introduced to model the joint dynamics of TB and HIV. The total population is divided into the following epidemiological subgroups: S, susceptible; L, latent with TB; I, infectious with TB; T, successfully treated with TB; J_1, HIV infectious; J_2, HIV infectious and TB latent; J_3, infectious with both TB and HIV; and A, full-blown AIDS. The compartmental diagram in Figure 8.3 illustrates the flow of individuals as they face the possibility of acquiring specific-disease infections or even coinfections.

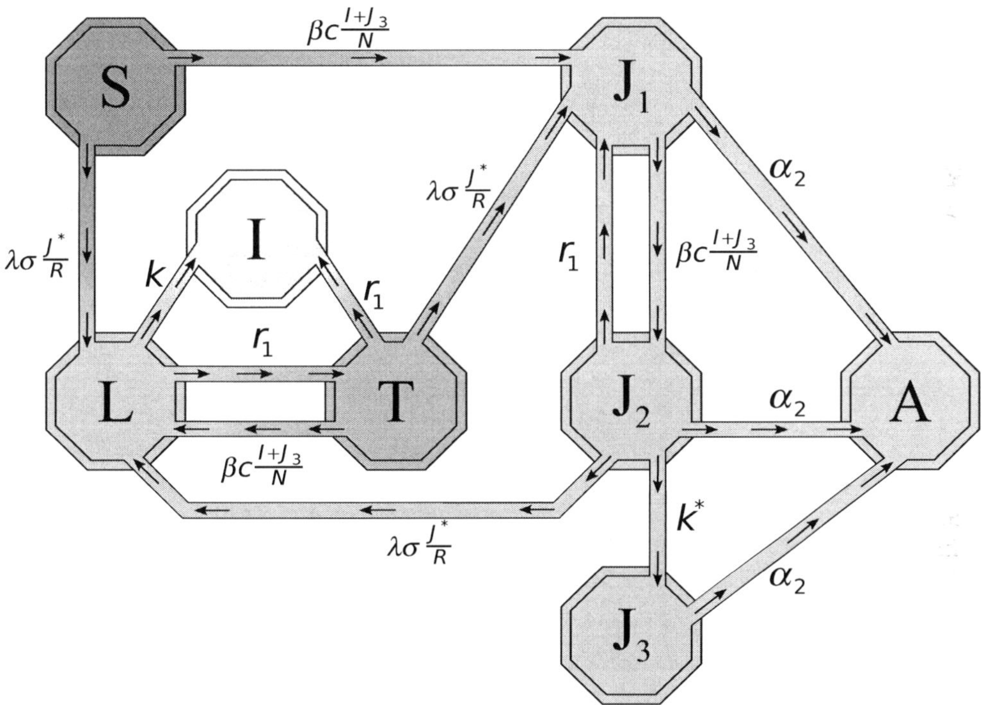

Figure 8.3. *Transition diagram between classes for the dynamics TB and HIV coinfections using per-capita rates (modified from* [76]*).*

The TB/HIV model is given by the following systems of eight ordinary differential equations:

$$
TB \begin{cases} \frac{dS}{dt} = \Lambda - \beta c S \frac{I+J_3}{N} - \lambda\sigma S \frac{J^*}{R} - \mu S, \\ \frac{dL}{dt} = \beta c (S+T) \frac{I+J_3}{N} - \lambda\sigma L \frac{J^*}{R} - (\mu + k + r_1) L, \\ \frac{dI}{dt} = kL - (\mu + d + r_2) I, \\ \frac{dT}{dt} = r_1 L + r_2 I - \beta c T \frac{I+J_3}{N} - \lambda\sigma T \frac{J^*}{R} - \mu T, \end{cases} \tag{8.28}
$$

Table 8.1. *Parameters and state variable definitions for the TB/HIV model as they appear in* [76] *and* (8.28).

Symbol	Definition
N	total population
R	total active population $(= N - I - J_3 - A = S + L + T + J_1 + J_2)$
J^*	individuals with HIV who have not developed AIDS $(= J_1 + J_2 + J_3)$
Λ	constant recruitment rate
β	probability of TB infection per contact with a person with active TB
λ	probability of HIV infection per contact with a person with HIV
c	per-capita contact rate for TB
σ	per-capita contact rate for HIV
μ	per-capita natural death rate
k	per-capita TB progression rate for individuals not infected with HIV
k^*	per-capita TB progression rate for individuals infected also with HIV
d	per-capita TB-induced death rate
d^*	per-capita HIV-induced death rate
f	per-capita AIDS-induced death rate
r_1	per-capita latent TB treatment rate for individuals with no HIV
r_2	per-capita active TB treatment rate for individuals with no HIV
r^*	per-capita latent TB treatment rate for individuals with HIV
α_i	per-capita AIDS progression rate for individuals in the J_i $(i = 1,2,3)$

$$HIV \begin{cases} \frac{dJ_1}{dt} = \lambda\sigma(S+T)\frac{J^*}{R} - \beta c J_1 \frac{I+J_3}{N} - (\alpha_1+\mu)J_1 + r^* J_2, \\ \frac{dJ_2}{dt} = \lambda\sigma L \frac{J^*}{R} + \beta c J_1 \frac{I+J_3}{N} - (\alpha_2+\mu+k^*+r^*)J_2, \\ \frac{dJ_3}{dt} = k^* J_2 - (\alpha_3+\mu+d^*)J_3, \\ \frac{dA}{dt} = \alpha_1 J_1 + \alpha_2 J_2 + \alpha_3 J_3 - (\mu+f)A, \end{cases}$$

where

$$\begin{aligned} N &= S+L+I+T+J_1+J_2+J_3+A, \\ R &= N-I-J_3-A = S+L+T+J_1+J_2, \\ J^* &= J_1+J_2+J_3. \end{aligned} \tag{8.29}$$

The variable R here collects noninfectious "circulating" individuals, that is, those who do not have active TB or AIDS. Definitions of model parameters are collected in Table 8.1.

The modeling and epidemiological class assumptions include the following: homogeneous mixing; HIV positive and TB infectious individuals (J_3) showing severe HIV symptoms that therefore cannot be effectively treated for active TB; the restriction that TB infections are acquired only through contacts with TB infectious individuals (I and J_3); and in addition that individuals may acquire HIV infections only through contacts with HIV infectious individuals (J^* group). Further, the "probability" of infection per contact is assumed to be the same for T and S classes (β and λ). Furthermore, I (TB infectious), J_3 (TB and HIV infectious), and A (AIDS) individuals are too ill to remain sexually active and, consequently, they do not transmit HIV through sexual activity. Hence, $R \equiv N - I - J_3 - A$ and the HIV incidence is modeled by $\lambda\sigma J^*/R$ (see [20, 61, 92]).

The probability of having contact with HIV infectious individuals is modeled as J^*/R, and the number of new HIV infections in a unit time is therefore $\lambda\sigma SJ^*/R$ (HIV transmission via IV drug injections, childbirth, or breast feeding are ignored). The most drastic in this model comes from the incorporation of sexual transmission as an indirect risk factor, a function of HIV prevalence. Further, demographic changes are ignored or, alternatively, it is assumed that the time scale under consideration is such that changes in population size are not too significant. The TB control reproduction number (under treatment) is given by the expression

$$\mathcal{R}_1 = \frac{\beta ck}{(\mu+k+r_1)(\mu+d+r_2)}, \tag{8.30}$$

while the HIV reproduction number is

$$\mathcal{R}_2 = \frac{\lambda\sigma}{\alpha_1+\mu}. \tag{8.31}$$

$\mathcal{R}_1$ is the product of [the average number of susceptible infected by one TB infectious individual over its effective infectious period, $\beta c/(\mu+d+r_2)$] $\times$ [the fraction of the population, $k/(\mu+k+r_1)$, that survives the TB latent period]. $\mathcal{R}_1$ denotes the number of secondary TB infectious cases generated by a typical TB infectious individual during its effective infectious period if introduced in a population of mostly TB-susceptible individuals, in a population where TB treatment is accessible. $\mathcal{R}_2$ is the HIV reproduction number in a TB-free society, the number of secondary HIV infectious produced by an HIV infectious (but not TB-infected) individual during its infectious period if introduced in a population of HIV-susceptible individuals (in a TB-free world). The reproductive numbers do not involve the parameters tied to the dynamics of TB/HIV coinfection, that is, k^* and α_3.

Consequently, the reproduction number for system (8.28) under TB treatment is given by

$$\mathcal{R} = \max\{\mathcal{R}_1, \mathcal{R}_2\}.$$

We have shown [76] that TB and HIV will die out if $\mathcal{R} < 1$, while either or both diseases may become endemic if $\mathcal{R} > 1$.

In [76], it was shown that system (8.28) is well-posed, that is, solutions that start in this octant where all the variables are nonnegative stay there. It was also shown that system (8.28) has three possible nonnegative boundary equilibria: the disease-free equilibrium (DFE) or E_0, the TB-only (HIV-free) equilibrium or E_T, and the HIV-only (TB-free) equilibrium or E_H. The components of E_0 are

$$S_0 = \frac{\Lambda}{\mu}, \quad L_0 = I_0 = T_0 = J_{01} = J_{02} = J_{03} = A_0 = 0.$$

The E_T components are

$$S_T = \frac{\Lambda}{\mu+\beta cI_T/N_T}, \quad L_T = \frac{I_T}{\mathcal{R}_{1b}}, \quad I_T = \frac{N_T(\mathcal{R}_1-1)}{\mathcal{R}_1+\mathcal{R}_{1a}}, \quad T_T = \frac{(r_1L+r_2I_T)S_T}{\Lambda},$$

$$J_{1T} = J_{2T} = J_{3T} = A_T = 0,$$

where

$$N_T = \frac{\Lambda}{\mu + d(\mathcal{R}_1 - 1)/(\mathcal{R}_1 + \mathcal{R}_{1a})},$$

with

$$\mathcal{R}_{1a} = \frac{c}{\mu + k + r_1}, \qquad \mathcal{R}_{1b} = \frac{k}{\mu + d + r_2}. \tag{8.32}$$

The E_H components are

$$S_H = \frac{\Lambda}{\mu \mathcal{R}_2 + \alpha_1(\mathcal{R}_2 - 1)}, \qquad L_H = I_H = T_H = 0,$$

$$J_{1H} = (\mathcal{R}_2 - 1)S_H, \qquad J_{2H} = J_{3H} = 0, \qquad A_H = \frac{\alpha_1 J_{1H}}{\mu + f}.$$

The following results were established in [76].

Theorem 8.8. *The disease-free equilibrium E_0 is locally asymptotically stable (LAS) if $\mathcal{R} < 1$, and it is unstable if $\mathcal{R} > 1$.*

Theorem 8.9. *The HIV-free equilibrium E_T is LAS if $\mathcal{R}_1 > 1$ and $\mathcal{R}_2 < 1$.*

We observe that E_H may not be LAS under the conditions $\mathcal{R}_1 < 1$ and $\mathcal{R}_2 > 1$. Our numerical studies show that when $\mathcal{R}_1 < 1$ and $\mathcal{R}_2 > 1$ it is possible that the equilibrium E_H is unstable and TB can coexist with HIV [76]. Further, whenever both reproduction numbers are greater than 1, that is, $\mathcal{R}_1 > 1$ and $\mathcal{R}_2 > 1$, E_T and E_H both exist and E_0 is unstable. Our numerical studies show that all three boundary equilibria are unstable and solutions converge to an interior equilibrium point. Furthermore, partial analytical results and numerical simulations support the existence of an interior equilibrium $\hat{E}$ when both reproduction numbers, $\mathcal{R}_1$ and $\mathcal{R}_2$, are greater than 1. The numerical simulations of the system further suggest that the interior equilibrium is LAS in most cases, although the possibility of stable periodic solutions seems likely [76].

8.5 Final Thoughts

In this chapter we revisited models for the transmission dynamics of HIV that focused on investigating the role of long incubation HIV periods within a single homogeneously mixing homosexually active population. The theory supports the view that the long incubation periods do not give rise to periodic outbreaks, that is, the disease either dies out or remains endemic. The *relative quantitative* effects of selecting alternative distributions to model the incubation period can be estimated. In [26] two extremes were compared.

First we assume that $P_I(x) = e^{-\alpha_I x}$, and $P_Y(x) = e^{-\alpha_Y x}$. The reproductive number, given by

$$\mathcal{R} = \lambda C \left(\frac{\Lambda}{\mu}\right) \int_0^\infty [pP_I(x) + (1-p)P_Y(x)]e^{-\mu x}dx,$$

reduces to

$$\mathcal{R}_1 = \lambda C\left(\frac{\Lambda}{\mu}\right)\left\{p\frac{1}{\mu+\alpha_I} + (1-p)\frac{1}{\mu+\alpha_Y}\right\}.$$

If we take the other extreme and assume that $P_I(x) = H(x) - H(x-\omega)$, $P_Y(x) = H(x) - H(x-\tau)$, where $H(x)$ denotes the Heaviside function (the fact that $P_I(x)$ and $P_Y(x)$ are not continuously differentiable is just a technical nuisance), then

$$\mathcal{R}_2 = \lambda C\left(\frac{\Lambda}{\mu}\right)\left\{p\frac{1-e^{-\mu\omega}}{\mu} + (1-p)\frac{1-e^{-\mu\tau}}{\mu}\right\}.$$

Hence, we have that

$$\frac{\mathcal{R}_1}{\mathcal{R}_2} = \frac{p\left(\frac{1}{\mu+\alpha_I}\right) + (1-p)\left(\frac{1}{\mu+\alpha_Y}\right)}{p\left(\frac{1-e^{-\mu\omega}}{\mu}\right) + (1-p)\left(\frac{1-e^{-\mu\tau}}{\mu}\right)} = f(p).$$

Therefore if we take $p = 0.5$, $\omega = 10$ years $(= 1/\alpha_I)$, $\tau = 30$ years $(= 1/\alpha_Y)$, $(1/\mu) = 30$ years, then $\mathcal{R}_1/\mathcal{R}_2 \approx 0.82$. If, for example, $\omega = 6$ years, $\tau = 30$ years $(= 1/\alpha_Y)$, $(1/\mu) = 30$ years, then

$$\frac{\mathcal{R}_1}{\mathcal{R}_2} = \frac{\frac{p}{6} + \frac{1-p}{2}}{p(1-e^{-2}) + (1-p)(1-e^{-1})}.$$

Hence $f(1/3)$, the ratio of the reproductive numbers, is approximately 0.81. A value of $p = 2/3$ gives a ratio of about 0.84, a value of $p = 8/9$ gives a ratio of about 0.88, and a value of $p = 1$ gives a ratio of about 0.92. In general, note that

$$f(p) = \frac{pD_{1,I} + (1-p)D_{1,Y}}{pD_{2,I} + (1-p)D_{2,Y}},$$

where the indices differentiate between the death-adjusted mean infectious periods for model 1 (exponential removal) and model 2 (fixed period of infectiousness). We further observe that $f(p)$ is an increasing function of p provided that

$$\frac{\mu + \frac{1}{\tau}}{\mu + \frac{1}{\omega}} > \frac{1-e^{-\mu\omega}}{1-e^{-\mu\tau}}$$

which holds whenever $\tau > \omega$. Hence whenever $\tau > \omega$, $f(p)$ satisfies

$$f(0) = \frac{D_{1,Y}}{D_{2,Y}} = \frac{\frac{1}{\mu+\alpha_Y}}{\frac{1-e^{-\mu\tau}}{\mu}} \le f(p) \le f(1) = \frac{D_{1,I}}{D_{2,I}} = \frac{\frac{1}{\mu+\alpha_I}}{\frac{1-e^{-\mu\omega}}{\mu}}, \quad 0 \le p \le 1.$$

Thus, even though the assumption of simple exponential removal underestimates the reproductive number, the above expression gives us a way to estimate the relative error because the above two distributions represent the two extremes. Hence, under the assumptions of the model, the "true" value of $\mathcal{R}$ lies somewhere in between. In addition, for a value p near unity (which unfortunately is not out of the realm of possibility), the qualitative dynamics predicted by these models are not very different. Furthermore, since the qualitative dynamics are governed largely by their reproductive numbers, and their values are not very different (at least for the realistic parameters chosen in the

> above examples), the effect of changing key parameters (once these are determined with higher accuracy) can be assessed readily. Note, however, that the transient dynamics could be quite different; this is partially due to the dimensionality of the system (finite versus infinite). If the infinite-dimensional model (that is, the distributed delay model) is more realistic, then it will be extremely difficult to predict the transient dynamics; that is, short-term predictions become more difficult. [26]

In [76] partial analytical results were obtained for the full 8-dimensional TB/HIV model (8.28). It was shown that the disease-free equilibrium is LAS whenever $\mathcal{R} < 1$, and that the HIV-free equilibrium with TB present is LAS if $\mathcal{R}_1 > 1$ and $\mathcal{R}_2 < 1$. Simulation showed disease coexistence when $\mathcal{R}_1 < 1$ and $\mathcal{R}_2 > 1$. No explicit expression for possible interior equilibrium $\hat{E}$ was obtained, but a pair of equations were derived in [76] that can be used to determine the existence of $\hat{E}$. Numerical studies support the view that the system has a unique interior equilibrium whenever $\mathcal{R} > 1$. As noted in [76]:

> The simulation results provided many interesting insights into the effect of the dynamical interactions between TB and HIV. For example, the results ... show that, when the progression from latent to active TB is faster in people with HIV than in people without (i.e., $k^* > k$), the presence of HIV can lead to the coexistence of TB and HIV even if the TB reproduction number ($\mathcal{R}_1$) is below 1 (i.e., TB infection would not be able to establish itself in the absence of HIV). However, the condition $k^* > k$ does not always lead to a significant increase in TB in the presence of HIV.... [Additional] results suggest that if $\alpha_3 >> \alpha_1$ (i.e., the development of HIV to AIDS is much faster in individuals co-infected with TB than without) then the effect of k^* will be diminished or not dramatic. However, simulation results ... suggest that when $\alpha_i > \alpha_1$, $i = 2,3$), the presence of TB may have a significant influence on HIV dynamics. Moreover, increasing α_2 and α_3 may lead to oscillatory behaviors of the system.
>
> Numerical results suggest that to reduce or control the impact of TB, investing more in reducing the prevalence of HIV can be an effective option. Such reductions would not be easy due to the lack of effective vaccine and medication. However, significant reductions may be obtained through programs that accelerate the treatment of active TB cases. Since there are about 8 million new cases of active TB per year, a program may be feasible. It has worked in countries that allocate substantial resources to public health. Naturally, accelerating the treatment rate of individuals with active TB is more critical in areas where HIV prevalence is high. Unfortunately, the areas with the highest prevalence of co-infections have limited resources and cannot implement accelerated TB treatment programs. [76]

Bibliography

[1] Anderson, R.M., R.M. May, G.F. Medley, and A. Johnson (1986) *A preliminary study of the transmission dynamics of the human immunodeficiency virus (HIV), the causative agent of AIDS*, IMA J. Math. Med. Bio. **3**: 229–263.

[2] Anderson, R.M. and R.M. May (1987) *Transmission dynamics of HIV infection*, Nature **326**: 137–142.

[3] Anderson, R.M. (1988) *The epidemiology of HIV infection: Variable incubation plus infectious periods and heterogeneity in sexual activity*, J. Roy. Stat. Soc. A **151**: 66–93.

[4] Anderson, R.M., D.R. Cox, and H.C. Hillier (1989) *Epidemiological and statistical aspects of the AIDS epidemic: Introduction*, Phil. Trans. Roy. Soc. Lond. B **325**: 39–44.

[5] Anderson, R.M., S.P. Blythe, S. Gupta, and E. Konings (1989) *The transmission dynamics of the Human Immunodeficiency Virus Type* 1 *in the male homosexual community in the United Kingdom: The influence of changes in sexual behavior*, Phil. Trans. R. Soc. Lond. B **325**: 145–198.

[6] Anderson, R.M. and R.M. May (1991) *Infectious Diseases of Humans*, Oxford Science Publications, Oxford.

[7] Aparicio, J.P., A.F. Capurro, and C. Castillo-Chavez (2002) *Markers of disease evolution: The case of tuberculosis*, J. Theor. Biol. **215**: 227–237.

[8] Bailey, N.T.J. (1988) *Statistical problems in the modeling and prediction of HIV/AIDS*, Aust. J. Stat. **3OA**: 41–55.

[9] Barré-Sinoussi, F., J.C. Chermann, F. Rey, M.T. Nugeyre, S. Chamaret, J. Gruest, C. Dauguet, C. Axler-Blin, F. Vézinet-Brun, C. Rouzioux et al. (1983) *Isolation of a T-lymphotropic retrovirus from a patient at risk for acquired immune deficiency syndrome (AIDS)*, Science **220**: 868–870.

[10] Blower, S., P. Small, and P. Hopewell (1996) *Control strategies for tuberculosis epidemics: New models for old problems*, Science **273**: 497–500.

[11] Blythe, S.P. and R.M. Anderson (1988) *Distributed incubation and infectious periods in models of the transmission dynamics of the human immunodeficiency virus (HIV)*, IMA J. Math. Med. Bio. **5**: 1–19.

[12] Blythe, S.P. and C. Castillo-Chavez (1989) *Like-with-like preference and sexual mixing models*, Math. Biosc. **96**: 221–238.

[13] Blythe, S.P., C. Castillo-Chavez, J. Palmer, and M. Cheng (1991) *Towards a unified theory of mixing and pair formation*, Math. Biosc. **107**: 379–405.

[14] Blythe S.P., K.L. Cooke, and C. Castillo-Chavez (1991) *Autonomous Risk-Behavior Change, and Non-linear Incidence Rate, in Models of Sexually Transmitted Diseases*, Biometrics Unit Technical Report B-1048-M.

[15] Blythe, S.P., C. Castillo-Chavez, and G. Casella (1992) *Empirical methods for the estimation of the mixing probabilities for socially structured populations from a single survey sample*, Mathematical Population Studies **3**: 199–225.

[16] Blythe, S.P., S. Busenberg, and C. Castillo-Chavez (1995) *Affinity and paired-event probability*, Math. Biosc. **128**: 265–284.

[17] Brookmeyer, R. and M.H. Gail (1988) *A method for obtaining short-term projections and lower bounds on the size of the AIDS epidemic*, J. Am. Stat. Assoc. **83**: 301–308.

[18] Busenberg, S. and C. Castillo-Chavez (1989) *Interaction, Pair Formation and Force of Infection Terms in Sexually Transmitted Diseases*, Lect. Notes in Biomath. **83**, Springer-Verlag, New York.

[19] Busenberg, S. and C. Castillo-Chavez (1991) *A general solution of the problem of mixing subpopulations, and its application to risk- and age-structured epidemic models for the spread of AIDS*, IMA J. of Mathematics Applied in Med. and Biol. **8**: 1–29.

[20] Castillo-Chavez, C., H.W. Hethcote, V. Andreasen, S.A. Levin, and W.M. Liu (1988) *Cross-Immunity in the Dynamics of Homogeneous and Heterogeneous Populations, Mathematical Ecology*, T.G. Hallam, L.G. Gross, and S.A. Levin, eds., World Scientific, Singapore: 303–316.

[21] Castillo-Chavez, C., ed. (1989) *Mathematical and Statistical Approaches to AIDS Epidemiology*, Lect. Notes in Biomath. **83**, Springer-Verlag, Berlin, Heidelberg, New York.

[22] Castillo-Chavez, C. (1989) *Review of recent models of HIV/AIDS transmission*, in Applied Mathematical Ecology, S. Levin, ed., Biomathematics Texts **18**, Springer-Verlag: 253–262.

[23] Castillo-Chavez, C., K. Cooke, W. Huang, and S.A. Levin (1989) *The role of long periods of infectiousness in the dynamics of acquired immunodeficiency syndrome*, in Mathematical approaches to resource management and epidemiology, C. Castillo-Chavez, S.A. Levin, and C. Shoemaker, eds., Lect. Notes in Biomath. **81**, Springer-Verlag, Berlin, Heidelberg, New York, London, Paris, Tokyo, Hong Kong: 177–189.

[24] Castillo-Chavez, C., K.L. Cooke, W. Huang, and S.A. Levin (1989) *Results on the dynamics for models for the sexual transmission of the human immunodeficiency virus*, Appl. Math. Letters **2**: 327–331.

[25] Castillo-Chavez, C., K. Cooke, W. Huang, and S.A. Levin (1989) *On the role of long incubation periods in the dynamics of HIV/AIDS. Part* 2*: Multiple group models*, in Mathematical and Statistical Approaches to AIDS Epidemiology, C. Castillo-Chavez, ed., Lect. Notes in Biomath. **83**, Springer-Verlag, Berlin, Heidelberg, New York: 200–217.

[26] Castillo-Chavez, C., K. Cooke, W. Huang, and S.A. Levin (1989) *The role of long incubation periods in the dynamics of HIV/AIDS. Part* 1*: Single populations models,* J. Math. Biol. **27**: 373–398.

[27] Castillo-Chavez, C. and S. Busenberg (1990) *On the solution of the two-sex mixing problem,* in Proceedings of the International Conference on Differential Equations and Applications to Biology and Population Dynamics, S. Busenberg and M. Martelli, eds., Lect. Notes in Biomath. **92,** Springer-Verlag, Berlin, Heidelberg, New York: 80–98.

[28] Castillo-Chavez, C., S. Busenberg, and K. Gerow (1990) *Pair formation in structured populations,* in Differential Equations with Applications in Biology, Physics and Engineering, J. Goldstein, F. Kappel, W. Schappacher, eds., Marcel Dekker, New York: 47–65.

[29] Castillo-Chavez, C., J.X. Velasco-Hernández, and S. Fridman (1993) *Modeling Contact Structures in Biology*, Lect. Notes in Biomath. **100**, Springer-Verlag.

[30] Castillo-Chavez, C., W. Huang, and J. Li (1996) *On the existence of stable pair distributions*, J. Math. Biol. **34**: 413–441.

[31] Castillo-Chavez, C. and Z. Feng (1998) *Mathematical models for the disease dynamics of tuberculosis*, in Advances in Mathematical Population Dynamics-Molecules, Cells and Man, M.A. Horn, G. Simonett, and G. Webb, eds., Vanderbilt University Press: 117–128.

[32] Castillo-Chavez, C. and S.-F. Hsu Schmitz (1997) *The evolution of age-structured marriage functions: It takes two to tango*, in Structured-Population Models Marine, Terrestrial, and Freshwater Systems, S. Tuljapurkar and H. Caswell, eds., Chapman and Hall, New York: 533–550.

[33] Castillo-Chavez, C. and Z. Feng (1997) *To treat or not to treat: The case of tuberculosis*, J. Math. Biol. **35**: 629–656.

[34] Castillo-Chavez, C. and Z. Feng (1998) *Global stability of an age-structure model for TB and its applications to optimal vaccination*, Math. Biosc. **151**: 135–154.

[35] Castillo-Chavez, C. and B. Song (2004) *Dynamical models of tuberculosis and their applications*, Math. Biosc. & Eng. **1**: 361–404.

[36] Cox, D.R. and G.F. Medley (1989) *A process of events with notification delay and the forecasting of AIDS*, Phil. Trans. Roy. Soc. Lond. B **325**: 135–145.

[37] Crawford, C.M., S.J. Schwager, and C. Castillo-Chavez (1990) *A Methodology for Asking Sensitive Questions among College Undergraduates*, Technical Report BU-1105-M in the Biometrics Unit series, Cornell University, Ithaca, NY.

[38] Dietz, K. (1988) *On the transmission dynamics of HIV*, Math. Biosci. **90**: 397–414.

[39] Dietz, K. and K.P. Hadeler (1988) *Epidemiological models for sexually transmitted diseases*, J. Math. Biol. **26**: 1–25.

[40] Feng, Z. and C. Castillo-Chavez (2000) *A model for tuberculosis with exogenous reinfection*, Theor. Pop. Biol. **57**: 235–247.

[41] Feng, Z., W. Huang, and C. Castillo-Chavez (2001) *On the role of variable latent periods in mathematical models for tuberculosis*, J. Dynam. Differential Equations **13**: 425–452.

[42] Gallo, R.C., S.Z. Salahuddin, M. Popovic, G.M. Shearer, M. Kaplan, B.F. Haynes, T. Palker, R. Redfield, J. Oleske, B. Safai, G. White, P. Foster, and P.D. Markhamet (1984) *Frequent detection and isolation of sytopathic retroviruses (HTLV-III) from patients with AIDS and at risk for AIDS*, Science **224**: 500–503.

[43] Gallo, R.C. (1986) *The first human retrovirus*, Scientific American **255**: 88–98.

[44] Godfrey-Faussett, P., D. Maher, Y. Mukadi, P. Nunn, J. Perriens, and M. Raviglione (2002) *How human immunodeficiency virus voluntary testing can contribute to tuberculosis control*, Bulletin of the World Health Organization **80**: 939–945.

[45] Gupta S., R.M. Anderson, and R.M. May (1989) *Networks of sexual contacts: Implications for the pattern of spread of HIV*, AIDS **3**: 1–11.

[46] Francis, D.P., P.M. Feorino, J.R. Broderson, H.M. Mcclure, J.P. Getchell, C.R. Mcgrath, B. Swenson, J.S. Mcdougal, E.L. Palmer, and A.K. Harrison (1984) *Infection of chimpanzees with lymphadenopathy-associated virus*, Lancet **2**: 1276–1277.

[47] Hadeler, K.P. (1989) *Modeling AIDS in structured populations*, in Proceedings of the 47th Session of the International Statistical Institute, Paris, **C1-2**: 83–99.

[48] Hadeler, K.P. and C. Castillo-Chavez (1995) *A core group model for disease transmission*, Math. Biosc. **128**: 41–55.

[49] Hethcote, H.W., H.W. Stech, and P. van den Driessche (1981) *Nonlinear oscillations in epidemic models*, SIAM J. Appl. Math. **40**: 1–9.

[50] Hethcote, H.W. and J.W. van Ark (1987) *Epidemiological methods for heterogeneous populations: Proportional mixing, parameter estimation, and immunization programs*, Math. Biosc. **84**: 85–118.

[51] Hethcote, H.W. and J.W. Van Ark (1992) *Modeling HIV Transmission and AIDS in the United States*, Lect. Notes in Biomath. **95**, Springer-Verlag, Berlin, Heidelberg, New York.

[52] Hsu Schmitz, S.F. (1993) *Some Theories, Estimation Methods and Applications of Marriage Functions and Two-Sex Mixing Functions in Demography and Epidemiology*, Unpublished doctoral dissertation, Cornell University, Ithaca, New York.

[53] Hsu Schmitz, S.F. and C. Castillo-Chavez (1994) *Parameter estimation in non-closed social networks related to dynamics of sexually transmitted diseases*, in Modeling the AIDS Epidemic: Planning, Policy, and Prediction, E.H. Kaplan and M.L. Brandeau, eds., Raven Press, New York: 533–559.

[54] Huang, W., K.L. Cooke, and C. Castillo-Chavez (1992) *Stability and bifurcation for a multiple-group model for the dynamics of HIV/AIDS transmission*, SIAM J. Appl. Math. **52**: 835–854.

[55] Hyman, J.M. and E.A. Stanley (1988) *A risk base model for the spread of the AIDS virus*, Math. Biosc. **90**: 415–473.

[56] Hyman, J.M. and E.A. Stanley (1989) *The effects of social mixing patterns on the spread of AIDS*, in Mathematical Approaches to Problems in Resource Management and Epidemiology, C. Castillo-Chavez, S.A. Levin, and C.A. Shoemaker, eds., Lect. Notes in Biomath. **81**, Springer-Verlag, Berlin: 190–219.

[57] Isham, V. (1989) *Estimation of the incidence of HIV infection*, Phil. Trans. Roy. Soc. Lond. B **325**: 113–121.

[58] Kaplan, E.H. (1989) *What Are the Risks of Risky Sex?*, Operations Research.

[59] Kingsley, R.A., R. Kaslow, C.R. Rinaldo Jr., K. Detre, N. Odaka, M. VanRaden, R. Detels, B.F. Polk, J. Chimel, S.F. Kersey, D. Ostrow, and B. Visscher (1987) *Risk factors for seroconversion to human immunodeficiency virus among male homosexuals*, Lancet **1**: 345–348.

[60] Kirschner, D. (1999) *Dynamics of co-infection with M. tuberculosis and HIV*-1, Theor. Pop. Biol. **55**: 94–109.

[61] Koelle, K., S. Cobey, B. Grenfell, and M. Pascual (2006) *Epochal evolution shapes the phylodynamics of interpandemic influenza A (H3N2) in humans*, Science **314**: 1898–1903.

[62] Koopman, J., C.P. Simon, J.A. Jacquez, J. Joseph, L. Sattenspiel, and T. Park (1988) *Sexual partner selectiveness effects on homosexual HIV transmission dynamics*, Journal of AIDS **1**: 486–504.

[63] Lange, J.M., D.A. Paul, H.G. Huisman, F. De Wolf, H. van den Berg, R.A. Coutinho, S.A. Danner, J. van der Noordaa, and J. Goudsmit (1986) *Persistent HIV antigenaemia and decline of HIV core antibodies associated with transition to AIDS*. Brit. Med. J. **293**: 1459–1462.

[64] Lagakos, S.W., L.M. Barraj, and V. de Gruttola (1988) *Nonparametric analysis of truncated survival data, with applications to AIDS*, Biometrika **75**: 515–523.

[65] Luo, X., and C. Castillo-Chavez (1991) *Limit behavior of pair formation for a large dissolution rate*, Journal of Mathematical Systems, Estimation, and Control **3**: 247–264.

[66] May, R.M. and R.M. Anderson (1989) *Possible demographic consequence of HIV/AIDS epidemics: II. Assuming HIV infection does not necessarily lead to AIDS*, in Mathematical Approaches to Problems in Resource Management and Epidemiology C. Castillo-Chavez, S.A. Levin, and C.A. Shoemaker, eds., Lect. Notes in Biomath. **81**, Springer-Verlag, Berlin, Heidelberg, New York, London, Paris, Tokyo, Hong Kong: 220–248.

[67] May, R.M. and R.M. Anderson (1989) *The transmission dynamics of human immunodeficiency virus (HIV)*, in Applied Mathematical Ecology, S. Levin, ed., Biomathematics Texts **18**, Springer-Verlag, New York.

[68] Medley, G.F., R.M. Anderson, D.R. Cox, and L. Billiard (1987) *Incubation period of AIDS in patients infected via blood transfusions*, Nature **328**: 719–721.

[69] Miller, R.K. (1971) *Nonlinear Volterra Integral Equations*, Benjamin, Menlo Park, CA.

[70] Morin, B., C. Castillo-Chavez, S.F. Hsu Schmitz, A. Mubayi, and X. Wang (2010) *Notes from the heterogeneous: A few observations on the implications and necessity of affinity*, Journal of Biological Dynamics **4**: 456–477.

[71] Naresh, R. and A. Tripathi (2005) *Modelling and analysis of HIV-TB Co-infection in a variable size population*, Mathematical Modelling and Analysis **10**: 275–286.

[72] Pickering, J., J.A. Wiley, N.S. Padian et al. (1986) *Modeling the incidence of acquired immunodeficiency syndrome (AIDS) in San Francisco, Los Angeles, and New York*, Math. Modelling **7**: 661–688.

[73] Porco, T. and S. Blower (1998) *Quantifying the intrinsic transmission dynamics of tuberculosis*, Theor. Pop. Biol. **54**: 117–132.

[74] Porco, T., P. Small, and S. Blower (2001) *Amplification dynamics: Predicting the effect of HIV on tuberculosis outbreaks*, Journal of Acquired Immune Deficiency Syndromes **28**: 437–444.

[75] Raimundo, S.M., A.B. Engel, H.M. Yang, and R.C. Bassanezi (2003) *An approach to estimating the transmission coefficients for AIDS and for tuberculosis using mathematical models*, Systems Analysis Modelling Simulation **43**: 423–442.

[76] Roeger, L.-I.W., Z. Feng, and C. Castillo-Chavez (2009) *The impact of HIV infection on tuberculosis*, Math. Biosc. & Eng. **6**: 815–837.

[77] Rubin, G., D. Umbauch, S.-F. Shyu, and C. Castillo-Chavez (1992) *Application of capture-recapture methodology to estimation of size of population at risk of AIDS and/or other sexually-transmitted diseases*, Statistics in Medicine **11**: 1533–1549.

[78] Salahuddin, S.Z., J.E. Groopman, P.D. Markham, M.G. Sarngaharan, R.R. Redfield, M.F. McLane, M. Essex, A. Sliski, and R.C. Gallo (1984) *HTLV-III in symptom-free seronegative persons*, Lancet **2**: 1418–1420.

[79] Sattenspiel, L. (1989) *The structure and context of social interactions and the spread of HIV*, in Mathematical and Statistical Approaches to AIDS Epidemiology, C. Castillo-Chavez, ed., Lect. Notes in Biomath. **83**, Springer-Verlag, Berlin: 242–259.

[80] Sattenspiel, L., J. Koopman, C.P. Simon, and J.A. Jacquez (1990) *The effects of population subdivision on the spread of the HIV infection*, American Journal of Physical Anthropology **82**: 421–429.

[81] Sattenspiel, L. and C. Castillo-Chavez (1990) *Environmental context, social interactions, and the spread of HIV*, American J. of Human Biology **2**: 397–417.

[82] Schinazi, R.B. (2003) *Can HIV invade a population which is already sick?*, Bull. Braz. Math. Soc. (N.S.) **34**: 479–488.

[83] Schulzer, M., M.P. Radhamani, S. Grybowski, E. Mak, and J.M. Fitzgerald (1994) *A mathematical model for the prediction of the impact of HIV infection on tuberculosis*, Int. J. Epidemiol. **23**: 400–407.

[84] Schwager, S., C. Castillo-Chavez, and H.W. Hethcote (1989) *Statistical and mathematical approaches to AIDS epidemiology: A review*, in Mathematical and Statistical Approaches to AIDS Epidemiology, C. Castillo-Chavez, ed., Lect. Notes in Biomath. **83**, Springer-Verlag, Berlin: 2–35.

[85] Thieme, H. and C. Castillo-Chavez (1989) *On the role of variable infectivity in the dynamics of the human immunodeficiency virus epidemic*, in Mathematical and Statistical Approaches to AIDS Epidemiology, C. Castillo-Chavez, ed., Lect. Notes in Biomath. **83**, Springer-Verlag, Berlin, Heidelberg, New York, London, Paris, Tokyo, Hong Kong: 157–176.

[86] Thieme, H.R. and C. Castillo-Chavez (1993) *How may infection-age dependent infectivity affect the dynamics of HIV/AIDS?*, SIAM J. Appl. Math. **53**: 1447–1479.

[87] UNAIDS (1997) *Tuberculosis and AIDS: UNAIDS Point of View*, UNAIDS, Geneva.

[88] West, R. and J. Thompson (1996) *Modeling the impact of HIV on the spread of tuberculosis in the United States*, Math. Biosc. **143**: 35–60.

[89] WHO (World Health Organization) (2006) *Global Summary of the AIDS Epidemic*, http://www.who.int/hiv/mediacentre/02-Global/Summary/2006/EpiUpdate/eng.pdf.

[90] WHO (World Health Organization) (2007) *Tuberculosis Facts*, http://www.who.int/tb/publications/2007/factsheet/2007.pdf.

[91] Wong-Staal, F. and R.C. Gallo (1985) *Human T-lymphotropic retroviruses*, Nature **317**: 395–403.

[92] Wu, L.-I. and Z. Feng (2000) *Homoclinic bifurcation in an SIQR model for childhood diseases*, J. Diff. Equations **168**: 150–167.

Lecture 9

Dynamical Models of Tuberculosis and Applications

9.1 Introduction

The success of deterministic and stochastic mathematical models in advancing population dynamics theory is connected to the development of effective paradigms or frameworks built under specific, oversimplified, mechanistic, or phenomenological assumptions by theoreticians or mathematicians. The "mean" field models revisited in this lecture are characteristic of such efforts, and their analyses increase our understanding of, for example, the dynamics of coevolving processes, like demography and disease. The success of the computational, modeling, and theoretical enterprise depends on the flexibility of a framework to capture key (question-specific) features with a minimal number of (hopefully) measurable parameters.

Mycobacterium tuberculosis is the etiological agent of tuberculosis (TB), an organism capable of supporting huge levels of TB (high disease prevalence) in populations across the world particular, in areas dominated by coexisting "neglected" human diseases like malaria or HIV. Overpopulated economically challenged regions of the world facilitate or reinforce the success of coinfections, increased disease morbidity, or mortality. Urbanization, a process that exploded after the Industrial Revolution, has been considered a major driver of TB spread [27, 28, 29].

The historical reduction in TB progression rates (from latent to active TB) are connected to demographic, epidemiological, and social factors operating over multiple organizational and/or temporal scales, and teasing out their relative importance is being carried out with the aid of mathematical models that incorporate epidemiological forces (exogenous and endogenous reinfections), demographic changes, and human mobility. This lecture provides an overview of some of the questions raised and associated models used to study the transmission dynamics and control of tuberculosis [1, 3, 6]. The underlying goals of these chapters are still ambitious. Specifically, we hope that mathematicians may find challenges in the study of frameworks used to build evidence-based and model-driven public health policies [1, 3, 6, 18, 20, 21, 24, 52, 60, 61, 69]. It is estimated that one in three individuals in the world are infected with TB, although most carry TB as a latent inactive infection. Models for studying TB dynamics are introduced. They are used to explore the potential role of identified transmission mechanisms on disease dynamics at the population level. Population structure, including age structure, is included because heterogeneity is most often at the heart of issues like susceptibility, mobility, and mortality, processes that are important in the study of TB disease dynamics (see [6]). This chapter provides an overview of TB models using as its platform our decade-old review (see [17]). The discussion in this chapter is based on prior modeling and mathematical work, including [1, 3, 6, 18, 20, 21, 24, 52, 60, 61, 69].

9.2 Intrinsic Mechanics of Transmission

Tuberculosis is primarily transmitted through the air (coughing) from sources that include individuals with active TB infections, particularly pulmonary tuberculosis. The probability of transmission per contact, per unit of time, may be in general quite low today, a conclusion based on the fact that active TB is "rare" (roughly 8–9 million cases per year in a population of 2 billion latent cases). Individuals at high risk of infection include those exposed for long period of times to infectious individuals, for example, those living within a small group of individuals with active TB infections. Medical personnel in TB hospitals may face continuous risk of acquiring an active infection. Assessing TB levels (prevalence) is not simple since most infected individuals today remain asymptomatic (latent TB) over their entire lifetimes. Active TB infections (clinical disease) may or may not progress into pulmonary or extrapulmonary forms. Extrapulmonary TB is most common in children, while pulmonary TB is seen primarily among adults. *Mycobacterium tuberculosis* is transmitted *almost* exclusively via pulmonary cases (exceptions may include laryngeal TB). Cases activated within five years following infection are classified as *primary*, while cases that emerge in some parts of the world five years after the initial infection are referred to as *secondary*. Endogenous reactivation (exacerbation of an old infection) or exogenous tuberculosis (the result of reinfection) are classified as secondary cases of TB activation. The number of new TB-active cases has been seen to decline more or less exponentially as a function of the age of infection [63] (see Figure 9.1). Styblo [63] reviews the results of a ten-year follow-up study that concludes that (i) nearly 60% of new active TB infections emerge over the first year following infection; and (ii) the cumulative number of cases over the first five years, following an primary infection, account for nearly 95% of total observed cases. From Figure 9.1, we detect exponential decline in progression risk. If such a trend were to continue over the lifetime of individuals, then endogenous reactivation contributions to progression would be small, possibly less than 5% (higher increases on the risk of endogenous reactivation in the elderly may include immune system depression). Smear positive pulmonary tuberculosis cases have turned out to be more infectious than smear negative (culture positive or culture negative cases), signaling the possibility that differences in infectiousness also play a role [53, 63], while the rise in infections has enhanced the role of endogenous reactivation. We observe that untreated pulmonary TB-case fatality is not uniform and around 50% variability arises from sources that include length of the infectious period, the strength of the hosts' immunological responses following primary infections, and the likelihood of early TB activation [7]. Recovered individuals, naturally or from treatment, may develop active TB again, that is, TB relapse is also a possible outcome.

9.2.1 Towards the development of TB models

Different models have been used to study the long-term dynamics of TB and an overview of some of them are discussed in this lecture, including simple standard-incidence

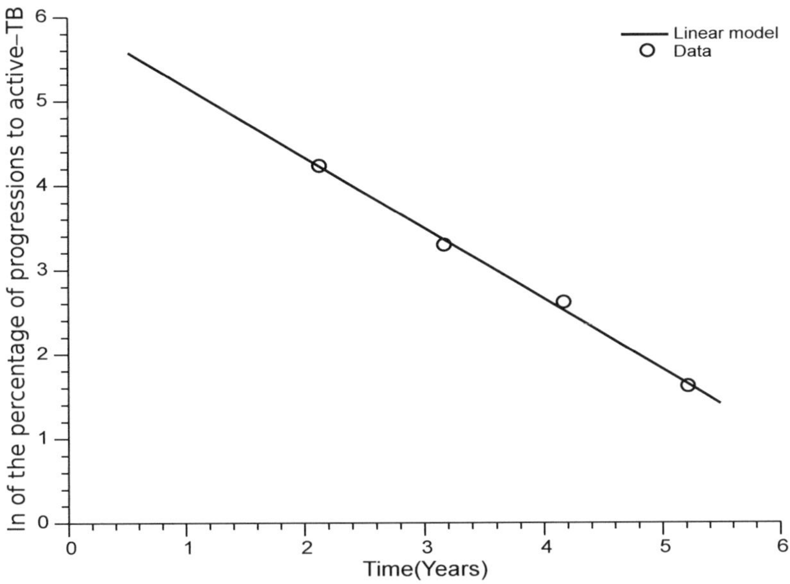

Figure 9.1. *New TB-active cases have declined almost exponentially as a function of the age of infection. Modified from Styblo* [63].

compartmental models (extensions of the models in [3, 4, 5]), aggregated cluster models (extensions of the models in [1, 6, 60]), and age-structured models [6]. The risks posed by TB are typically assessed over long windows of time since disease progression is extremely slow. Transmission most likely takes place primarily within small groups of close acquaintances. That is, infection and progression outcomes depend on local, regional, social, and environmental conditions. In the U.S., TB is in a declining phase. TB peaked roughly around the middle of the 19th century. We have not seen upward trends within the U.S., except for a small period of re-emergence at the start of the U.S. HIV epidemic. A full description of U.S. TB trends and the causes behind the actual long-term U.S. TB dynamics decline makes use of a model that factors in U.S. historical epidemic patterns and substantial U.S. demographic shifts [1, 3, 4, 6]. Relevant references, including additional mathematical and modeling details quite similar to those highlighted in this volume, can be found in [17].

9.2.2 Slow and fast modes of TB transmission

It is believed that exposed individuals, infected hosts with no symptoms, have initially a higher risk of developing active or symptomatic TB than those who have managed a latent-TB infection for some time. Individuals who escape the initial risk-progression stage, that is, those with asymptomatic (latent) infections, still face the possibility of progressing to the infectious TB stage. It is believed that the rate of TB progression dramatically slows down among healthy individuals. In other words, the likelihood of becoming TB symptomatic (active infection) decreases with age of the infection.

We review simple models and modeling approaches in the context of TB progression. We focus on those found in [9, 10, 11, 19, 25, 47]. The population is partitioned into three

Table 9.1. *Symbols and definitions of parameters (from* [17]*).*

Symbol	Explanation
Λ	recruitment rate
β	transmission rate (meaning varies)
c	average number of contacts per person per unit time
k	per-capita regular progression rate
μ	per-capita natural mortality rate
d	per-capita excess death rate due to TB
r_0	per-capita treatment rate for recently latently infected
r_1	per-capita treatment rate for latently infected
r_2	per-capita treatment rate for actively infected
ω	per-capita progression rate for early latent-TB progression

epidemiological classes: susceptible, latent, and infectious (as in [9, 10, 11]). The infection rate modeled, via βSI (mass-action law), is budgeted (a priori) as follows: the portion $p\beta SI$ is assumed to give rise to active cases immediately, while the rest, $(1-p)\beta SI$, gives rise to latent asymptomatic TB cases. The progression rate, slow TB, from the latent to the active TB stage, is assumed to be proportional to the number of latent TB cases; kE, where k is a positive constant (the range, 0.00256 to 0.00527, slow progression, is reasonable). The total incidence rate, new cases of active TB per unit of time, is given by $p\beta SI + kE$. The version in [9] is given by the following system of nonlinear differential equations:

$$\frac{dS}{dt} = \Lambda - \beta SI - \mu S, \tag{9.1}$$

$$\frac{dE}{dt} = (1-p)\beta SI - kE - \mu E, \tag{9.2}$$

$$\frac{dI}{dt} = p\beta SI + kE - dI - \mu I, \tag{9.3}$$

with parameters defined in Table 9.1. The qualitative dynamics of model (9.1)–(9.3) are rather straightforward and, naturally, governed by the basic reproductive number $\mathcal{R}_0$, which has been discussed often in this volume. Specifically, we have that

$$\mathcal{R}_0 = p\frac{\Lambda}{\mu}\frac{\beta}{\mu+d} + (1-p)\frac{\Lambda}{\mu}\frac{k}{\mu+k}. \tag{9.4}$$

This dimensionless number or ratio quantifies the average number of secondary infectious cases produced by a "typical" infectious individual in a population of susceptibles, at a demographic steady state. The first term in (9.4) gives the number of new cases generated via fast progression, while the second those arising from slow progression. The analysis of this model is straightforward. Simulation of system (9.4) shows that TB dynamics are quite slow for acceptable TB parameter ranges (similar models, like Waaler's [67], also supported slow TB dynamics). Model drawbacks include the fact that p, a fixed proportion, must be known a priori. In addition, $\mathcal{R}_0$ as defined depends linearly on population size, an important fact that cannot be overlooked given that the model includes the impact of TB on mortality.

9.2.3 Variable latent period

Information on the development of clinical or active TB in tuberculin converters in the general population can be found in, for example, the British Medical Research Council's TB vaccines trial. This trial involved 243 cases, initially tuberculin-negative, among the participating population, who developed the (active) disease within 8 years. This study reports that 54% developed the disease within a year; 29% during the next 3 years; and 17% during the last 4 years. The data over the past century show that TB has evolved a "friendly" relationship with human hosts. This observation arises from the fact that only a *relatively small proportion* of infected individuals go on to develop clinical disease (active TB). Today, most individuals seem capable of mounting an effective immune response to infection, the kind of response that limits proliferation of the bacilli and leads to long-lasting partial immunity to further active infections and/or to the reactivation of the latent bacilli. As is often the case, the risk of disease is highest shortly after infection, declining thereafter. The inclusion of typical TB epidemiological features is considered via the generalization of the model introduced that assumed that a prespecified a priori proportion (p) of infected individuals would get active TB (on a fast time scale) per unit of time. The most general version of the model incorporates a distributed delay that accounts for the effects of variable periods of latency (rather than exponentially distributed) on TB dynamics, the topic of this section.

We let $p(s)$ denote a function that represents the proportion of individuals who become exposed at time t and that, if alive, remain infected (but not infectious) at time $t+s$, that is, the proportion of individuals who survive as infected but not infectious. We naturally assume that

$$p(s) \geq 0, \quad \dot{p}(s) \leq 0, \quad p(0) = 1,$$

and

$$\int_0^\infty p(s)ds < \infty.$$

The total number of TB-exposed individuals from the initial time $t = 0$ to the current time t, who are still in the E class, is therefore given by the integral

$$\int_0^t \sigma S(s)\frac{I(s)}{N(s)}p(t-s)e^{-(\mu+r_1)(t-s)}ds.$$

Since $-\dot{p}(\tau)$ is the rate of removal of individuals from the L class into the I class τ units of time after effective exposure, then the number of individuals becoming infectious from time 0 to t that survive (alive) now in the I class is given by the double integral

$$\int_0^t \int_0^\tau \sigma S(s)\frac{I(s)}{N(s)}e^{-(\mu+r_1)(\tau-s)}\left(-\dot{p}(\tau-s)e^{-(\mu+r_2+d)(t-\tau)}\right)dsd\tau.$$

Hence, a model that includes arbitrarily distributed latency periods [24] via the introduction of the function $p(s)$ and, therefore, with $-\dot{p}(\tau)$ denoting the removal rate from the E into the I class τ units of time after exposure, is given by the following system of nonlinear integro-differential equations:

$$\frac{dS}{dt} = \Lambda - \sigma S \frac{I}{N} - \mu S + r_1 E + r_2 I, \tag{9.5}$$

$$E(t) = E_0(t) + \int_0^t \sigma S(s) \frac{I(s)}{N(s)} p(t-s) e^{-(\mu+r_1)(t-s)} ds, \tag{9.6}$$

$$\begin{aligned} I(t) &= \int_0^t \int_0^\tau \sigma S(s) \frac{I(s)}{N(s)} e^{-(\mu+r_1)(\tau-s)} \left(-\dot{p}(\tau-s) e^{-(\mu+r_2+d)(t-\tau)}\right) ds d\tau \\ &\quad + I_0 e^{-(\mu+r_2+d)t} + I_0(t), \qquad (9.7) \\ N &= S + E + I, \end{aligned}$$

with $\sigma = \beta c$ denoting the force of infection per susceptible and per infective; r_1 and r_2 model the (assumed constant) per-capita treatment rates for the E and I classes, respectively; μ is the natural per-capita mortality rate; d is the added per-capita death rate due to TB; $E_0(t)$ denotes the individuals in the E class at time $t = 0$ still in the latent class at time t; $I_0(t)$ denotes the individuals initially in the E class who moved to the I class and are still alive at time t; and $I_0 e^{-(\mu+r_2+d)t}$, with $I_0 = I(0)$ representing individuals infectious at time 0, denotes individuals still alive in the I class at time t. It is assumed that $E_0(t)$ and $I_0(t)$ have compact support.

The introduction of an arbitrary latency period distribution does not change the qualitative local dynamics of TB. That is, the dynamics are qualitatively equivalent (locally) to those generated from the simplest model. In fact, a forward bifurcation characterizes the dynamics of both of these models (see [24] and Figure 9.2) (9.5)–(9.7).

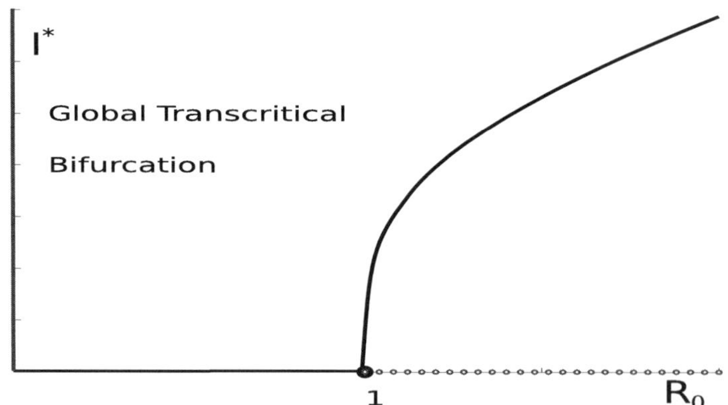

Figure 9.2. *Forward bifurcation diagram for TB models (modified from Figure 7 of* [17, p. 380]*). We see that if $\mathcal{R}_0 > 1$, the disease grows and reaches an endemic equilibrium; otherwise it dies out. The analysis is local for the distributed delay case but global for system* (9.1)–(9.3).

9.2.4 Multiple strains—competitive interference and coexistence

Exploring the joint dynamics of drug-resistant and drug-sensitive TB strains is certainly of interest, particularly since incomplete drug treatment and/or coinfections, especially but not exclusively with HIV, facilitate or accelerate the emergence of drug-resistant TB strains (multiple drug resistant, or MDR, strains). It is certainly in our interest to quantify the risks posed by scenarios where drug-resistant TB strains survive (coexisting with drug-sensitive strains). Multiple TB-strain models have been introduce to study the competitive dynamics of diseases [12]. In the context of influenza, possibly the most (mathematically) studied multistrain disease, substantial theoretical work has been carried out (see, for example, [14, 15, 31, 44, 45, 46]). In the context of prevalent intestinal infections, caused by coexisting *rotavirus* strains, vaccines have been developed to address transmission challenges. Monovalent (making use of the most prevalent rotavirus type) and multivalent vaccines (built around multiple strains) have been deployed over the past few years. Through the use of our models, we found that the study of the rotavirus' vaccine dynamics in a population where rotavirus infections are highly prevalent are somewhat similar to those found in the literature under "dynamics of competing disease strains." Here, we deal with a situation in which one severe strain (real disease) and one mild strain (vaccine) are in competition (see [57, 58, 59]). Research that explores the joint dynamics of drug-resistant and sensitive TB strains, under the assumption that such strains compete for hosts (interference competition), has also been carried out [10, 18, 20]. The emerging outcomes that arise when drug-resistant and drug-sensitive strains compete are studied here [18, 20]. We observe that the focus in this chapter is on the study of mathematical scenarios that involve a large number of individuals facing drug-sensitive and *naturally or mutationally driven* drug-resistant TB strains. If the subscripts s and r are used to denote drug-sensitive and drug-resistant strains, then the multistrain TB model used is given by the following nonlinear system:

$$\frac{dS}{dt} = \Lambda - \beta_s cS\frac{I_s}{N} - \beta_r cS\frac{I_r}{N} - \mu S, \tag{9.8}$$

$$\frac{dE_s}{dt} = \beta_s cS\frac{I_s}{N} - (\mu + k_s)E_s - r_{1s}E_s + pr_{2s}I_s - \beta_s cE_s\frac{I_r}{N}, \tag{9.9}$$

$$\frac{dI_s}{dt} = k_s E_s - (\mu + d_s)I_s - r_{2s}I_s, \tag{9.10}$$

$$\frac{dT}{dt} = r_{1s}E_s + (1-p-q)r_{2s} - \beta_s cT\frac{I_s}{N} - \beta_r cT\frac{I_r}{N} - \mu T, \tag{9.11}$$

$$\frac{dE_r}{dt} = qr_{2s}I_s - (\mu + k_r)E_r + \beta_r c(S + E_s + T)\frac{I_r}{N}, \tag{9.12}$$

$$\frac{dI_r}{dt} = k_r E_r - (\mu + d_r)I_r, \tag{9.13}$$

$$N = S + E_s + I_s + T + E_r + I_r.$$

Since treatment is not an option for the I_r class, the treatment rate is set at zero ($q = 0$ in (9.12)). The proportion p modifies the rate at which untreated individuals depart from the latent class; $p + q$ represents the proportion of treated infectious individuals who do not complete treatment; and $qr_{2s}I_s$ denotes the rate at which individuals develop resistant TB from lack of compliance with treatment. Consequently, $1 - p - q$ denotes the proportion of

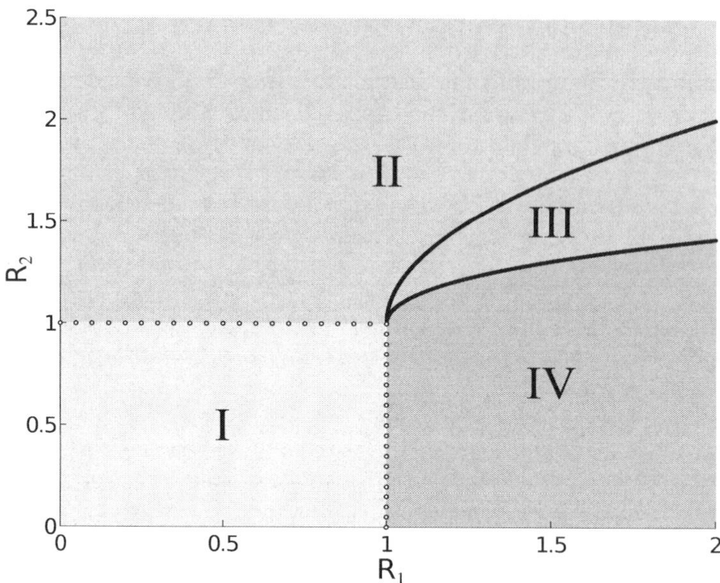

Figure 9.3. *Bifurcation diagram for model* (9.8)–(9.13) *when* $q = 0$ *(see* [20]*). In region I, the disease-free equilibrium is globally asymptotically stable; in regions II and IV, one of strains disappears; III represents the region of strain coexistence (modified from Figure* 3 *of* [17, p. 369]*).*

successfully treated individuals. The dimensionless quantities (numbers or ratios) given by

$$\mathcal{R}_1 = \left(\frac{\beta_s c + p r_{2s}}{\mu + d_s + r_{2s}}\right)\left(\frac{k_s}{\mu + k_s + d_s}\right)$$

and

$$\mathcal{R}_2 = \left(\frac{\beta_r c}{\mu + d_r}\right)\left(\frac{k_r}{\mu + k_r}\right)$$

represent the basic reproductive number of strains j, $j = 1,2$. It has been shown that $\mathcal{R}_j$ controls the asymptotic behavior of model (9.8)–(9.13), and Figures 9.3 and 9.4 provide a bifurcation diagram collecting the dynamical outcomes for the two-strain model when *naturally* resistant and wild strains (drug-sensitive) coexist. We see that the region of coexistence is small (region IV in Figure 9.3). On the other hand it has been established [20] that *antibiotic induced resistance* generates substantial expansions in the size of the region of coexistence. Specifically, regions IV and III fuse into a single *large* region of coexistence; that is, minimal levels of human-induced antibiotic resistance would virtually guarantee resistant strains' survival. The systematic lack of 100% population compliance with antibiotic regimes means that we must continue to deal with the emergence and reemergence of resistant TB strains (see also [10]). The development and implementation of effective policies that take into account imperfect (or nonexistent) access to treatment and deficient compliance regimes are central to public health policies that aim at minimizing the impact of TB or wish to prevent public health disasters.

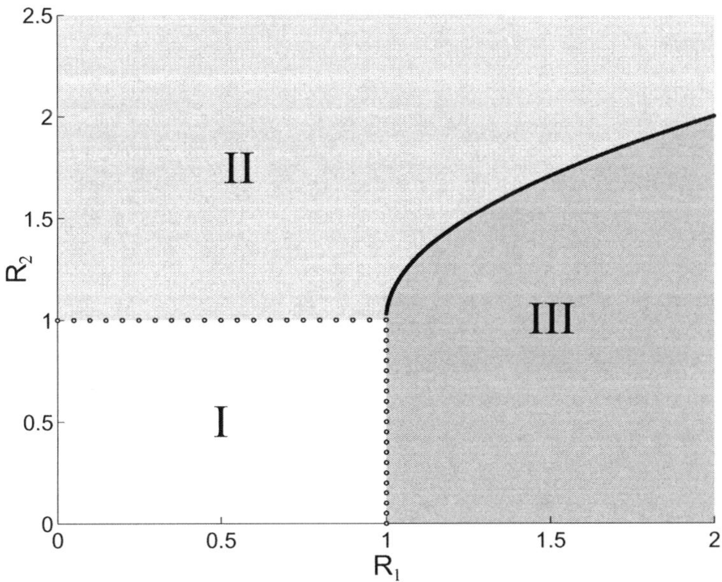

Figure 9.4. *Bifurcation diagram for model* (9.8)–(9.13) *when* $q > 0$. *The coexistence of the two strains is impossible (see* [20]*) (modified from Figure* 4 *of* [17, p. 369]*).*

9.2.5 Exogenous reinfection—novel mechanism for disease progression

The dynamical outcomes that follow the establishment of a TB infection vary from individual to individual. Right after a primary infection is settled, individuals on average tend to experience a higher risk of *fast* disease progression (becoming a TB-active case). Infected individuals who do not become infectious "quickly" (active TB) may nevertheless still develop active infections (naturally over a longer time scale) via alternative mechanisms that include exogenous or endogenous reinfections. The potential impact of exogenous reinfection on the dynamics of TB has been discussed in the past. The model in [25] has been used to highlight the potential impact of exogenous reinfection. We illustrate such a possibility [25] via the following model:

$$\frac{dS}{dt} = \Lambda - \beta c S \frac{I}{N} - \mu S, \tag{9.14}$$

$$\frac{dE}{dt} = \beta c S \frac{I}{N} - p\beta c E \frac{I}{N} - (\mu + k)E + \sigma \beta c T \frac{I}{N}, \tag{9.15}$$

$$\frac{dI}{dt} = p\beta c E \frac{I}{N} + kE - (\mu + r + d)I, \tag{9.16}$$

$$\frac{dT}{dt} = rI - \sigma \beta c T \frac{I}{N} - \mu T \tag{9.17}$$

$$N = S + E + I + T.$$

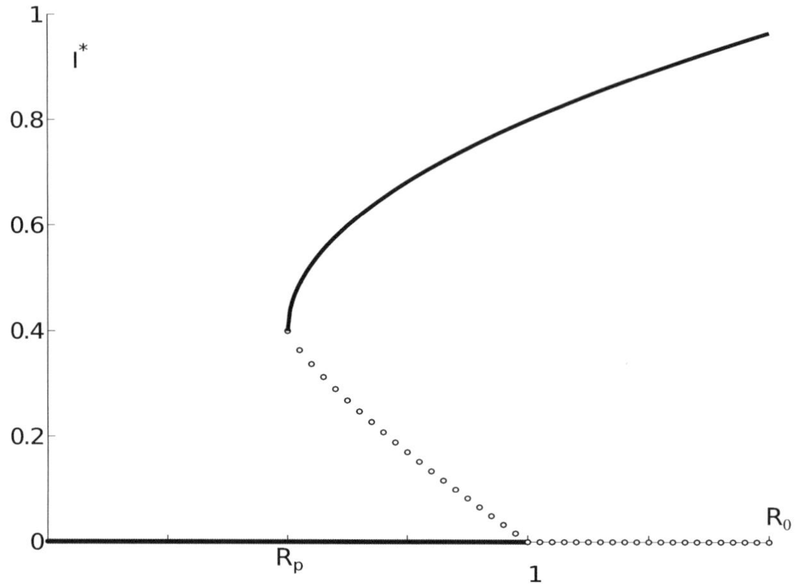

Figure 9.5. *Backward bifurcation diagram generated by exogenous reinfection, model* (9.14)–(9.17). *When $\mathcal{R}_0 < \mathcal{R}_p$, the disease-free equilibrium is globally asymptotically stable. However, when $\mathcal{R}_p < \mathcal{R}_0 < 1$, there are two endemic equilibria. The upper ones are stable and the lower ones are unstable (see* [25]*) (modified from Figure* 5 *of* [17, p. 371]*).*

The term $p\beta c E \frac{I}{N}$ has been added to the standard TB model as a way of incorporating exogenous reinfection, that is, the potential reactivation of TB that may result from continuous exposure to TB via contacts between latently infected and actively infected individuals.

An examination of the model (9.14)–(9.17) dynamics shows that $\mathcal{R}_0 = 1$ is not always the key threshold. In Figure 9.5, we see that exogenous reinfection is capable of supporting multiple steady states. It has been shown that system (9.14)–(9.17) does support two endemic ("positive") states as well as the TB-free equilibrium when $\mathcal{R}_0 < 1$. This kind of result brings into question the centrality that $\mathcal{R}_0$ has played in the development of disease control efforts. The existence of coexisting multiple states means that outcomes are tightly linked to initial conditions. Work on models that support multiple steady states via *backward* bifurcations has been carried out in multiple contexts [16, 23, 25, 30, 31, 33, 34, 40, 55, 62, 69]. This body of research suggests (who would be surprised?) that such behavior may be generic. If that is the case, then the robustness of current intervention or control models will have to be carefully scrutinized at least for some diseases.

9.2.6 Models with multiple epidemiological units

As reported in [43],

> Robert Koch, a German physician and scientist, presented his discovery of *Mycobacterium tuberculosis*, the bacterium that causes tuberculosis (TB), on the evening of

> March 24, 1882.... Koch's lecture, considered by many to be the most important in medical history, was so innovative, inspirational and thorough that it set the stage for the scientific procedures of the twentieth century.... Koch brought his entire laboratory to the lecture room: microscopes, test tubes with cultures, glass slides with stained bacteria, dyes, reagents, glass jars with tissue samples, etc.... Koch showed tissue dissections from guinea pigs which were infected with tuberculous material from the lungs of infected apes, from the brains and lungs of humans who had died from blood-borne tuberculosis, from the cheesy masses in lungs of chronically infected patients and from the abdominal cavities of cattle infected with TB. In all cases, the disease which had developed in the experimentally infected guinea pigs was the same, and the cultures of bacteria taken from the infected guinea pigs were identical.

Robert Koch was awarded the fifth Nobel prize in medicine in 1905 [42]. Soon after Koch identified the pathogen responsible for TB in the 19th century [43], it was learned that individuals exposed to TB over long windows of time would naturally face a *substantially* higher risk of acquiring a TB infection, and as a result the characterization of contacts as *close and casual* gained acceptance. Case studies supported the view that most new infections are directly linked to close contacts: (i) a teacher-librarian experiencing an active TB infection, generated secondary infections among the children in his/her classroom but not among students at the library [48]; or (ii) a tourist with active TB managed to infect at least six airline passengers while traveling within the United States [35, 39]. In response to the airline outbreak, the WHO declared that commercial flights lasting more than eight hours can pose a risk of TB infection [41].

A dynamical model that incorporates close and casual contacts (as if there were two epidemiological contact units) was developed and analyzed in order to address the role of heterogeneous contacts on TB transmission [1]. The *epidemiological unit* introduced in this context is a *generalized household* or an *epidemiologically (active or inactive) cluster* (see [1]). The resulting modeling framework involves two epidemiological units: individuals and generalized households. The assumptions and the use of the model in the study of the transmission dynamics of TB follow.

9.2.7 Generalized household model

The population is partitioned into TB-active and TB-inactive clusters. The term *generalized household* describes a group of persons (friends or relatives or coworkers) who have frequent close contact with each other. Although the probability of TB transmission per unit of time is believed to be in general low, the sharing of a closed environments between susceptible individuals and an actively infectious individual for *long periods of time* poses a significant risk of infection. As soon as a member of an inactive cluster develops active TB, the members of the cluster are placed at a relatively high risk of infection. This is signaled by relabeling the cluster as an epidemiologically active TB cluster or an *active* generalized household. In other words, a generalized household or cluster that includes an infectious individual is "infected" or "active."

We review the ideas behind a modeling approach for the study of the dynamics of infections generated via close contacts, within active generalized households, and at "random" via casual contacts anywhere [1]. The simplified framework does not incorporate specific contacts within epidemiologically active clusters. Instead, it assumes that infection within an epidemiological active cluster is just a matter of "time" and, consequently, a function of the average "life span" of the average active cluster (here assumed to be roughly that of the average length an individual's infection period).

The *mean* generalized household size, denoted by n, is assumed to be *significantly* smaller than the size of the population of clusters (that is, we have a large population of clusters). It is assumed that at *only one actively infectious individual is found per active generalized household*, an assumption justified by the existence of about 8 to 9 million active TB cases per year within a world population of roughly 2 billion latently TB-infected individuals. The extremely low recorded levels of active TB prevalence (I/N) and the extreme low progression rates, from latent to active TB, are used to assume that finding two active TB infections within a cluster is rare and hence "negligible." We have that I/N is under 100 per 100,000 in the population of most developing countries, and significantly lower in developed nations [22].

Individuals in the active generalized households, together with all the infectious individuals, constitute the "cluster population" (size $N_c(t)$). The per susceptible mean risk of infection within an active generalized households is given by β. In addition, infectious individual who recover or die (at the per-capita rate γ) reduce the risk of infection, within the corresponding suddenly inactive generalized household, naturally to zero. That is, when an infectious individual recovers or dies, in a cluster of size $n+1$ (or just n if the infectious individual dies), the noninfectious individuals are returned to the "general population" (of size $N_{nc}(t)$). Furthermore, the emergence of each new infectious individual leads to the movement of a cluster, n individuals, from the general population to the population of active clusters. Here, we use the subscript 1 for the (noninfectious) epidemiological classes in the cluster population and the subscript 2 for the corresponding classes in the general population. We further simplify matters by not following clusters through time, or, in other words, we follow the dynamics of only the aggregated populations $N_c(t)$ and $N_{nc}(t)$; that is, when latently infected individuals, members of the N_{nc} population, develop active TB (disease progression), they are moved, together with all the members of their clusters (susceptibles), into the N_c population. Naturally, when an infectious individual recovers, he/she is returned, with all the members to his/her associated (now inactive) cluster, to the N_{nc} population.

We let $N_1 = S_1 + E_1$ denote the noninfectious individuals in N_c and $N_2 = S_2 + E_2$ the individuals in the N_{nc} population. Hence, it is reasonable to assume further that the N_1 population is significantly smaller than the N_2 population. The definition of epidemiologically active cluster and the above assumptions imply that $N_1 = nI$ and that $N_c = (n+1)I$, where n is the mean generalized household size. In our efforts to build the simplest possible setting, it is assumed that the process of epidemiologically active cluster formation has *no memory*; that is, when a latent individual develops active TB, he or she has no prior information about the cluster from which he/she acquired TB, an assumption that gains additional justification due to the long periods of latency associated with TB, but an assumption that can be weakened (see [1]). The development of the system of nonlinear equations describing our version of a cluster or generalized household model, as schematically described in the flow chart shown in Figure 9.6, is given by

$$\frac{dS_1}{dt} = -(\beta+\gamma)S_1 + \frac{S_2}{N_2}nkE_2, \tag{9.18}$$

$$\frac{dE_1}{dt} = \beta S_1 - \gamma E_1 + \frac{E_2}{N_2}nkE_2, \tag{9.19}$$

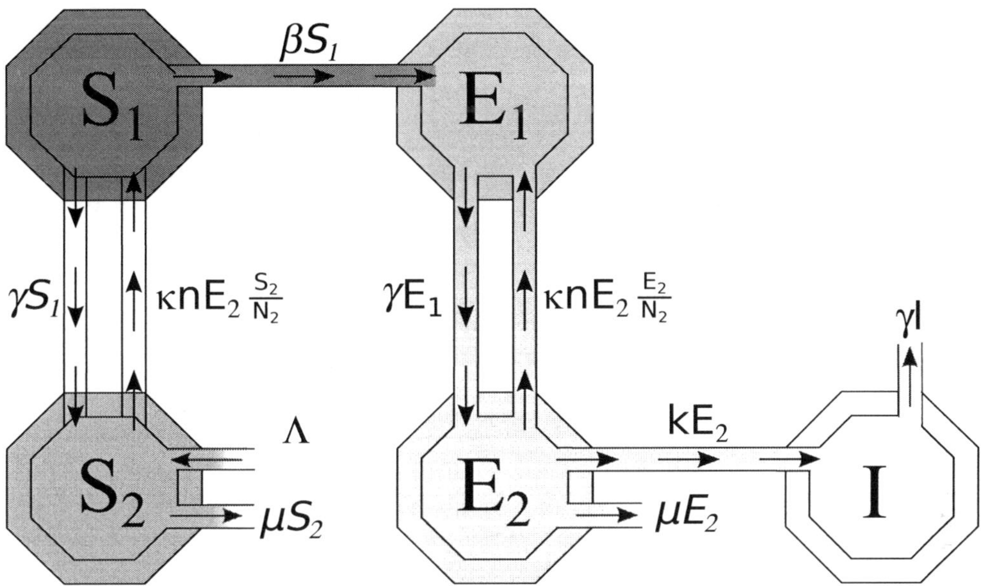

Figure 9.6. *Flow chart of the basic cluster model (modified from Figure 6 of [17, p. 377]).*

$$\frac{dI}{dt} = kE_2 - \gamma I, \tag{9.20}$$

$$\frac{dS_2}{dt} = \Lambda - \mu S_2 + \gamma S_1 - \frac{S_2}{N_2} nkE_2, \tag{9.21}$$

$$\frac{dE_2}{dt} = \gamma E_1 - (\mu + k)E_2 - \frac{E_2}{N_2} nkE_2. \tag{9.22}$$

To sum it up, our simplest cluster or generalized household model in [1] restates the following set of observations and assumptions for completeness:

- An exposed individual (member of the E_2 population) that becomes infectious as he or she joins the N_1 population increases the size of this population by n (the average cluster size) while decreasing the size of the N_2 population by $n+1$. Similarly, an infectious individual that recovers after treatment or dies (regardless of the causes) decreases the N_1 population by n while increasing the N_2 population n.

- Since k is the per-capita active TB progression rate, then kE_2 new infectious individuals are generated per unit of time resulting in an increase of $nkE2$ in the rate of change of the N_1 population also per unit of time. This rate is, by assumption, budgeted (distributed) into a susceptible and a latent component via the fractions S_2/N_2 and E_2/N_2, respectively. That is, the gain terms are $(S_2/N_2)nkE_2$ and $(E_2/N_2)nkE_2$ for the S_1 and E_1 classes.

- Since γ denotes the total per-capita removal rate in the infectious class, then $n\gamma I$ people leave the N_1 population per unit of time. In agreement with the modeling philosophy used above, it is assumed that the S_1/N_1 proportion of this rate is used to budget the return of individuals to the susceptible class, while the proportion E_1/N_1 budgets the return of individuals to the latent class, per unit of time. The relation $nI = N_1$ implies that $(S_1/N_1)n\gamma I = \gamma S_1$ and $(E_1/N_1)n\gamma I = \gamma E_1$, a most convenient outcome.

- Again, in agreement with the above modeling assumptions, the constant flux of susceptible individuals (Λ) is distributed proportionally into the populations $N_c = N_1 + I$ and $N_{nc} = N_2$.
- Further, as it is customary, the per-capita natural mortality (μ), disease-induced mortality (d), and treatment (r) rates are assumed to be constant. Therefore, the net per-capita removal rate of infectious individuals is $\gamma = b + d + r$.

The basic reproductive number is

$$\mathcal{R}_0 = \frac{\beta n}{(\beta+\gamma)} \frac{k}{(\mu+k)}.$$

$\mathcal{R}_0$ depends in a nonlinear fashion on the parameter β (risk of infection within an *epidemiologically active* cluster of size n) and linearly on the average generalized household size n. Model (9.18)–(9.22) has been generalized by removing or weakening some of the assumptions specified above. The specifics of the generalized version can be found in [64]. The associated system of equations is

$$\frac{dS_1}{dt} = -(p\beta(n)+\gamma)S_1 + \frac{S_2}{N_2} nkE_2 - (1-p)\beta^* \frac{I}{N-n} S_1, \tag{9.23}$$

$$\frac{dE_1}{dt} = p\beta(n)S_1 - \gamma E_1 + \frac{E_2}{N_2} nkE_2 + (1-p)\beta^* \frac{I}{N-n} S_1, \tag{9.24}$$

$$\frac{dI}{dt} = kE_2 - \gamma I, \tag{9.25}$$

$$\frac{dS_2}{dt} = \Lambda - \mu S_2 + \gamma S_1 - \frac{S_2}{N_2} nkE_2 - (1-p)\beta^* \frac{I}{N-n} S_2, \tag{9.26}$$

$$\frac{dE_2}{dt} = \gamma E_1 - (\mu+k)E_2 - \frac{E_2}{N_2} nkE_2 + (1-p)\beta^* \frac{I}{N-n} S_2, \tag{9.27}$$

where β depends on the *average* cluster size, n. The proportion p, the *average fraction of time* spent by a source case within his/her generalized household ($1-p$ denoting the average fraction of time spent by a source case outside the cluster), has also been incorporated so that the rate of infection within clusters becomes $p\beta(n)S_1$, while the rate of infection outside the cluster is $(1-p)\beta^* \frac{I}{N-n}(S_1+S_2)$, with N denoting the total population size and $N-n$ the average number of individuals outside this cluster. Consequently, $(1-p)\beta^* \frac{I}{N-n} S_1$ accounts for the number of new infections per unit of time in the N_1 population (the incidence from S_1 to E_1), while $(1-p)\beta^* \frac{I}{N-n} S_2$ accounts for the incidence from S_2 to E_2. Again, since no new cases of *active* TB are generated within epidemiologically active clusters, the infection rate, within such clusters, is just $p\beta(n)S_1$. New cases of infection generated via casual contacts (per unit of time) is described using standard incidence models. The extended cluster model (9.23)–(9.27) includes the basic cluster model (9.18)–(9.22) ($p = 1$ and $\beta(n)$ is independent of n). The basic reproductive number that corresponds to the generalized cluster model is

$$\mathcal{R}_0(n) = \left(\frac{p\beta(n)n}{p\beta(n)+\gamma} + (1-p)\frac{\beta^*}{\gamma}\frac{K}{K-n} \right) \frac{k}{(\mu+k)}, \tag{9.28}$$

where $K = \frac{\Lambda}{\mu}$ is the asymptotic carrying capacity of the total population.

Two specific forms of $\beta(n)$, discussed in [64], are revisited here:

Case 1. $\beta(n)$ is a piecewise continuous function given by

$$\beta(n) = \begin{cases} \beta_0 & \text{for } n \le n_L, \\ \frac{\beta_1}{n} & \text{for } n_L < n < n_M, \end{cases}$$

where n_L denotes the critical cluster size; that is, after the threshold is crossed, $\beta(n)$ decreases; and n_M is a cluster size upper bound. Consequently,

$$\mathcal{R}_0(n) = \begin{cases} \left(\frac{p\beta_0 n}{p\beta_0+\gamma} + (1-p)\frac{\beta^*}{\gamma}\frac{K}{K-n}\right)\frac{k}{(\mu+k)} & \text{for } n \le n_L, \\ \left(\frac{p\beta_1}{p\frac{\beta_1}{n}+\gamma} + (1-p)\frac{\beta^*}{\gamma}\frac{K}{K-n}\right)\frac{k}{(\mu+k)} & \text{for } n \ge n_L. \end{cases}$$

Given that the maximum cluster size n_M is significantly smaller than the carrying capacity K, we have that $\frac{K}{K-n} \approx 1$. Hence, as long as $n < n_L$, $\mathcal{R}_0$ increases linearly with the cluster size, that is, $Q_0 \approx \frac{p\beta_0}{p\beta_0+\gamma}n + (1-p)\frac{\beta^*}{\gamma}$, where Q_0 denotes the number of secondary infections generated by *one* infectious individual.

On the other hand, if $n > n_L$, $Q_0 \approx \frac{p\beta_1 n}{p\beta_1+n\gamma} + (1-p)\frac{\beta^*}{\gamma}\frac{K}{K-n}$, an expression that levels off at the value $p\frac{\beta_1}{\gamma} + (1-p))\frac{\beta^*}{\gamma}$. We observe that although increases in n translate to increases in TB transmission, the rate of increase is nonlinear. $\mathcal{R}_0(n)$ is bounded, a bound that limits TB prevalence size.

Case 2. $\beta(n)$ is now assumed to be inversely proportional to n: $\beta(n) = \frac{\beta_1}{n}$. $\mathcal{R}_0(n)$ is the sum of new secondary cases of infection contributions, generated from within and from outside the cluster. The ratio $E(n)$ given by

$$E(n) = \frac{\gamma\beta_1 p}{K\beta^*(1-p)}\frac{n(K-n)}{(p\beta_1+\gamma n)}$$

captures the relative contributions of within and between cluster transmission. $E(n)$ increases and reaches its maximum value at $n^* = \frac{K}{1+\sqrt{1+\frac{\gamma K}{p\beta_1}}}$, where n^* is by definition the *optimal cluster size*, the value that maximizes within to between cluster transmission.

Can cluster-model dynamics be characterized? Disease dynamics are often tied to whims of characteristic demographic or epidemiological time scales. Since the average infectious (active TB) period is roughly 3–4 months, that is, much shorter than the average latent period (which is comparable in magnitude to the life span of the host population), then rescaling time, using characteristic population or epidemiological time scales, provides ways of analyzing the long-term dynamics of TB. For example, if time is measured using the average latency period $1/k$ as the unit of time ($\tau = kt$); if the independent variables S_2 and E_2 are rescaled by Ω, the total asymptotic population size ($\Omega = \frac{\Lambda}{\mu}$); and if N_1 is rescaled using the balance factor $\frac{k}{\beta+\gamma}\Omega$, then new rescaled variables and nondimensional parameters help reduce the complexity of the model. Specifically, making use of $x_1 = \frac{S_2}{\Omega}$, $x_2 = \frac{E_2}{\Omega}$, $y_1 = \frac{\beta+\gamma}{k}\frac{S_1}{\Omega}$, $y_2 = \frac{\beta+\gamma}{k}\frac{E_1}{\Omega}$, and $y_3 = \frac{\beta+\gamma}{k}\frac{I}{\Omega}$ leads to the rescaled model equations

$$\frac{dx_1}{d\tau} = B(1-x_1)+(1-m)y_1 - n\frac{x_1x_2}{x_1+x_2}, \tag{9.29}$$

$$\frac{dx_2}{d\tau} = (1-m)y_2 - (1+B)x_2 - n\frac{x_2^2}{x_1+x_2}, \tag{9.30}$$

$$\epsilon\frac{dy_1}{d\tau} = -y_1 + n\frac{x_1x_2}{x_1+x_2}, \tag{9.31}$$

$$\epsilon\frac{dy_2}{d\tau} = my_1 - (1-m)y_2 + n\frac{x_2^2}{x_1+x_2}, \tag{9.32}$$

$$\epsilon\frac{dy_3}{d\tau} = x_2 - (1-m)y_3, \tag{9.33}$$

where $\epsilon = \frac{k}{\beta+\gamma}$, $m = \frac{\beta}{\beta+\gamma} < 1$, and $B = \frac{\mu}{k}$. The terms on the right-hand side of system (9.29)–(9.30) are of the same order of magnitude whenever $\epsilon \ll 1$. Under such assumption, y_1, y_2, and y_3 can be considered fast variables, while x_1 and x_2 would be considered slow variables. Hoppensteadt's early theorem [32] helped established the global stability of the endemic equilibrium of System (9.29)–(9.30) when ϵ is small. Lyapunov and a Dulac functions helped establish the global stability of the disease-free equilibrium. The forward bifurcation in Figure 9.2 turned out to capture the dynamics of the asymptotic dynamics of cluster models as well. The specifics used in the analyses (singular perturbation theory and multiple time scales techniques) can be found in [64].

9.3 Treatment of Latent TB—Theoretical Modeling Results

TB models have been used systematically in the evaluation of control strategies (see, e.g., [13, 51, 67, 68]). The emphasis has been on the evaluation of the effectiveness of TB-vaccination strategies—a good idea, except that data (from two decades ago) show that 12% of the U.S. GNP is spent on health care [8], with only a token amount on prevention. The WHO noted that if the amount of aid spent on TB treatment programs had been increased from \$15 to \$100 million yearly, 1.2 million deaths would have been avoided every year over the last two decades [50], a reduction then in deaths of over 30%. What strategies would lead to the elimination of TB? The simultaneous use of several carefully chosen options would likely prove most effective. Models make it abundantly clear that the inclusion of control measures that effectively reduce the size of the latently infected TB class are the most critical (see [17, 18, 20, 24, 52, 65, 70]), an evident result once we realize that the pool of latently infected TB individuals is possibly the *largest infection reservoir* of any human infectious disease in the world [49].

In addition, the emergence and re-emergence of human diseases can reduce the effectiveness of intervention efforts (HIV or malaria coinfections compromise the immune system). The importance of treating individuals, particularly those in the latent TB stage, has been addressed. The rest of this section focuses on the impact that latent infection interventions would have on the long-term dynamics of TB. Hence, we add early latent and long-term latent classes to the model proposed in (9.1)–(9.3), additions and modifications that lead to the following system:

$$\frac{dS}{dt} = \Lambda - \beta SI - \mu S, \tag{9.34}$$

$$\frac{dE_1}{dt} = \beta SI - (\mu + \omega + r_0)E_1, \tag{9.35}$$

$$\frac{dE_2}{dt} = (1-p)\omega E_1 - (k + \mu + r_1)E_2, \tag{9.36}$$

$$\frac{dI}{dt} = p\omega E_1 + kE - (\mu + d + r_2)I. \tag{9.37}$$

Early latently infected individuals progress to active TB at the rate $p\omega$, while the rest move at the rate $(1-p)\omega$ into the long-term latent TB cases. Long-term latent individuals are assumed to develop active TB at the per-capita rate k; the treatment rates for early latent, long-term latent, and active TB classes of individuals are r_0, r_1, and r_2, respectively. We use this two-stage latent TB model because it differentiates between the risk of progression to active TB following a primary infection and progression to active TB after a long-term latent infection. These assumptions are consistent with the fact that $p = 0.05 \gg k = 0.00256$. The results generated by the system (9.34)–(9.37) show that the treatment of 25% of early latent TB cases may be enough, that is, may lead to the elimination of TB as long as this effort is combined with the adequate treatment of 80% of individuals housing active TB infections.

9.4 Key to the Elimination of TB

Baojun Song asked the following question (see [66]): Is the self-imposed deadline set by the CDC to eliminate TB in the U.S. reasonable? Song, using a version of the models introduced above but with time-dependent parameters, addressed the above question using 50 years of U.S. data (TB incidence and U.S. demographic and mortality) to estimate key parameters from the best fit to the data. He showed in [66] that TB may be reduced to *one case of active TB per million* by the CDC's self-imposed deadline, *the year* 2020, provided that the treatment of at least 20% of latently infected individuals was accomplished (not clearly defined in their plans). The impact of HIV/AIDS prevalence on TB incidence (after 1983) was included in the analysis in a crude but effective way. An artificial function was introduced that accelerated TB progression just over the window of time when HIV contributed the most to the documented increases of TB incidence in the U.S. As it turned out, TB's case rate control was not too sensitive to U.S. HIV increases. That is, TB could be controlled under a policy that treats a good percentage of individuals with latent TB infections under U.S. HIV conditions.

The total population size $N(t)$ comes into the model as an external input (time series built from census and projection data). The latently infected classes included are a primary latent/exposed class (E_1) and a permanently latent class (E_2), leading to the model

$$\frac{dE_1}{dt} = \beta\left(N(t) - E_1 - E_2 - I\right)\frac{I}{N(t)} - (\mu(t) + k + r_1 + p + A(t))E_1, \tag{9.38}$$

$$\frac{dE_2}{dt} = pE_1 - (\mu(t) + r_2 + A(t))E_2, \tag{9.39}$$

$$\frac{dI}{dt} = kE_1 + A(t)(E_1 + E_2) - (\mu(t) + d(t) + r_3)I, \tag{9.40}$$

where $A(t)$ is given by the formula

$$A(t) = \begin{cases} \alpha_1(t-1983)^{\alpha_2} e^{-\alpha_3(t-1983)^{\alpha_4}} & \text{if } 1983 < t, \\ 0 & \text{otherwise.} \end{cases}$$

Here the α_i's are constants determined from fitting simulations to data. $N(t)$ is *assumed* to be independent of the disease and comes as a given "external" input. The values of $N(t)$ are generated from U.S. demographic data, sometimes extrapolated from published U.S. demographic data. The transmission rate, β, TB's activation rate k, and the treatment rates are assumed to be constant; r_i ($i = 1,2,3$), as well as p the fraction of the rate at which primary latent TB cases join the permanent latent TB class, are also assumed to be constant. However, $\mu(t)$ and $d(t)$ are functions of time. Estimates for some of theses parameters are listed in Table 9.2.

Table 9.2. *Estimated parameters of TB transmission for the U.S. as listed in* [17, 64, 65, 66], *(taken from* [17]*).*

Parameter	β	c	k	r_1	r_2	r_3	p
Estimation	0.22	10	0.01	0.05	0.05	0.65	0.1

The pattern in Figure 9.7 highlights the value of the excess progression rate function $A(t)$. The model fits the data well, capturing the history of TB in the U.S. The values of $r_1 = r_2 = 0.05$ used are based on the assumption that in the past only 5% of latently infected individuals have received treatment each year, our baseline assumption. We carried out several numerical experiments and found that the treatment of 100% of active TB cases per unit time ($r_3 = 1$, instead of 0.65) turned out to be insufficient to reach the CDC's goal (see Figure 9.8). We also found out that adequate increases in the rate of treatment of latently infected individuals (raising r_1 and r_2 to roughly 20% per year) would indeed help the CDC achieve its target of 1/1,000,000 active TB cases per year, within a reasonable period of time (see Figures 9.9 and 9.10). In this section, we have used simulations and a flexible model to highlight the role of models in a practical application. Figure 9.10 shows that the effect of HIV on TB prevalence is captured by our short-term phenomenological perturbation, the kind of local disturbance that helped us calibrate the model used to test the viability of the CDC's goal. We see that HIV, as expected, delays the ability of the CDC to achieve their

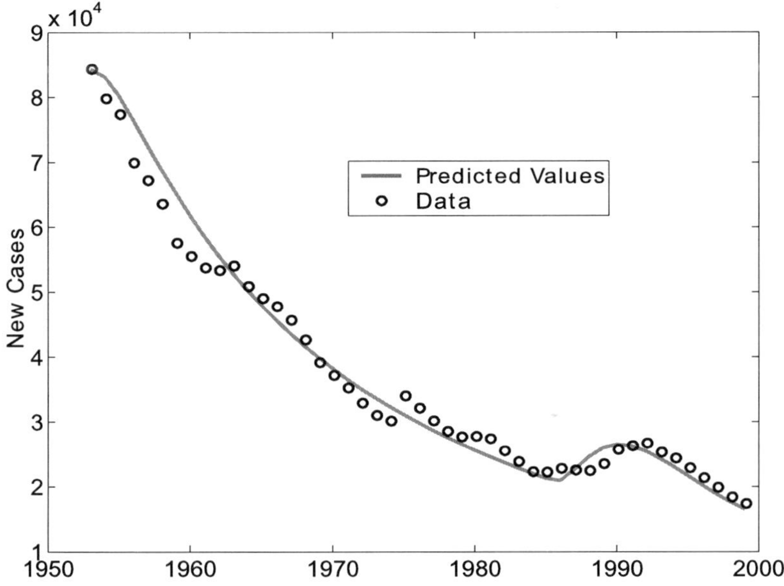

Figure 9.7. *New cases of TB and data models (modified from Figure* 9 *of* [17, p. 393]*).*

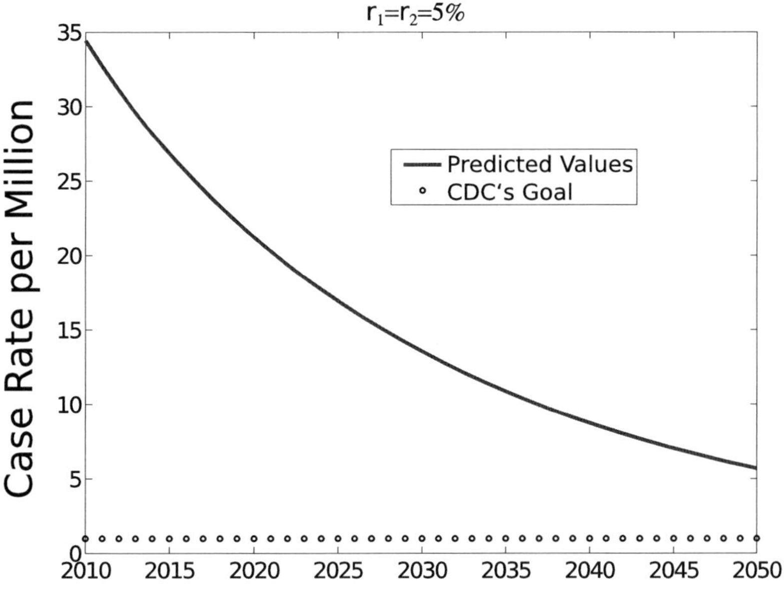

Figure 9.8. $r_1 = r_2 = 5\%$*; the CDC's "TB elimination" cannot be achieved by* 2020 *(modified from Figure* 10 *of* [17, p. 394]*).*

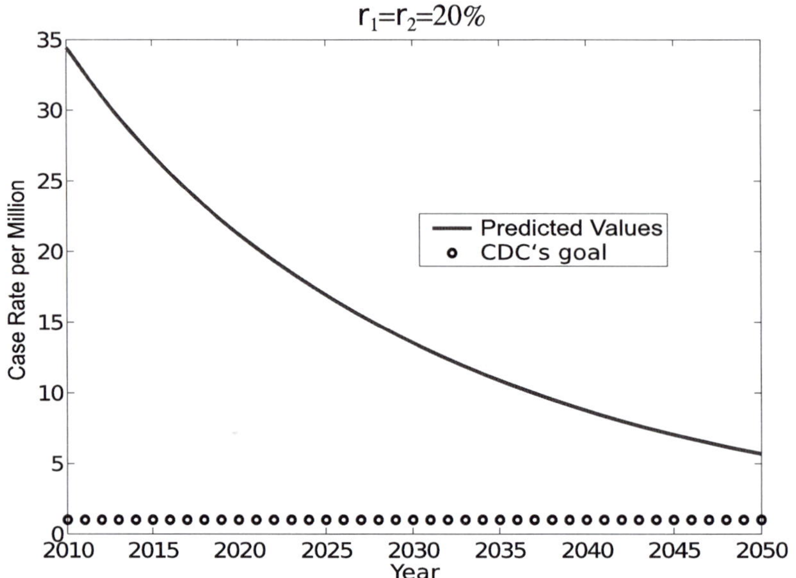

Figure 9.9. $r_1 = r_2 = 20\%$; *the CDC's "TB elimination" can be achieved by* 2020 *(modified from Figure* 11 *of* [17, p. 394]*).*

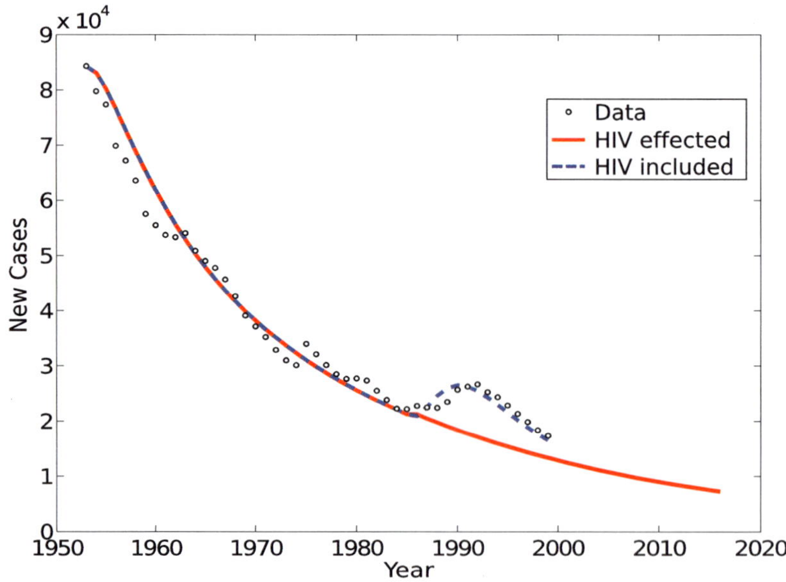

Figure 9.10. *Impact of HIV TB prevalence. The lower curve represents no HIV effect; the upper curve represents the case rate when HIV is included; both are the same before* 1983*. Dots represent real data (modified from Figure* 12 *of* [17, p. 395]*).*

goal but, fortunately, has not had a long-term impact on the decreasing persistence of TB in the U.S. Model results support the perspective that emphasis on treating at least 20% of the latently infected individuals (per unit of time) offers the best strategy if one wishes to try to meet—*partially at best* the CDC's target by 2020. Finally, we remark that the content of this last section has deliberately ignored an important problem, namely, the study of the coevolutionary or joint dynamics of coinfections (but see [52]).

9.5 Thoughts and Conclusions

Sir Ronald Ross, awarded the second Nobel Prize in Medicine and Physiology for his fundamental research in the field of malaria, proceeded to create the field of *mathematical epidemiology* through the introduction of his celebrated model in an appendix [54]. His work had a deep impact on Kermack and McKendrick, who in 1927, in work motivated by Ross's models, not only put in print their textbook SIR model but also brought into play the concept of a "tipping point," most often referred to as the *basic reproduction number or ratio* ($\mathcal{R}_0$) [36]. In the context of TB, *a slow disease* at the population level, $\mathcal{R}_0$ plays a central role in the study of its dynamics and, consequently, in the design and evaluation of control measures aimed at reducing its prevalence and morbidity (see [21]). The characterization of the dynamics in simple terms, a transcritical bifurcation, has facilitated and highlighted the role that mathematical models plays in the identification, development, and implementation of public health policies, strongly influencing the field of population-level epidemiology. The importance of $\mathcal{R}_0$ in the context of TB was already transparent in 1937 when Johns Hopkins epidemiologist W. H. Frost [26] used the definition of *basic reproduction number* to make the following observation:

> However, for the eventual eradication of tuberculosis it is not necessary that transmission be *immediately* and *completely* prevented. It is necessary only that the rate of transmission be held permanently below the level at which a given number of infection spreading (*i.e.*, open) cases succeed in establishing an equivalent number to carry on the succession. If in successive periods of time, the number of infectious hosts is continuously reduced, the end-result of this diminishing ratio, if continued long enough, must be extermination of tubercle bacillus.... This means that under present conditions of human resistance and environment the tubercle bacillus is losing ground, and that the eventual eradication of tuberculosis requires only that the present balance against it be maintained.

Frost's observation was probably driven by the fact that long-term downward TB mortality and incidence trends had been recorded already over many decades, a trend that has continued in most parts of the world. However, it is precisely, over the time scales that most likely drove Frost's thinking that the concept of $\mathcal{R}_0$, as it is most often used today, fails to capture the dynamics. Models over long time scales, highlighted by the efforts described above to assess the likelihood that the CDC would meet its self-imposed TB reduction goals, must include demographic growth over a long time. Hence, model parameters cannot be assumed to be constant; they must *naturally* change over time. Nonautonomous models, involving time-dependent parameters and external functions, must therefore be systematically used to assess public health goals [17, 66]. The use of nonautonomous models in studies to evaluate the role of mechanisms that may have been responsible for the observed *TB-active incidence and mortality* declining trends, in a world where TB manages to infect roughly a third of its population, is but another example of the importance of carrying out studies that goes beyond the power of autonomous models [1, 2, 3, 4, 6].

In addition, the general perception that disease dynamics are, in general, well (nearly completely) characterized by transcritical bifurcations, for the purposes of developing control/intervention efforts, needs to be scrutinized since levels of robustness attributed to epidemiological models are unlikely to be supported within scales that involve high levels of heterogeneity, a common pattern in the world that we live in [16, 25]. In addition, the past decades have seen a tremendous growth in the number of articles that highlight and explore the joint role of epidemiological and social factors, including host mobility, on the dynamics of TB, at the population level [17, 18, 19]. Finally, the use of epidemiological frameworks in the study of TB is not limited to questions at the population level; in fact, a series of ongoing efforts on the use of epidemiological frameworks that address questions at the immunological level have been carried out systematically as well (see [37, 38, 56]).

Bibliography

[1] Aparicio J., A. Capurro, and C. Castillo-Chavez (2000) *Transmission and dynamics of tuberculosis on generalized households*, J. Theor. Biol. **206**: 327–341.

[2] Aparicio, J.P., A.F. Capurro, and C. Castillo-Chavez (2002) *Frequency dependent risk of infection and the spread of infectious diseases*, in Mathematical Approaches for Emerging and Reemerging Infectious Diseases: An Introduction, C. Castillo-Chavez, with S.M. Blower, P. van den Driessche, D. Kirschner, and A.A. Yakubu, eds., IMA Vol. Math. Appl. **125**, Springer-Verlag, New York: 341–350.

[3] Aparicio, J., A. Capurro, and C. Castillo-Chavez (2002) *Markers of disease evolution: The case of tuberculosis*, J. Theor. Biol. **215**: 227–237.

[4] Aparicio, J., A. Capurro, and C. Castillo-Chavez (2002) *On the long-term dynamics and re-emergence of tuberculosis*, in Mathematical Approaches for Emerging and Reemerging Infectious Diseases: An Introduction, C. Castillo-Chavez, with P. van den Driessche, D. Kirschner, and A.-A. Yakubu, IMA Vol. Math. Appl. **125**, Springer-Verlag, New York: 351–360.

[5] Aparicio, J.P. and M. Pascual (2007) *Building epidemiological models from R_0: An implicit treatment of transmission in networks*, Proc. Roy. Soc. B **274**: 505–512.

[6] Aparicio, J. and C. Castillo-Chavez (2009) *Mathematical modeling of tuberculosis epidemics*, Math. Biosc. & Eng. **6**: 209–237.

[7] Barnes, D.S. (1995) *The Making of a Social Disease: Tuberculosis in the Nineteenth-Century France*, University of California Press: 5–13.

[8] Bloom, B.R. and C.J.L. Murray (1992) *Tuberculosis: Commentary on a reemergent killer*, Science, **257**: 1055–1064.

[9] Blower, S.M., A.R. McLean, T.C. Porco, P.M. Small, P.C. Hopwell, M.A. Sanchez, and A.R. Moss (1995) *The intrinsic transmission dynamics of tuberculosis epidemics*, Nature Medicine **1**: 815–821.

[10] Blower, S.M., P.M. Small, and P.C. Hopwell (1996) *Control strategies for tuberculosis epidemics: New models for old problems*, Science **273**: 497–500.

[11] Blower, S.M. and J.L. Gerberding (1998) *Understanding, predicting and controlling the emergence of drug-resistant tuberculosis: A theoretical framework*, J. Mod. Med. **76**: 624–636.

[12] Brauer, F. and C. Castillo-Chavez (2012) *Mathematical Models in Population Biology and Epidemiology*, 2nd ed., Texts in Applied Mathematics **40,** Springer-Verlag.

[13] Brogger, S. (1967) *Systems analysis in tuberculosis control: A model*, Amer. Rev. Resp. Dis. **95**: 419–434.

[14] Castillo-Chavez, C., H. Hethcote, V. Andreasen, S.A. Levin, and W.-M., Liu (1988) *Cross-immunity in the dynamics of homogeneous and heterogeneous populations*, in Mathematical Ecology, T.G. Hallam, L.G. Gross, and S.A. Levin, eds., World Scientific Publishing, Singapore: 303–316.

[15] Castillo-Chavez, C., H. Hethcote, V. Andreasen, S.A. Levin, and W.-M., Liu (1989) *Epidemiological models with age structure, proportionate mixing, and cross-immunity*, J. Math. Biol. **27**: 233–258.

[16] Castillo-Chavez, C., Z. Feng, and W. Huang (2002) *On the computation of $\mathcal{R}_0$ and its role on global stability*, in Mathematical Approaches for Emerging and Reemerging Infectious Diseases: Models, Methods and Theory, Volume I, C. Castillo-Chavez, S. Blower, P. van den Driessche, D. Kirschner, and A.A. Yakubu, eds., Springer-Verlag, Berlin, Heidelberg, New York: 229–256.

[17] Castillo-Chavez, C. and B. Song (2004) *Dynamical models of tuberculosis and their applications*, J. Math. Biosc. & Eng. **1**: 361–404.

[18] Castillo-Chavez, C. and Z. Feng (1998) *Mathematical models for the disease dynamics of tuberculosis*, in Advances in Mathematical Population Dynamics - Molecules, Cells and Man, O. Arino, D. Axelrod, and M. Kimmel, eds., World Scientific: 629–656.

[19] Castillo-Chavez, C., A.F. Capurro, M. Zellner, and J.X. Velasco-Hernandez (1998) *El transporte publico y la dinamica de la tuberculosis a nivel poblacional*, Aportaciones Matematicas, Serie Comunicaciones **22**: 209–225.

[20] Castillo-Chavez, C. and Z. Feng (1997) *To treat or not to treat: The case of tuberculosis*, J. Math. Biol. **35**: 629–656.

[21] Castillo-Chavez, C. and Z. Feng (1998) *Global stability of an age-structure model for TB and its application to optimal vaccination strategies*, Math. Biosc. **151**: 135–154.

[22] Davis, P.D.O., ed. (1998) *Clinical Tuberculosis*, Chapman and Hall, London.

[23] Dushoff, J., W. Huang, and C. Castillo-Chavez (1998) *Backward bifurcations and catastrophe in simple models of fatal diseases*, J. Math. Biol. **36**: 227–248.

[24] Feng, Z., W. Huang, and C. Castillo-Chavez (2001) *On the role of variable latent periods in mathematical models for tuberculosis*, Journal of Dynamics and Differential Equations **13**: 425–452.

[25] Feng, Z., C. Castillo-Chavez, and A.F. Capurro (2000) *A model for tuberculosis with exogenous reinfection*, Theor. Pop. Biol. **57**: 235–247.

[26] Frost, W. H. (1937) *How much control of tuberculosis*, American Journal of Public Health and the Nation's Health **27**: 759–766.

[27] Grigg, E.R.N. (1958) *The arcana of tuberculosis*, Am. Rev. Tuberculosis and Pulmonary Diseases **78**: 151–172.

[28] Grigg, E.R.N. (1958) *The arcana of tuberculosis III*, Am. Rev. Tuberculosis and Pulmonary Diseases **78**: 426–453.

[29] Grigg, E.R.N. (1958) *The arcana of tuberculosis IV*, Am. Rev. Tuberculosis and Pulmonary Diseases **78**: 583–608.

[30] Hadeler, K.P. and C. Castillo-Chavez (1995) *A core group model for disease transmission*, J. Math. Biosc. **128**: 41–55.

[31] Hethcote, H.W. (2000) *The mathematics of infectious diseases*, SIAM Rev. **42**: 599–653.

[32] Hoppensteadt, F. (1974) *Asymptotic stability in singular perturbation problems. II: Problems having matched asymptotic expansion solutions*, J. Differential Equations **15**: 510–521.

[33] Huang, W., K.L. Cooke, and C. Castillo-Chavez (1992) *Stability and bifurcation for a multiple-group model for the dynamics of HIV/AIDS transmission*, SIAM J. Appl. Math. **52**: 835–854.

[34] Huang, W. and C. Castillo-Chavez (2002) *Age-structured core groups and their impact on HIV dynamics*, in Mathematical Approaches for Emerging and Reemerging Infectious Diseases: Models, Methods and Theory, C. Castillo-Chavez, with P. van den Driessche, D. Kirschner, and A.-A. Yakubu, eds., IMA Vol. Math. Appl. **126**, Springer-Verlag, Berlin, Heidelberg, New York: 261–273.

[35] Kenyon, T.A., S.E. Valway, and W.W. Ihle (1996) *Transmission of multidrug-resistant Mycobacterium tuberculosis during a long airplane flight*, New England J. Medicine **334**: 933–938.

[36] Kermack, W.O. and A.G. McKendrick (1927) *A contribution to the mathematical theory of epidemics*, Proc. R. Soc. A **115**: 700–721.

[37] Kirschner, D. (1999) *Dynamics of co-infection with M. tuberculosis and HIV-1*, Theoretical population Biology **55**: 94–109.

[38] Kirschner, D.E. and J.J. Linderman (2009) *Mathematical and computational approaches can complement experimental studies of host pathogen interactions*, Cellular Microbiology **11**: 531–539.

[39] Kolata, G. (1995) *First documented cases of TB passed on airliner is reported by U.S.*, The New York Times, March 3.

[40] Kribs-Zaleta, C.M. and J.X. Velasco-Hernandez (2001) *A simple vaccination model with multiple endemic states*, Math. Biosc. **164**: 183–201.

[41] News in Brief (1999) *WHO warning for air passengers*, Lancet **353**: 305.

[42] Nobel Prize Organization (2012) *List of Nobel Laureates in Medicine and Physiology*, http://www.nobelprize.org/nobel/prizes/medicine/laureates/.

[43] Nobel Prize Organization (2012) *Robert Koch and Tuberculosis*, Description of Koch's Famous Lecture, http://www.nobelprize.org/educational/medicine/tuberculosis/readmore.html.

[44] Nuño, M., Z. Feng, M. Martcheva, and C. Castillo-Chavez (2005) *Dynamics of two-strains influenza with isolation and partial cross-immunity*, SIAM J. Appl. Math. **65**: 964–982.

[45] Nuño, M., C. Castillo-Chavez, Z. Feng, and M. Martcheva (2008) *Mathematical model of influenza: The role of cross-immunity, quarantine and age-structure*, in Mathematical Epidemiology, P. van den Driessche, J. Wu, and F. Brauer, eds., Springer-Verlag.

[46] Nuño, M., M. Martcheva, and C. Castillo-Chavez (2009) *Immune level structure model for influenza strains*, Journal of Biological Systems **17**: 713–737.

[47] Porco, T.C. and S.M. Blower (1998) *Quantifying the intrinsic transmission dynamics of tuberculosis*, Theor. Pop. Biol. **54**: 117–132.

[48] Raffalli, J., K.A. Sepkowitz, and D. Armstrong (1996) *Community-based outbreaks of tuberculosis*, Arch. Intern. Med. **156**: 1053–1060.

[49] Reichman, L.B. and J.H. Tanne (2002) *Timebomb: The Global Epidemic of Multi-drug-resistant Tuberculosis*, McGraw-Hill, New York.

[50] Reuters (1993) *Agency cities urgent need to fight increase in TB*, The New York Times, November 16: C8.

[51] ReVelle, C.S., W.R. Lynn, and F. Feldmann (1967) *Mathematical models for the economic allocation of tuberculosis control activities in developing nations*, Am. Rev. Respir. Dis. **96**: 893–909.

[52] Roeger, L.-I.W., Z. Feng, and C. Castillo-Chavez (2009) *Modeling TB and HIV co-infections*, Math. Biosc. & Eng. **6**: 815–837.

[53] Rose, D.E., G.O. Zerbe, S.O. Lantz, and W.C. Bailey (1979) *Establishing priority during investigation of tuberculosis contacts*, Am. Rev. Respir. Dis. **119**: 603–609.

[54] Ross, R. (1911) *The Prevention of Malaria*, 2nd ed. (with Addendum), John Murray, London.

[55] Sanchez, F., X. Wang, C. Castillo-Chavez, P. Gruenewald, and D. Gorman (2007) *Drinking as an epidemic—a simple mathematical model with recovery and relapse*, in Therapist's Guide to Evidence Based Relapse Prevention, K. Witkiewitz and G.A. Marlatt, eds., Elsevier: 353–368.

[56] Segovia-Juarez, J.L., S. Ganguli, and D. Kirschner (2004) *Identifying control mechanism of granuloma formation during M. tuberculosis infection using an agent based model*, J. Theor. Biol. **231**: 357–376.

[57] Shim, E., H.T. Banks, and C. Castillo-Chavez (2006) *Seasonality of rotavirus infection with its vaccination*, in Mathematical Studies on Human Disease Dynamics, A. Gumel, C. Castillo-Chavez, D.F. Clemence, and R.E. Mickens, eds., Contemp Math. **410**, American Mathematical Society, Providence, RI: 327–348.

[58] Shim, E., Z. Feng, M. Martcheva, and C. Castillo-Chavez (2006) *An age-structured epidemic model of rotavirus with vaccination*, J. Math. Biol. **53**: 719–746.

[59] Shim, E. and C. Castillo-Chavez (2009) *The epidemiological impact of rotavirus vaccination programs in the United States and Mexico*, in Mathematical and Statistical Estimation Approaches in Epidemiology, G. Chowell, J.M. Hyman, L.M.A. Bettencourt, and C. Castillo-Chavez, eds., Springer-Verlag.

[60] Song, B., C. Castillo-Chavez, and J.A. Aparicio (2002) *Tuberculosis models with fast and slow dynamics: The role of close and casual contacts*, Math. Biosc. **180**: 187–205.

[61] Song, B., C. Castillo-Chavez, and J.P. Aparicio (2002) *Global dynamics of tuberculosis models with density dependent demography*, in Mathematical Approaches for Emerging and Reemerging Infectious Diseases: Models, Methods and Theory, C. Castillo-Chavez, with S.M. Blower, P. van den Driessche, D. Kirschner, A.-A. Yakubu, eds., IMA Vol. Math. Appl. **126**, Springer-Verlag, New York: 275–294.

[62] Song, B., M. Garsow-Castillo, K. Rios-Soto, M. Mejran, L. Henso, and C. Castillo-Chavez (2006) *Raves, clubs, and ecstasy: The impact of peer pressure*, J. Math. Biosc. & Eng. **3**: 1–18.

[63] Styblo, K. (1991) *Epidemiology of Tuberculosis*, Selected Papers, **24**, Royal Netherlands Tuberculosis Association, The Hague.

[64] Song, B., J.P. Aparicio, and C. Castillo-Chavez (2002) *Tuberculosis models with fast and slow dynamics*: *The role of close and casual contacts*, Math. Biosc. **180**: 187–205.

[65] Song, B. and C. Castillo-Chavez (2001) *Tuberculosis Control in the U.S.*: *A Strategy to Meet CDC's Goal*, Technical Report Series BU-1562-M, Biometrics Department, Cornell University.

[66] Song, B. (2002) *Dynamical Epidemical Models and Their Applications*, Ph.D. Thesis, Cornell University.

[67] Waaler, H.T., A. Gese, and S. Anderson (1962) *The use of mathematical models in the study of the epidemiology of tuberculosis*, Am. J. Publ. Health **52**: 1002–1013.

[68] Waaler, H.T. and M.A. Piot (1970) *Use of an epidemiological model for estimating the effectiveness of tuberculosis control measures*, Bull. World Health. Org. **43**: 1–16.

[69] Wang, X., Z. Feng, J. Aparicio, and C. Castillo-Chavez (2010) *On the dynamics reinfection: The case of tuberculosis*, in BIOMAT 2009, International; Symposium on Mathematical and Computational Biology, R. P. Mondaini, ed., World Scientific: 304–330.

[70] Ziv, E., C.L. Daley, and S.M. Blower (2001) *Early therapy for latent tuberculosis infection*, Am. J. Epidemiol. **153**: 381–385.

Lecture 10

Models for Sexually Transmitted Diseases

10.1 Single and Two-Sex STD Models

The emergence of antibiotic-resistant STD strains has motivated the study of the joint dynamics of competing strains in heterosexually active populations. The competition for pathogen strains for hosts is revisited first in this lecture in as simple a setting as possible, that is, under a two-sex susceptible-infected-susceptible (*SIS*) models [30, 31, 32, 35].

Mathematical studies of the dynamics and evolution of STDs using *individuals* as the *unit of selection* are often reduced to the study of nonlinear systems. The resulting models are rather complex as they need to incorporate mechanisms tied to the role of mate availability, preference, and competition as well as demographic and epidemiological processes. This lecture focuses on the study of the dynamics of competing STD strains in the simplest setting possible. The role of *core* populations [56] on the dynamics of sexually transmitted HIV are also revisited [63] in a setting built to evaluate, in a rather crude way, the joint HIV dynamics of sex workers and truck drivers in Nigeria.

10.2 Sir Ronald Ross and STD Models

Sir Ronald Ross, second Nobel Laureate in Medicine, introduced the first nonlinear system of differential equations for the *dynamics* of vector-transmitted diseases [89]. Ross instantly recognized that his framework could also be used to study the dynamics of STDs since vector-host interactions are formally *equivalent* to male-female STD dynamics [89, p. 678]. In 1973, the first population-level gonorrhea model appeared [40]. Cooke and Yorke's mathematical and modeling work reinvigorated the use of nonlinear differential equations in the study of the transmission dynamics and control of STDs. Hethcote and Yorke [56] introduced the concept of *core group* and used it to highlight the importance of heterogeneity on STD dynamics and control. The research of these individuals has had a tremendous impact not only on applied mathematicians but also on U.S. policies aimed at controlling gonorrhea. Their 1984 monograph is one of the most important mathematical/modeling contributions in epidemiology [56].

Over time, Ross's observations became important modeling elements, not always explicitly acknowledged, of the dynamics of vector and sexually transmitted diseases. He used the fact that the average total rate of contacts between host and vectors must be conserved [89, p. 667]. This is now a basic assumption used by researchers on the construction of heterogeneous contact/mixing structures and therefore in their applications to epidemiology [16, 17, 19, 23, 24, 29, 73, 79].

Mathematical models for STDs have often incorporated (modeling) restrictions aimed at facilitating the mathematical analyses. For example, in the study of the role of heterogeneity in STD dynamics, the population of interest is often divided into groups or subpopulations made up of "identical" individuals under the assumption that the sizes of interacting sexually active subpopulations remain *essentially* constant. This assumption means that the disease does not have an impact on the size of each "homogeneous" subpopulation (an assumption that implies that the overall interacting group dynamics remains essentially unchanged; see [56, 65] and the references therein). This assumption, a priori, precludes the role of disease pathogens as agents of selection. Models where disease-induced mortality is allowed to alter population size have shown to generate significantly different qualitative dynamics than STD models that do not [21, 22, 44, 59, 60].

Sir Ronald Ross was also aware of the role of frequency-dependent dynamics. Hence, he did not restrict his models to situations where the sizes of the interacting subpopulations were unable to change (see [89, p. 678] or Lotka's review of Ross's work in [72]). Clearly, the study of population-level evolutionary dynamics of STDs must allow for the possibility of selection, and therefore the disease's impact on population size cannot be routinely ignored, as Ross knew quite well.

Studies that account for the role of selection in disease dynamics have always been of interests to evolutionary biologists and mathematicians; see, for example, [46, 47, 67, 68, 69, 70, 71, 76, 78, 79, 82, 83, 84, 101] and the references therein. The view, for example, that pathogen evolution selects for reduced levels of virulence has been challenged, not only in field studies but also via the mathematical analyses of host-parasite models [45, 49, 50, 68, 69, 76, 77]. In addition, as a result of the HIV epidemic, studies focusing on the role of social dynamics and behavior have significantly expanded, as can be seen in [2, 8, 10, 11, 12, 27, 30, 31, 33, 34, 38, 52, 54, 60, 77] and the references therein. Multiple modes of transmission or genetic variability are but some of the mechanisms that keep and maintain heterogeneity. In order to facilitate the study of the role of such mechanisms, hosts are often modeled as patches which may be colonized by infectious pathogens. In this setup, for example, studies of the role of patch quality or desirability or susceptibility to colonization to real or theoretical diseases have been carried out [1, 2, 4, 13, 14, 18, 20, 43, 45, 49, 50, 67, 68, 69, 76, 78, 81, 82, 83, 84, 98, 101].

This final lecture focuses on the study of the dynamics of multistrain STDs in homosexually and heterosexually active mixing communities. In Sections 10.3 and 10.4, we first revisit the dynamics of STDs in populations unaffected by disease-induced mortality, that is, where the effects of changing social dynamics are mathematically precluded a priori (see [56, 65] and the references in [55]). Section 10.3 introduces and analyzes an SIS model for the dynamics of STD infections in homogeneously mixing, homosexually active populations, while Section 10.4 highlights the mathematical analyses using a simplified two-sex model [30, 31, 32, 35]. Section 10.5 revisits a two-sex HIV model and its sensitivity to changes on key HIV-reduction control parameters [63]. Section 10.6 addresses, under a multitude of *crude simplifying* assumptions, the impact of core populations (sex workers and men that systematically visit sex workers) on the dynamics of HIV, within sexually active *noncore* populations [63]. Section 10.7 provides a brief discussion that revisits some of the points discussed in this lecture. As with all the lectures in this volume, we have been revisiting our published work and relevant publications in the literature, with the audience of this NSF-sponsored workshop in mind, that is, mathematics students, epidemiologists, biologists, and more.

10.3 Two-Strain Multigroup Single-Sex Model

An *SIS* STD model involving two groups of homosexually active individuals, susceptible and infected, and two strains are introduced. Individuals are assumed to respond differently to each strain for reasons that may possibly include their level and type of sexual activity, genetic susceptibility, immune response, and other factors. Infected (here assumed to be also infectious) individuals can only house a single pathogen strain, that is, coinfections are assumed to be impossible or so rare that they are neglected. S_k, $k = 1,2$, denotes the susceptible subpopulation with sexual-activity level, the average number of new sexual partners per unit time, b_k. Further, I_k and J_k denote the strain-specific strain 1 and strain 2 infected classes with sexual activity k. The STD dynamics are assumed to be governed by the following system of equations:

$$\begin{aligned} \dot{S}_k =& \Lambda_k - \mu_k S_k - \sum_{u=I,J} B_k^u(t) + \gamma_k^I I_k + \gamma_k^J J_k, \\ \dot{I}_k =& B_k^I - \left(\mu_k + \gamma_k^I\right) I_k, \\ \dot{J}_k =& B_k^J - \left(\mu_k + \gamma_k^J\right) J_k, \end{aligned} \tag{10.1}$$

where

$$B_k^I = S_k b_k \beta^I \frac{\sum\limits_j b_j I_j}{\sum\limits_j b_j T_j}, \qquad B_k^J = S_k b_k \beta^J \frac{\sum\limits_j b_j J_j}{\sum\limits_j b_j T_j}$$

denote the incidence rates, that is, new cases of infection per unit of time, with

$$T_j = S_j + I_j + J_j$$

denoting the population size of group j, $j = 1,2$.

The term Λ_k (input flows entering the sexually active subpopulations, $k = 1,2$) models the recruitment/arrival of homosexually active individuals to the susceptible population; that is, it is assumed that infections do not come from the outside. The constant terms $1/\mu_k$ ($k = 1,2$) denote the average sexual life spans of individuals in group k; β_k denotes the rates of infection; and γ_k^u, $u = I,J$, denotes the distinct recovery rates of individuals in classes I_k and J_k, respectively. That is, it is assumed that individuals with different sexual-activity levels have distinct rates of recovery for a multitude of factors that may include the fact that among some highly sexually active populations the most active individuals get diagnosed and treated more often.

Following the work in [27, 29, 30, 32, 97, 99] and using the fact that $\lim_{t\to\infty} T_k = \frac{\Lambda_k}{\mu_k} := p_k$, we see that the dynamics of Section 10.3.5 can be qualitatively determined by those of the appropriate limiting system given by

$$\begin{aligned} \dot{I}_k &= \sigma_k^I (p_k - I_k - J_k) \sum_j b_j I_j - \nu_k^I I_k, \\ \dot{J}_k &= \sigma_k^J (p_k - I_k - J_k) \sum_j b_j J_j - \nu_k^J J_k, \end{aligned} \tag{10.2}$$

where

$$\sigma_k^u := \frac{b_k \beta^u}{\sum_j b_j p_j}$$

and

$$\nu_k^u := \mu_k + \gamma_k^u, \quad u = I, J.$$

On the set

$$\mathbb{R}_+^4 := \{(x_1, x_2, x_3, x_4); \quad x_i \geq 0, \quad i = 1, \cdot, 4\},$$

we define the subset Ω of $\mathbb{R}_+^4$,

$$\Omega := \left\{(I_1, I_2, J_1, J_2) \in \mathbb{R}_+^4; \quad I_k + J_k \leq p_k, k = 1, 2\right\},$$

and observe that on Ω the flow generated by (10.2) is positively invariant. In fact, the flow is monotone under the following *special order* (introduced in [30]).

Definition 10.1. *Let* $x = (x_1, \ldots, x_4)^T \in \mathbb{R}^4$ *and* $K = \{x \in \mathbb{R}^4; x_1, x_2 \geq 0, \quad x_3, x_4 \leq 0\}$. *A type K order, denoted by "* $\leq_K$ *", is defined in such a way that*

$$x \leq_K y \qquad \text{if and only if} \quad x - y \in K. \tag{10.3}$$

Under the order (10.1), the flow generated by (10.2) is monotone. Specifically, we have the following lemma.

Lemma 10.2. *Let* $U = (I_1, I_2, J_1, J_2)^T$ *and let* $U(t, U_0)$ *be a solution of* $U(0, U_0) = U_0$. *Then*

$$U\left(t, U_0^a\right) \leq_K U\left(t, U_0^b\right), \quad t \geq 0,$$

if $U_0^a, U_0^b \in \Omega$ *and* $U_0^a \leq_K U_0^b$.

10.3.1 Identification of Key Thresholds

Linearization of (10.2) about the infection-free equilibrium results in

$$\begin{aligned} \dot{I}_k &= -\nu_k^I I_k + \sigma_k^I p_k \sum_j b_j I_j, \\ \dot{J}_k &= -\nu_k^J J_k + \sigma_k^J p_k \sum_j b_j J_j, \end{aligned} \tag{10.4}$$

that is, two decoupled systems of equations. It is observed that if

$$\nu_1^u \nu_2^u > \nu_1^u \sigma_2^u p_2 b_2 + \nu_2^u \sigma_1^u p_1 b_1,$$

then the infection-free state (with $u = I$ and J) is stable.

Further, under the reverse inequality,

$$\nu_1^u \nu_2^u \leq \nu_1^u \sigma_2^u p_2 b_2 + \nu_2^u \sigma_1^u p_1 b_1,$$

taking $u = I$ or J, we have that the infection-free state is unstable.

The above computations are used to define the reproductive numbers $\mathcal{R}^I$ and $\mathcal{R}^J$ for the classes under strain 1 and 2, respectively. We get

$$\mathcal{R}^u = \frac{\nu_2^u \sigma_1^u p_1 b_1 + \nu_1^u \sigma_2^u p_2 b_2}{\nu_1^u \nu_2^u} = p_1 b_1 \frac{\sigma_1^u}{\nu_1^u} + p_2 b_2 \frac{\sigma_2^u}{\nu_2^u}, \qquad u = I, J. \tag{10.5}$$

Letting

$$\mathcal{R}_k^u = \frac{\sigma_k^u}{\nu_k^u}, \qquad k = 1,2, \quad u = I, J,$$

denote the "reproductive numbers" of the disease in the corresponding subpopulations allows us to write $\mathcal{R}^u$ as

$$\mathcal{R}^u = p_1 b_1 \mathcal{R}_1^u + p_2 b_2 \mathcal{R}_2^u, \qquad u = I, J.$$

The approach in [30, 31, 32, 35] can be used to show that infection-free and boundary equilibria are globally stable. We state an appropriate subset of the results in [30, 31, 32, 35].

Lemma 10.3. *Let* $E_1 = (I_1, I_2, 0, 0)$ *and* $E_2 = (0, 0, J_1, J_2)$ *be equilibria of* (2.2)*, where* $I_i, J_i > 0$ *if* $\mathcal{R}^I > 1$ *and* $\mathcal{R}^J > 1$*, and* $I_i = J_i = 0$ *if* $\mathcal{R}^I \leq 1$ *and* $\mathcal{R}^J \leq 1$*. Let* $\xi^1 = (p_1, p_2, 0, 0)$ *and* $\xi^2 = (0, 0, p_1, p_2)$*. Then*

$$\lim_{t\to\infty} I\left(t, \xi^i\right) = E_i, \qquad i = 1,2.$$

Theorem 10.4. *Let the reproductive number* $\mathcal{R}^I$ *and* $\mathcal{R}^J$ *for each class be defined in* (3.2)*. Then if* $\mathcal{R}^I \leq 1$ *and* $\mathcal{R}^J \leq 1$*, the epidemic goes extinct regardless of the initial levels of infection . If* $\mathcal{R}^I > 1$ *or* $\mathcal{R}^J > 1$*, then the epidemic spreads in the population.*

10.3.2 Boundary Equilibria, Stability, and Competitive Exclusion

The reduced model supports two types of endemic equilibria: nontrivial boundary equilibria, namely, $(I_1, I_2, 0, 0)$ and $(0, 0, J_1, J_2)$, and a coexistence (endemic) equilibrium (all positive entries). Boundary equilibria always exist whenever the disease takes off in the population. We have the following result.

Theorem 10.5. *The equilibrium* $(I_1, I_2, 0, 0)$ *exists if and only if* $\mathcal{R}^I > 1$*, and the equilibrium* $(0, 0, J_1, J_2)$ *exists if and only if* $\mathcal{R}^J > 1$.

Proof. We only outline the proof of existence of $(I_1, I_2, 0, 0)$. From

$$\sigma_k^I(p_k - I_k)(b_1 I_1 + b_2 I_2) = \nu_k^I I_k,$$

it follows that

$$\mathcal{R}_k^I(p_k - I_k)(b_1 I_1 + b_2 I_2) = I_k, \tag{10.6}$$

$$\frac{\mathcal{R}_1^I(p_1 - I_1)}{I_1} = \frac{\mathcal{R}_2^I(p_2 - I_2)}{I_2}. \tag{10.7}$$

Solving (10.7) for I_2 gives

$$I_2 = \frac{p_2 \mathcal{R}_2^I I_1}{\mathcal{R}_1^I(p_1 - I_1) + \mathcal{R}_2^I I_1}. \tag{10.8}$$

Substituting (10.8) into (10.6) with $k = 1$ leads to the following equation for I_1:

$$\frac{1}{\mathcal{R}_1^I(p_1 - I_1)} - b_1 - \frac{b_2 p_2 \mathcal{R}_2^I}{\mathcal{R}_1^I(p_1 - I_1) + \mathcal{R}_2^I I_1} = 0. \tag{10.9}$$

Defining the left-hand side of (10.9) as $f(I_1)$ we see that $f'(I_1) > 0$ and, since

$$\lim_{I_1 \to \infty} f(I_1) = +\infty,$$

there exists a unique positive solution I_1 if and only if $f(0) < 0$. However,

$$f(0) = \frac{1 - \mathcal{R}^I}{\mathcal{R}_1^I p_1} < 0$$

if and only if $\mathcal{R}^I > 1$. □

10.3.3 Stability of the Boundary Equilibrium

It is easy to verify that the Jacobian of the linearization at the equilibrium $(I_k > 0, J_k = 0)$ has the form of

$$\begin{pmatrix} A_{11} & A_{12} \\ 0 & A_{22} \end{pmatrix},$$

where

$$A_{11} = \begin{pmatrix} -\nu_1^I + b_1\sigma_1^I(p_1 - I_1) - \sigma_1^I(b_1 I_1 + b_2 I_2) & b_2\sigma_1^I(p_1 - I_1) \\ b_1\sigma_2^I(p_2 - I_2) & -\nu_2^I + b_2\sigma_2^I(p_2 - I_2) - \sigma_2^I(b_1 I_1 + b_2 I_2) \end{pmatrix},$$

$$A_{12} = \begin{pmatrix} -\sigma_1^I(b_1 I_1 + b_2 I_2) & 0 \\ 0 & -\sigma_2^I(b_1 I_1 + b_2 I_2) \end{pmatrix},$$

and

$$A_{22} = \begin{pmatrix} -\nu_1^J + b_1\sigma_1^J(p_1 - I_1) & b_2\sigma_1^J(p_1 - I_1) \\ b_1\sigma_2^J(p_2 - I_2) & -\nu_2^J + b_2\sigma_2^J(p_2 - I_2) \end{pmatrix}.$$

Further, since

$$-\nu_1^I + b_1\sigma_1^I(p_1 - I_1) = -\nu_1^I\left(1 - b_1\mathcal{R}_1^I(p_1 - I_1)\right) = -\nu_1^I b_2\mathcal{R}_2^I(p_2 - I_2),$$
$$-\nu_2^I + b_2\sigma_2^I(p_2 - I_2) = -\nu_2^I\left(1 - b_2\mathcal{R}_2^I(p_2 - I_2)\right) = -\nu_2^I b_1\mathcal{R}_1^I(p_1 - I_1),$$

$$\begin{aligned} A_{11} &= \begin{pmatrix} -\nu_1^I I b_2\mathcal{R}_2^I(p_2 - I_2) & b_2\sigma_1^I(p_1 - I_1) \\ b_1\sigma_2^I(p_2 - I_2) & -\nu_2^I I b_2\mathcal{R}_2^I(p_2 - I_2) \end{pmatrix} \\ &+ \begin{pmatrix} -\sigma_1^I(b_1 I_1 + b_2 I_2) & 0 \\ 0 & -\sigma_2^I(b_1 I_1 + b_2 I_2) \end{pmatrix} := G_1 + G_2. \end{aligned} \tag{10.10}$$

Lemma 10.6. *Let P and Q denote $n \times n$ matrices with $Q = \operatorname{diag}(q_j)$, where $q_j < 0$, $j = 1,\ldots,n$. If all eigenvalues of P have nonpositive real parts, then all eigenvalues of $P + Q$ have negative real parts.*

It follows from the facts that $\det G_1 = 0$ and that the diagonal elements are negative that all eigenvalues of G_1 have nonpositive real parts. Hence from Lemma 10.6 it follows that A_{11} is stable. In addition, we have that

$$\begin{aligned} \det A_{22} &= \nu_1^J \nu_2^J\left(1 - \left(\mathcal{R}_1^J b_1(p_1 - I_1) + \mathcal{R}_2^J b_2(p_2 - I_2)\right)\right) \\ &= \nu_1^J \nu_2^J\left(1 - \left(\frac{\mathcal{R}_1^J}{\mathcal{R}_1^I}\frac{b_1 I_1}{b_1 I_1 + b_2 I_2} + \frac{\mathcal{R}_2^J}{\mathcal{R}_2^I}\frac{b_2 I_2}{b_1 I_1 + b_2 I_2}\right)\right) \\ &= \nu_1^J \nu_2^J\left(\frac{\mathcal{R}_1^J - \mathcal{R}_1^I}{\mathcal{R}_1^I}\frac{b_1 I_1}{b_1 I_1 + b_2 I_2} + \frac{\mathcal{R}_2^J - \mathcal{R}_2^I}{\mathcal{R}_2^I}\frac{b_2 I_2}{b_1 I_1 + b_2 I_2}\right). \end{aligned}$$

Thus, if $\mathcal{R}_k^J < \mathcal{R}_k^I$, $k = 1,2$, therefore the equilibrium $(I_k > 0, J_k = 0)$ is stable. Further if $\mathcal{R}_k^J > \mathcal{R}_k^I$, then it follows that $(I_k = 0, J_k > 0)$ is unstable, and under these assumptions there is no other endemic (disease present) equilibrium. Since system (10.2) is monotone under type K order we can conclude that the asymptotically locally stable boundary equilibrium is globally stable. (The proof follows that in [30].)

We summarize the results on boundary equilibria as follows.

Theorem 10.7. *Let $\mathcal{R}^u > 1$, $u = I, J$. If $\mathcal{R}_k^I > \mathcal{R}_k^J$, $k = 1,2$, then the boundary equilibrium $(I_k > 0, J_k = 0)$ is globally stable, while $(I_k = 0, J_k > 0)$ is unstable. In other words, strain 1 persists in the population globally, while strain 2 goes extinct. Similarly, if $\mathcal{R}_k^J > \mathcal{R}_k^I$, $k = 1,2$, then strain 2 persists in the population globally, while strain 1 goes extinct. We have what is called competitive exclusion.*

10.3.4 Existence of the Coexistence Equilibrium

Establishing coexistence corresponds to finding solutions to the system

$$\begin{aligned} \nu_k^I I_k^* &= \sigma_k^I(p_k - I_k^* - J_k^*)(b_1 I_1^* + b_2 I_2^*), \\ \nu_k^J J_k^* &= \sigma_k^J(p_k - I_k^* - J_k^*)(b_1 J_1^* + b_2 J_2^*), \end{aligned} \tag{10.11}$$

with $I_k^* > 0$ and $J_k^* > 0$ (that is, all positive entries). It follows from (10.11) that

$$\frac{\nu_k^I}{\sigma_k^I}\frac{\nu_k^J}{\sigma_k^J}\frac{I_k^*}{J_k^*} = \frac{b_1 I_1^* + b_2 I_2^*}{b_1 J_1^* + b_2 J_2^*}. \tag{10.12}$$

Setting

$$D_k = \frac{\mathcal{R}_k^J}{\mathcal{R}_k^I}$$

leads to

$$D_1 \frac{I_1^*}{I_2^*} = D_2 \frac{J_1^*}{J_2^*}. \tag{10.13}$$

Substituting (10.13) into (10.12) leads to

$$\begin{aligned}\frac{I_1^*}{I_2^*} &= \frac{b_2(1-D_2)}{b_1(D_1-1)},\\ \frac{J_1^*}{J_2^*} &= \frac{D_1 b_2(1-D_2)}{D_2 b_1(D_1-1)}.\end{aligned} \tag{10.14}$$

Hence whenever we have that $D_k > 1$, $k = 1,2$, no endemic equilibrium with all components positive is possible. The following conditions for coexistence are therefore necessary.

Theorem 10.8. *It is not possible to have coexistence if $\mathcal{R}_k^I > \mathcal{R}_k^J$ or $\mathcal{R}_k^J > \mathcal{R}_k^I$ for all $k = 1,2$.*

Two-pathogen strain coexistence requires that

$$\mathcal{R}_2^u > \mathcal{R}_2^v > \mathcal{R}_1^v > \mathcal{R}_1^u, \quad u,v = I,J, \quad u \neq v. \tag{10.15}$$

The computation of a coexistence equilibrium follows from (10.14) and solving (10.11) for $k = 1,2$, respectively. We get the following expressions for I_2^* and J_2^*:

$$\begin{aligned} I_2^* &= \frac{D_1(1-D_2)p_2b_2 - D_2(D_1-1)p_1b_1}{b_2(1-D_2)(D_1-D_2)} + \frac{D_1D_2(D_1-1)}{b_2(D_1-D_2)^2}\left(\frac{1}{\mathcal{R}_1^J} - \frac{1}{\mathcal{R}_2^J}\right),\\ J_2^* &= \frac{D_2((D_1-1)p_1b_1 - (1-D_2)p_2b_2)}{b_2(1-D_2)(D_1-D_2)} + \frac{D_2(D_1-1)}{b_2(D_1-D_2)^2\mathcal{R}_2^I}\left(\frac{1}{\mathcal{R}_2^I} - \frac{1}{\mathcal{R}_1^I}\right). \end{aligned} \tag{10.16}$$

It follows from (10.16), after some algebraic manipulations, that $I_k^* > 0$ and $J_k^* > 0$, $k = 1,2$, if and only if

$$\begin{aligned} &\frac{\mathcal{R}_2^u(\mathcal{R}_1^v - \mathcal{R}_1^u)p_1b_1 - \mathcal{R}_1^u(\mathcal{R}_2^u - \mathcal{R}_2^v)p_2b_2}{\mathcal{R}_2^u - \mathcal{R}_1^u} > \frac{(\mathcal{R}_1^v - \mathcal{R}_1^u)(\mathcal{R}_2^u - \mathcal{R}_2^v)}{\mathcal{R}_2^u\mathcal{R}_1^v - \mathcal{R}_1^u\mathcal{R}_2^v}\\ &\quad > \frac{\mathcal{R}_2^v(\mathcal{R}_1^v - \mathcal{R}_1^u)p_1b_1 - \mathcal{R}_1^v(\mathcal{R}_2^u - \mathcal{R}_2^v)p_2b_2}{\mathcal{R}_2^v - \mathcal{R}_1^v}. \end{aligned} \tag{10.17}$$

Therefore, we conclude the following.

Theorem 10.9. *As long as* (10.15) *and* (10.17) *are satisfied, there always exists a unique coexistence equilibrium. The equilibrium is given by* (10.14) *and* (10.16).

10.3.5 Stability of the Coexistence Equilibrium

The Jacobian matrix at the equilibrium (I_k^*, J_k^*) has the form

$$W := \begin{pmatrix} w_{11} & w_{12} & w_{13} & 0 \\ w_{21} & w_{22} & 0 & w_{24} \\ w_{31} & 0 & w_{33} & w_{34} \\ 0 & w_{42} & w_{43} & w_{44} \end{pmatrix},$$

where

$$\begin{aligned}
w_{11} &:= -\nu_1^I + \sigma_1^I b_1(p_1 - I_1^* - J_1^*) - \sigma_1^I(b_1 I_1^* + b_2 I_2^*), \quad w_{12} := \sigma_1^I b_2(p_1 - I_1^* - J_1^*), \\
w_{13} &:= -\sigma_1^I(b_1 I_1^* + b_2 I_2^*), \quad w_{21} := \sigma_1^I b_1(p_2 - I_2^* - J_2^*), \\
w_{22} &:= -\nu_2^I + \sigma_2^I b_2(p_2 - I_2^* - J_2^*) - \sigma_2^I(b_1 I_1^* + b_2 I_2^*), \quad w_{24} := -\sigma_2^I(b_1 I_1^* + b_2 I_2^*), \\
w_{31} &:= -\sigma_1^J(b_1 J_1^* + b_2 J_2^*), \quad w_{33} := -\nu_1^J + \sigma_1^J b_1(p_1 - I_1^* - J_1^*) - \sigma_1^J(b_1 J_1^* + b_2 J_2^*), \\
w_{34} &:= \sigma_1^J b_2(p_1 - I_1^* - J_1^*), \quad w_{42} := -\sigma_2^J(b_1 J_1^* + b_2 J_2^*), \\
w_{43} &:= \sigma_2^J b_1(p_2 - I_2^* - J_2^*), \quad w_{44} := -\nu_2^J + \sigma_2^J b_2(p_2 - I_2^* - J_2^*)\sigma_2^J(b_1 J_1^* + b_2 J_2^*).
\end{aligned}$$

Since

$$\sigma_k^I(p_k - I_k^* - J_k^*) = \frac{\nu_k^I I_k^*}{b_1 I_1^* + b_2 I_2^*}, \quad \sigma_k^J(p_k - I_k^* - J_k^*) = \frac{\nu_k^J J_k^*}{b_1 J_1^* + b_2 J_2^*},$$

w_{ij}, $i, j = 1, 2$, and w_{ij}, $i, j = 3, 4$, can be rewritten as

$$\begin{aligned}
w_{11} &= -\frac{\nu_1^I b_2 I_2^*}{b_1 I_1^* + b_2 I_2^*} - \sigma_1^I(b_1 I_1^* + b_2 I_2^*), \quad w_{12} = \frac{\nu_1^I b_2 I_1^*}{b_1 I_1^* + b_2 I_2^*}, \\
w_{21} &= \frac{\nu_2^I b_1 I_2^*}{b_1 I_1^* + b_2 I_2^*}, \quad w_{22} = -\frac{\nu_2^I b_1 I_1^*}{b_1 I_1^* + b_2 I_2^*} - \sigma_2^I(b_1 I_1^* + b_2 I_2^*), \\
w_{33} &= -\frac{\nu_1^J b_2 J_2^*}{b_1 J_1^* + b_2 J_2^*} - \sigma_1^J(b_1 J_1^* + b_2 J_2^*), \quad w_{34} = \frac{\nu_1^J b_2 J_1^*}{b_1 J_1^* + b_2 J_2^*}, \\
w_{43} &= \frac{\nu_2^J b_1 J_2^*}{b_1 J_1^* + b_2 J_2^*}, \quad w_{44} = -\frac{\nu_2^J b_1 J_1^*}{b_1 J_1^* + b_2 J_2^*} - \sigma_2^J(b_1 J_1^* + b_2 J_2^*).
\end{aligned}$$

Since W and the matrix

$$\widehat{W} := \begin{pmatrix} w_{11} & w_{12} & |w_{13}| & 0 \\ w_{21} & w_{22} & 0 & |w_{24}| \\ |w_{31}| & 0 & w_{33} & w_{34} \\ 0 & |w_{42}| & w_{43} & w_{44} \end{pmatrix}$$

have the same stability behavior, we let W_i, $i = 2,3,4$, denote the leading principal minors of $\widehat{W}$ with i rows. Long algebraic calculation leads to

$$\begin{aligned}
W_2 &= \sigma_1^I \nu_2^I b_1 I_1^* + \sigma_2^I \nu_1^I b_2 I_2^* + \sigma_1^I \sigma_2^I (b_1 I_1^* + b_2 I_2^*)^2 > 0, \\
W_3 &= -\frac{\left(\sigma_1^I \nu_2^I b_1 I_1^* + \sigma_2^I \nu_1^I b_2 I_2^* + \sigma_1^I \sigma_2^I (b_1 I_1^* + b_2 I_2^*)^2\right) \nu_1^J b_2 J_2^*}{b_1 J_1^* + b_2 J_2^*} \\
&\quad - \sigma_2^I \sigma_1^J \nu_1^I b_2 I_2^* (b_1 J_1^* + b_2 J_2^*) < 0, \\
W_4 &= \nu_1^I \nu_2^I \nu_1^J \nu_2^J b_1 b_2 I_2^* J_1^* \left(\frac{I_1^*}{I_2^*}\frac{J_2^*}{J_1^*} - 1\right)\left(\mathcal{R}_1^I \mathcal{R}_2^J - \mathcal{R}_1^J \mathcal{R}_2^I\right),
\end{aligned} \tag{10.18}$$

from which we observe that the stability of the coexistence equilibrium is determined by the sign of W_4. The use of (10.13) and (10.15) leads to

$$\frac{I_1^*}{I_2^*}\frac{J_2^*}{J_1^*} = \frac{D_2}{D_1}$$

and

$$\mathcal{R}_1^I \mathcal{R}_2^J - \mathcal{R}_1^J \mathcal{R}_2^I = \mathcal{R}_1^I \mathcal{R}_2^I \left(\frac{\mathcal{R}_2^J}{\mathcal{R}_2^I} - \frac{\mathcal{R}_1^J}{\mathcal{R}_1^I}\right) = D_1 \mathcal{R}_1^I \mathcal{R}_2^I \left(\frac{D_2}{D_1} - 1\right).$$

It follows that

$$W_4 = \nu_1^I \nu_2^I \nu_1^J \nu_2^J b_1 b_2 I_2^* J_1^* D_1 \mathcal{R}_1^I \mathcal{R}_2^I \left(\frac{D_2}{D_1} - 1\right)^2 > 0,$$

and therefore W_4 is always positive, a property that implies that the coexistence equilibrium is stable if it exists (M-matrix theory). Finally, since the flow generated is monotone, local stability of the coexistence equilibrium implies its global stability [95].

A nongeneric biological result also follows. We can see that if

$$\mathcal{R}_1^J \mathcal{R}_2^I = \mathcal{R}_1^I \mathcal{R}_2^J, \tag{10.19}$$

that is, if $D_1 = D_2$, then we have a one-dimensional continuum of equilibria. In fact, we have the following result.

Theorem 10.10. *If* (10.15) *and* (10.17) *are met, then there exists a globally stable coexistence equilibrium. Further, if* (10.19) *holds, unlikely in the biological world, then there exists a stable, one-dimensional continuum of equilibria.*

It follows that every point on the continuum is (neutrally) stable.

Hypotheses (10.15) and (10.17) can be rewritten as follows:

$$\begin{aligned}
&\mu_1 + \gamma_1^v < \mu_2 + \gamma_2^v, \\
&\mu_1 + \gamma_1^u < \mu_2 + \gamma_2^u, \\
&(\mu_1 + \gamma_1^v)(\mu_2 + \gamma_2^u) < (\mu_1 + \gamma_1^u)(\mu_2 + \gamma_2^v),
\end{aligned} \tag{10.20}$$

$$\frac{p_2 b_2}{p_1 b_1} < \frac{1 - \dfrac{\beta^u}{\beta^v} \dfrac{\mu_1 + \gamma_1^v}{\mu_1 + \gamma_1^u}}{\dfrac{\beta^u}{\beta^v} \dfrac{\mu_2 + \gamma_2^v}{\mu_2 + \gamma_2^u} - 1}, \tag{10.21}$$

$u, v = I, J,\ u \neq v.$

We can see that in some special cases, the conditions set in the theory are met. For example, (10.15) is satisfied if $\mu_1 = \mu_2$, $b_1 = b_2$, $\lambda_1 = \lambda_2$, and $\beta^I = \beta^J$ as long as we have that

$$\gamma_1^I < \gamma_2^I, \qquad \gamma_1^J < \gamma_2^J,$$
$$\frac{\mu + \gamma_1^J}{\mu + \gamma_1^I} < \frac{\mu + \gamma_2^J}{\mu + \gamma_2^I},$$

while (10.17) is satisfied if

$$\frac{\mu + \gamma_1^J}{\mu + \gamma_1^I} + \frac{\mu + \gamma_2^J}{\mu + \gamma_2^I} < 2.$$

Variation in the rates of recovery would be rather important to guarantee pathogen coexistence, since if, for example, we had that $(\mu_1 + \gamma_1^I)/(\mu_1 + \gamma_1^J) = (\mu_2 + \gamma_2^I)/(\mu_2 + \gamma_2^J)$, then (10.17) would not satisfied.

10.4 Two-Sex STD Models

The modeling of two-sex contact structures have been addressed by a variety of researchers, with our contributions found in [5, 6, 9, 16, 17, 23, 24, 28, 29, 33, 53, 94, 60, 79]. Efforts to ground two-sex frameworks on data have been carried out as well [7, 21, 25, 28, 29, 41, 92, 93, 60, 79, 91].

The results outlined in Section 10.3 were carried out in the context of single-sex *SIS* STD models using or adapting the results published in [30, 31, 32, 35, 37]. In this section, we revisit the concepts in Section 10.3 within a model that includes two-sex interactions.

We start with the premise that a heterosexually active population is being simultaneously invaded by n competing strains of a sexually transmitted pathogen. It is assumed that each host cannot simultaneously house more than one strain; that individuals recover naturally or through treatment; and that no immunity is gained in the process of recovery or treatment. The superscripts m and f are used throughout this section to differentiate between male and female members of the heterosexually active population under study.

Further, we let Λ^k, $k = m, f$, denote the "recruitment" rates into each of the sexually active populations; μ^k, $k = m, f$, denotes the natural death rates for males and females, respectively (rates that include removal from sexual activity); γ_i^k, $k = m, f$, denotes the rates of recovery (including the time it takes to become symptomatic); β_i^k, $k = m, f$, denotes the transmission rates of infection; T^m and T^f denote the total number of males and females, respectively; and, finally, functions of T^m and T^f, r^k, $k = m, f$, are used to model the average rates of partner acquisition per male and per female, respectively. The dynamics of n competing STD strains are therefore governed by the following system of nonlinear equations:

$$\begin{aligned}
\dot{S}^m &= \Lambda^m - B^m - \mu^m S^m + \sum_{i=1}^{n} \gamma_i^m I_i^m, \\
\dot{I}_i^m &= B_i^m - (\mu^m + \gamma_i^m) I_i^m, \\
\dot{S}^f &= \Lambda^f - B^f - \mu^f S^f + \sum_{i=1}^{n} \gamma_i^f I_i^f, \\
\dot{I}_i^f &= B_i^f - \left(\mu^f + \gamma_i^f\right) I_i^f,
\end{aligned} \tag{10.22}$$

where

$$B_i^m = r^m \left(T^m, T^f\right) S^m \beta_i^f \frac{I_i^f}{T^f}, \tag{10.23}$$

$$B_i^f = r^f \left(T^m, T^f\right) S^f \beta_i^m \frac{I_i^m}{T^m}, \tag{10.24}$$

$$B^m = \frac{r^m \left(T^m, T^f\right) S^m}{T^f} \sum_{j=1}^{n} \beta_j^f I_j^f, \tag{10.25}$$

$$B^f = \frac{r^f \left(T^m, T^f\right) S^f}{T^m} \sum_{j=1}^{n} \beta_j^m I_j^m. \tag{10.26}$$

We have that r^k must satisfy the "pairing" or "mixing" two-sex constraint [17, 23, 24, 25, 29, 33, 53, 94, 60, 79] given by the identity

$$r^m \left(T^m, T^f\right) T^m = r^f \left(T^m, T^f\right) T^f. \tag{10.27}$$

This identity states that the total average contact rate of females equals the total average contact rate of males.

Furthermore, since $T^k = S^k + \sum_{i=1}^{n} I_i^k$, we can replace model (10.22) by the following equivalent system:

$$\begin{aligned}
\dot{T}^m &= \Lambda^m - \mu^m T^m, \\
\dot{T}^f &= \Lambda^f - \mu^f T^f, \\
\dot{I}_i^m &= -(\mu^m + \gamma_i^m) I_i^m + r^m \left(T^m, T^f\right) \frac{\beta_i^f I_i^f}{T^f} \left(T^m - \sum_{j=1}^{n} I_j^m\right), \\
\dot{I}_i^f &= -\left(\mu^f + \gamma_i^f\right) I_i^f + r^f \left(T^m, T^f\right) \frac{\beta_i^m I_i^m}{T^m} \left(T^f - \sum_{j=1}^{n} I_j^f\right).
\end{aligned} \tag{10.28}$$

It is easily shown that the equilibrium solution for T^k, $k = m, f$, are

$$T^m = \frac{\Lambda^m}{\mu^m}, \qquad T^f = \frac{\Lambda^f}{\mu^f},$$

and therefore the corresponding equilibrium values for the contact rates are given by

$$c^m := r^m\left(\Lambda^m/\mu^m, \Lambda^f/\mu^f\right), \qquad c^f := r^f\left(\Lambda^m/\mu^m, \Lambda^f/\mu^f\right).$$

From constraint (10.27), it follows that

$$c^m \Lambda^m = c^f \Lambda^f$$

as $t \to \infty$.

Using these computations and the results in [27, 97, 99], we conclude that a dynamically equivalent limiting system to (10.28) is given by the following reduced set of equations:

$$\begin{aligned} \dot{I}_i^m &= -\left(\mu^m + \gamma_i^m\right) I_i^m + \frac{\mu^f c^m \beta_i^f}{\Lambda^f}\left(\frac{\Lambda^m}{\mu^m} - \sum_{j=1}^n I_j^m\right) I_i^f, \\ \dot{I}_i^f &= -\left(\mu^f + \gamma_i^f\right) I_i^f + \frac{\mu^m c^f \beta_i^m}{\Lambda^m}\left(\frac{\Lambda^f}{\mu^f} - \sum_{j=1}^n I_j^f\right) I_i^m. \end{aligned} \tag{10.29}$$

Setting

$$\sigma_i^k := \left(\mu^k + \gamma_i^k\right), \quad a_i^m := \frac{\mu^f c^m \beta_i^f}{\Lambda^f}, \quad a_i^f := \frac{\mu^m c^f \beta_i^m}{\Lambda^m}, \quad \text{and } p^k := \frac{\Lambda^k}{\mu^k}$$

allows us to rewrite system (10.29) as follows:

$$\begin{aligned} \dot{I}_i^m &= -\sigma_i^m I_i^m + a_i^m \left(p^m - \sum_{j=1}^n I_j^m\right) I_i^f, \\ \dot{I}_i^f &= -\sigma_i^f I_i^f + a_i^f \left(p^f - \sum_{j=1}^n I_j^f\right) I_i^m. \end{aligned} \tag{10.30}$$

Finally, we observed that since the dynamics of (10.22) or (10.28) are qualitatively equivalent to those of system (10.30), then we can focus on the study of system (10.30).

10.4.1 Thresholds and Global Stability

Strain-specific reproductive numbers provide a measure of the ability of a disease strain to invade a population. Strain-specific reproductive numbers can be derived from the linearization of system (10.30) about the infection-free equilibrium, namely, from the system

$$\begin{aligned} \dot{I}_i^m &= -\sigma_i^m I_i^m + a_i^m p^m I_i^f, \\ \dot{I}_i^f &= -\sigma_i^f I_i^f + a_i^f p^f I_i^m, \qquad i = 1, \ldots, n. \end{aligned} \tag{10.31}$$

Since the n equations in system (10.31) are decoupled, it follows that if

$$\sigma_i^m \sigma_i^f > a_i^m a_i^f p^m p^f, \qquad i = 1,\ldots,n,$$

then the infection-free equilibrium is stable. If, on the other hand, there exists an index i $(1 \le i \le n)$ such that

$$\sigma_i^m \sigma_i^f < a_i^m a_i^f p^m p^f,$$

then we must conclude that the infection-free equilibrium is unstable.

We define the ith subgroup reproductive number by the expression

$$\mathcal{R}_i := \frac{c^m c^f \beta_i^m \beta_i^f}{\left(\mu + \gamma_i^m\right)\left(\mu + \gamma_i^f\right)}, \tag{10.32}$$

and observe that if $\mathcal{R}_i \le 1$, then $(I_i^m, I_i^f) \to (0,0)$. Therefore, if $\mathcal{R}_i \le 1$ for all i, then it follows that the infection-free equilibrium is (locally) stable; all the strains of the disease go extinct in this case. If, however, there exists at least one subgroup (let's say i) for which $\mathcal{R}_i > 1$, then we have, for this subgroup, that $(I_i^m, I_i^f) \not\to (0,0)$. Hence, strain i will spread in the population.

Finally, it can be shown that under appropriate conditions the infection-free state is globally asymptotically stable. The proof of the global stability of the infection-free state makes use of the following lemma.

Lemma 10.11 (see [30, Theorem 4.1.2]). *Consider the following system of differential equations:*

$$\begin{aligned}
\dot{\widehat{I}}_i^m &= -\sigma_i^m \widehat{I}_i^m + a_i^m \left(p^m - \sum_{j=1}^{2} \widehat{I}_j^m \right) \widehat{I}_i^f, \\
\dot{\widehat{I}}_i^f &= -\sigma_i^f \widehat{I}_i^f + a_i^f \left(p^f - \sum_{j=1}^{2} \widehat{I}_j^f \right) \widehat{I}_i^m, \qquad i = 1,2.
\end{aligned}$$

Let

$$\widehat{\mathcal{R}}_i := \frac{a_i^m a_i^f p^m p^f}{\sigma_i^m \sigma_i^f}, \qquad i = 1,2.$$

If $\widehat{\mathcal{R}}_i \le 1$, then $\lim_{t\to\infty} \widehat{I}_i^k(t) = 0$ for all $I_i^k(0) > 0$, $i = 1,2$, $k = m,f$. If $\widehat{\mathcal{R}}_j > \widehat{\mathcal{R}}_l > 1$, $j,l = 1,2$, $j \ne l$, then $\lim_{t\to\infty} \widehat{I}_l^k(t) = 0$ for all $I_l^k(0) > 0$ and $k = m,f$.

The proof of the global stability of the infection-free equilibrium if $\mathcal{R}_i \le 1$ for all i follows from Lemma 10.11 and goes as follows:

For any $1 \le j,l \le n,\ j \ne l$, consider the system

$$\begin{aligned}
\dot{\widehat{I}_j^m} &= -\sigma_j^m \widehat{I}_j^m + a_j^m \left(p^m - \left(\widehat{I}_j^m + \widehat{I}_l^m\right)\right)\widehat{I}_j^f,\\
\dot{\widehat{I}_j^f} &= -\sigma_j^f \widehat{I}_j^f + a_j^f \left(p^f - \left(\widehat{I}_j^f + \widehat{I}_l^f\right)\right)\widehat{I}_j^m,\\
\dot{\widehat{I}_l^m} &= -\sigma_l^m \widehat{I}_l^m + a_l^m \left(p^m - \left(\widehat{I}_j^m + \widehat{I}_l^m\right)\right)\widehat{I}_l^f,\\
\dot{\widehat{I}_l^f} &= -\sigma_l^f \widehat{I}_l^f + a_l^f \left(p^f - \left(\widehat{I}_j^f + \widehat{I}_l^f\right)\right)\widehat{I}_l^m.
\end{aligned}$$

If $\widehat{\mathcal{R}}_j$ and $\widehat{\mathcal{R}}_l$ denotes the reproductive numbers for group j and group l respectively, then $\widehat{\mathcal{R}}_j = \mathcal{R}_j$ and $\widehat{\mathcal{R}}_l = \mathcal{R}_l$. Since by assumption $\mathcal{R}_i \le 1$ for all i (which implies $\widehat{\mathcal{R}}_j \le 1$ and $\widehat{\mathcal{R}}_l \le 1$) it follows from Lemma 10.11 that $\lim_{t\to\infty} \widehat{I}_j^k(t) \to 0$ and $\lim_{t\to\infty} \widehat{I}_l^k(t) \to 0$, as $t \to \infty$ for all $\widehat{I}_j^k(0) > 0$ and $\widehat{I}_l^k(0) > 0$, $k = m, f$. In addition, the comparison principle implies that $I_j^k(t) \le \widehat{I}_j^k(t)$, $I_l^k(t) \le \widehat{I}_l^k(t)$, $k = m, f$, for all $t \ge 0$. Thus, the infection-free equilibrium is globally stable. Therefore, we have established the following.

Theorem 10.12. *Let the reproductive number $\mathcal{R}_i$ for each group be defined in* (10.12). *Then if $\mathcal{R}_i \le 1$ for all $1 \le i \le n$, the epidemic goes extinct regardless of the initial levels of infection. If $\mathcal{R}_i > 1$ for some $1 \le i \le n$, then the epidemic spreads in the population.*

Remark. We reiterate that the mathematical results in this section have appeared in one form or another in [30, 31, 32, 35].

10.4.2 Endemic equilibria

The approach and methods used in [30] can be used to establish the following results.

Theorem 10.13. *Assume that $\mathcal{R}_i > 1,\ 1 \le i \le n$. Then a unique nontrivial equilibrium $(S^k > 0, I_i^k > 0, I_j^k = 0, j \ne i)$ exists.*

Proof. We proceed to solve

$$\sigma_i^m I_i^m = a_i^m \left(p^m - I_i^m\right) I_i^f, \qquad \sigma_i^f I_i^f = a_i^f \left(p^f - I_i^f\right) I_i^m$$

for I_i^k, $0 < I_i^k < p^k$, and after some algebra we arrive at

$$\begin{aligned}
I_i^m &= \frac{a_i^m a_i^f p^m p^f - \sigma_i^m \sigma_i^f}{a_i^f \left(\sigma_i^m + a_i^m p^f\right)} = \frac{(\mathcal{R}_i - 1)\sigma_i^m \sigma_i^f}{a_i^f \left(\sigma_i^m + a_i^m p^f\right)},\\
I_i^f &= \frac{a_i^m a_i^f p^m p^f - \sigma_i^m \sigma_i^f}{a_i^m \left(\sigma_i^f + a_i^f p^m\right)} = \frac{(\mathcal{R}_i - 1)\sigma_i^m \sigma_i^f}{a_i^m \left(\sigma_i^f + a_i^f p^m\right)}.
\end{aligned}$$

Hence, we conclude that $I_i^k > 0$ if and only if $\mathcal{R}_i > 1$. $\square$

Among all these equilibria, there exists only one which is globally stable, with the other equilibria unstable. As expected the stability is totally determined by the reproductive numbers. In fact, an application of Lemma 10.11 leads to the following result.

Theorem 10.14. *Let there be more than one reproductive number that is greater than one; assume that they are all distinct. Further, if we let $\mathcal{R}_i$ denote the largest reproductive number, then it follows that the nontrivial equilibrium ($S^k > 0, I_i^k > 0, I_j^k = 0, j \neq i$, $k = m, f$) is stable while the other equilibria ($S^k > 0, I_j^k > 0, I_l^k = 0, l \neq j, k = m, f$), $j \neq i$, are unstable.*

Proof. We assume that $\mathcal{R}_1 > \mathcal{R}_j$ for all $j \neq 1$, and for any $j > 1$ consider the system

$$\begin{aligned}
\dot{\widehat{I_1^m}} &= -\sigma_1^m \widehat{I_1^m} + a_1^m \left(p^m - \left(\widehat{I_1^m} + \widehat{I_j^m}\right)\right)\widehat{I_1^f}, \\
\dot{\widehat{I_1^f}} &= -\sigma_1^f \widehat{I_1^f} + a_1^f \left(p^f - \left(\widehat{I_1^f} + \widehat{I_j^f}\right)\right)\widehat{I_1^m}, \\
\dot{\widehat{I_j^m}} &= -\sigma_j^m \widehat{I_j^m} + a_j^m \left(p^m - \left(\widehat{I_1^m} + \widehat{I_j^m}\right)\right)\widehat{I_j^f}, \\
\dot{\widehat{I_j^f}} &= -\sigma_j^f \widehat{I_j^f} + a_j^f \left(p^f - \left(\widehat{I_1^f} + \widehat{I_j^f}\right)\right)\widehat{I_j^m}.
\end{aligned}$$

If we let $\widehat{\mathcal{R}}_1$ and $\widehat{\mathcal{R}}_j$ denote the reproductive numbers for group 1 and group j, respectively, then $\widehat{\mathcal{R}}_1 = \mathcal{R}_1$ and $\widehat{\mathcal{R}}_j = \mathcal{R}_j$. It follows that $\widehat{\mathcal{R}}_1 > \widehat{\mathcal{R}}_j$, and from Lemma 10.11 we have that $\lim_{t\to\infty} \widehat{I_j^k}(t) = 0$ for all $\widehat{I_j^k}(0) > 0$, $k = m, f$. Use of the comparison principle allows us to conclude that $I_j^k(t) \leq \widehat{I_j^k}(t)$, $k = m, f$, for all $t \geq 0$. Hence, $\lim_{t\to\infty} I_j^k(t) = 0$, $k = m, f$ and therefore all solutions approach the equilibrium ($S^k > 0, I_1^k > 0, I_j^k = 0, j \neq 1$, $k = m, f$). □

Coexistence occurs in the nongeneric case when all strains have the same reproductive numbers.

Theorem 10.15. *Let Ω be a nonempty subset of $\{1,2,\ldots,n\}$; then there exists a nontrivial equilibrium $\left(S^k > 0, I_l^k > 0, l \in \Omega, I_u^k = 0, u \notin \Omega\right)$ if*

$$\mathcal{R}_i = \mathcal{R}_j \qquad \textit{for all } i, j \in \Omega.$$

Proof. If we assume that such a nontrivial equilibrium exists, then

$$\begin{aligned}
\sigma_i^m I_i^m &= a_i^m \left(p^m - \sum_{l\in\Omega} I_l^m\right) I_i^f, \\
\sigma_i^f I_i^f &= a_i^f \left(p^f - \sum_{l\in\Omega} I_l^f\right) I_i^m,
\end{aligned}$$

that is,

$$I_i^m = \frac{a_i^m}{\sigma_i^m}\left(p^m - \sum_{l\in\Omega} I_l^m\right) I_i^f,$$

$$I_i^f = \frac{a_i^f}{\sigma_i^f}\left(p^f - \sum_{l\in\Omega} I_l^m\right) I_i^m.$$

Hence

$$\frac{a_i^m a_i^f}{\sigma_i^m \sigma_i^f}\left(p^m - \sum_{l\in\Omega} I_l^m\right)\left(p^f - \sum_{l\in\Omega} I_l^f\right) = 1,$$

or

$$\frac{\mu^2}{\Lambda^m \Lambda^f}\left(p^m - \sum_{l\in\Omega} I_l^m\right)\left(p^f - \sum_{l\in\Omega} I_l^f\right)\frac{c^m c^f \beta_i^m \beta_i^f}{(\mu+\gamma_i^m)\left(\mu+\gamma_i^f\right)} = 1,$$

which holds for all $i \in \Omega$. This completes the proof. □

If it is now assumed that there are q subgroups with identical reproductive numbers and proceed to relabel them 1 to q (with no loss of generality), that is, $\mathcal{R}_i = \mathcal{R}_j$, $1 \le i, j \le q$, then we can proceed to identify explicitly a continuum of coexistence equilibria; $I_i^k > 0$ for all $1 \le i \le q$. In other words, we get the following result.

Theorem 10.16. *If it is assumed that there are q subgroups such that $\mathcal{R}_i = \mathcal{R}$ for all $1 \le i \le q$, then there exists a q-dimensional continuum of equilibria*

$$\begin{aligned}
I_i^m &= \frac{p^m\left(\mathcal{R}\sigma_l^m + p^f a_l^m\right) a_i^m \alpha_i}{\mathcal{R}\sigma_i^m\left(p^f a_l^m + \sigma_l^m\left(1 - \sum_{j\in U}\left(a_l^m/\sigma_l^m - a_j^m/\sigma_j^m\right)\right)\alpha_j\right)}, \qquad i \in U,\\
I_i^f &= \alpha_i, \qquad i \in U, \qquad\qquad (10.33)\\
I_l^m &= \frac{p^m a_l^m\left(p^f \sigma_l^m(\mathcal{R}-1) - \sigma_l^m \sum_{j\in U}\left(\mathcal{R} + p^f a_j^m/\sigma_j^m\right)\alpha_j\right)}{\mathcal{R}\sigma_i^m\left(p^f a_l^m + \sigma_l^m\left(1 - \sum_{j\in U}\left(a_l^m/\sigma_l^m - a_j^m/\sigma_j^m\right)\right)\alpha_j\right)}, \qquad l \notin U,\\
I_l^f &= \frac{p^f \sigma_l^m(\mathcal{R}-1) - \sigma_l^m \sum_{j\in U}\left(\mathcal{R} + p^f a_j^m/\sigma_j^m\right)\alpha_j}{\mathcal{R}\sigma_l^m + p^f a_l^m},
\end{aligned}$$

where $U := \{i_1, \ldots, i_{q-1}\} \subset \{1, \ldots, q\}$; $\alpha_i > 0$ are $q-1$ arbitrary constants satisfying

$$\sum_{j\in U}\left(\mathcal{R} + p^f \frac{a_j^m}{\sigma_j^m}\right)\alpha_j < p^f(\mathcal{R}-1). \qquad (10.34)$$

Proof. We proceed to solve the system

$$\sigma_i^m I_i^m = a_i^m \left(p^m - \sum_{j=1}^{q} I_j^m \right) I_i^f,$$

$$\sigma_i^f I_i^f = a_i^f \left(p^f - \sum_{j=1}^{q} I_j^f \right) I_i^m \tag{10.35}$$

for $I_i^k > 0$ with $\sum_{j=1}^q I_j^m < p^m$ and $\sum_{j=1}^q I_j^f < p^f$. Using (10.35) and solving for I_i^m, we have that

$$I_i^m = \frac{p^m a_i^m I_i^f}{\sigma_i^m \left(1 + \sum_{j=1}^q \frac{a_j^m}{\sigma_j^m} I_j^f \right)}. \tag{10.36}$$

The substitution of (10.36) into $(10.35)_2$ after some algebra leads to

$$\sum_{j=1}^{q} \left(\mathcal{R} + p^f \frac{a_j^m}{\sigma_j^m} \right) I_j^f = p^f (\mathcal{R} - 1).$$

Choosing $q-1$ $I_j^f = \alpha_j > 0$, satisfying (10.34), leads to I_l^f as in $(10.33)_4$. The expressions $(10.33)_1$ and $(10.33)_3$ follow from (10.36). This continuum is actually stable but its structural instability limits its biological importance. □

Next, we highlight an application of the modeling and thinking approaches discussed in Section 10.4, specifically a mathematical study of the dynamics of HIV driven by scenarios that incorporate some of the elements characterizing HIV in Nigeria (see [63]).

Remark. The mathematical results in this subsection have appeared in one form or another in [30, 31, 32, 35].

10.5 Transactional Sex and HIV in Nigeria

Estimates of HIV-infected individuals in sub-Saharan Africa have reached 23 million [3], with Nigeria and South Africa maintaining unprecedented high levels [3, 48]. In 2001, 170,000 adults and children died of AIDS in Nigeria according to [100]. New estimates report increases of over fifty percent [3]. Not surprisingly, the sex industry has been identified as a major force behind these increases in Nigeria. Studies like [62] have specifically evaluated the role of long-distance truck drivers, commercial motorcycle riders, and related groups—the primary clients of female sex workers—on HIV dynamics.

Researchers have observed that truck drivers and itinerant sex workers in Nigeria are members of a large network of individuals involved with multiple sex partners along the Ilorin-Ibadan-Lagos highway [86]. Despite the stigma that engulfs sex workers and the risks of HIV, the sex industry continues to thrive in Nigeria due to extreme poverty in large segments of the population. Truck driving, a lucrative profession, is particularly appealing to young males with limited skills or education. Drivers spend multiple nights on the road, becoming quite often involved with female sex workers in stopover towns that shadow major transportation routes. As a result of economic and lifestyle factors, truck drivers are highly connected nodes of networks that facilitate the spread of HIV among large segments of the Nigerian population [58, 86, 87, 85]. The interactions between these two core groups increase HIV risk levels significantly among individuals that otherwise would be classified as low-risk HIV targets.

Data highlight many of the challenges posed by the transmission dynamics of HIV in highly sexually active populations. In a 1991 study, for example, track drivers reported an average of 6.3 concurrent sexual partners (sex workers), 12 sexual partners during the prior year, and 25 sexual partners besides their mates (wives) over their lifetimes [86]. It was also reported in [85] that the prevalence of HIV infections among Nigerian truck drivers in transit towns was 400 times higher (54% instead of 17%) than in nontransit towns. Studies along a major Ugandan highway have estimated truck driver HIV prevalence at 35%, with roughly 37% of these individuals having more than 50 female sexual partners during their lifetimes [102]. In addition studies on the sexual practices and customary barriers associated with condom use among truck drivers in Nigeria report that truck drivers' condom use is at 9% level, even though roughly 70% of these individuals are aware of the role of condoms in preventing HIV infections [96]. On the other hand, condom use seems to be in general well accepted by female sex workers [87], although it is not always enforced due to customers' reluctance to protect the women and themselves.

The material reintroduced in the next sections comes from [63]. That is, the models and model results, revisited in this lecture, come from our preliminary efforts to assess HIV dynamics in Nigeria, where the prevalence of HIV within the general population is in the 3.5 to 8% range (ages 15–49), an approximate 5% average between 1999 and 2003. Data show that the rates among men and women are approximately the same within this age window [100]. However, the percentages among adult men who hire at least one commercial sex workers per year have been estimated to be between 8 and 11%. The problem is quite serious since, in fact, the percentage of truck drivers who have reported extramarital (including casual) sexual activity (assumed here to be primarily with sex workers) has been estimated to be 72–92% [80, 88]. For sub-Saharan Africa the fraction of the female population that are sex workers is highly variable over local scales, low in cities and high in rural towns along major transportation routes. The percentage of the population that are truck drivers is around 2–4%, while the overall estimated population average of HIV-infected individuals falls in the 1–2% range in Nigeria [80, 86, 87, 88].

In the remaining sections of this chapter, the role of transactional sex on the dynamics of HIV spread within the two core groups is revisited [63]. The models presented are not the first models that address these issues. In fact, the core model reported in [64] was used to study the effects of the HIV/AIDS epidemic on Africa's truck drivers from estimates in the reported losses of truck drivers. The goal in [63], the basis of these last sections, is different. It starts by studying the dynamics of HIV spread in high-risk groups and proceeds to focus on developing models that help us generate rough estimates of the influence that core groups have on HIV spread in the entire sexually active population.

Remark. The models and mathematical results in this sections appeared in [63].

10.5.1 Core group model and dynamics

We start with a simplified scenario involving two interacting core groups. Individuals are removed from the core due to retirement from risky sexual activity or natural mortality. AIDS-diagnosed individuals are replaced immediately in the core via the recruitment of new members from a nonspecified general population. The economic conditions are such that it is assumed that the supply of workers (sex workers and truck drivers) exceeds the demand. In this subsection, only sexual activity between truck drivers and sex workers is considered; both groups select partners at random; transmission rates are constant over the life of the disease; recruitment brings only uninfected persons to the core the size of core groups does not change since lost truck drivers and sex workers are immediately replaced; AIDS cases are assumed to be highly symptomatic; and progression from HIV to AIDS guarantees the removal of individuals from the sexually active core.

Here S_m and S_f denote the number of susceptible truck drivers and female sex workers, respectively; I_m and I_f denote the number of infected male truck drivers and female sex workers, respectively. Truck drivers and sex workers are recruited at the same rate as they are lost; in other words, it is assumed that the supply of workers is always sufficient. Losses from the system can be traced back to natural mortality (μ's), non-AIDS related retirement (ρ's), and removal or death due to progression from HIV to AIDS (γ's). The onset of AIDS makes it impossible (in this framework) for a person to continue to be employed as a truck driver or sex worker. New infections are generated exclusively via heterosexual contacts between susceptible and infected individuals in the core (the transmission coefficients given by the β's). The rate of new infections among sex workers (for instance) is the product $\beta_{mf}\nu_m\frac{I_m}{N_m}S_f$, where $\frac{I_m}{N_m}$ is the fraction of truck drivers infected, and ν_m is the fraction of the adult male population of Nigeria that are truck drivers. The product of the two terms ($\nu_m\frac{I_m}{N_m}$) then gives the probability that a male client selected at random will actually be a infected. The force of infection, therefore, is given by $\beta_{mf}\nu_m\frac{I_m}{N_m}$. The exact description of the parameters used is in Table 10.1. We observe that the contact rates between sex workers and truck drivers must conform to the "conservation of contacts law." Hence, if ξ_{fm} denotes the probability that a susceptible male contracts the disease from

Table 10.1. *Model parameters as given in* [63].

Symbol	Description
β_{fm}	rate at which female sex workers infect truck drivers per susceptible truck driver
β_{mf}	rate at which truck drivers infect commercial sex workers per susceptible sex worker
μ_m (μ_f)	natural mortality rate of truck drivers (sex workers)
ρ_m (ρ_f)	retirement rate of truck drivers (sex workers)
ψ_m	turnover rate of uninfected truck drivers ($=\mu_m+\rho_m$)
ψ_f	turnover rate of uninfected sex workers $(=\mu_f+\rho_f)$
γ_m (γ_f)	rate at which infected men (women) progress to AIDS
ν_m (ν_f)	fraction of *all* adult males (females) that are truck drivers (sex workers)

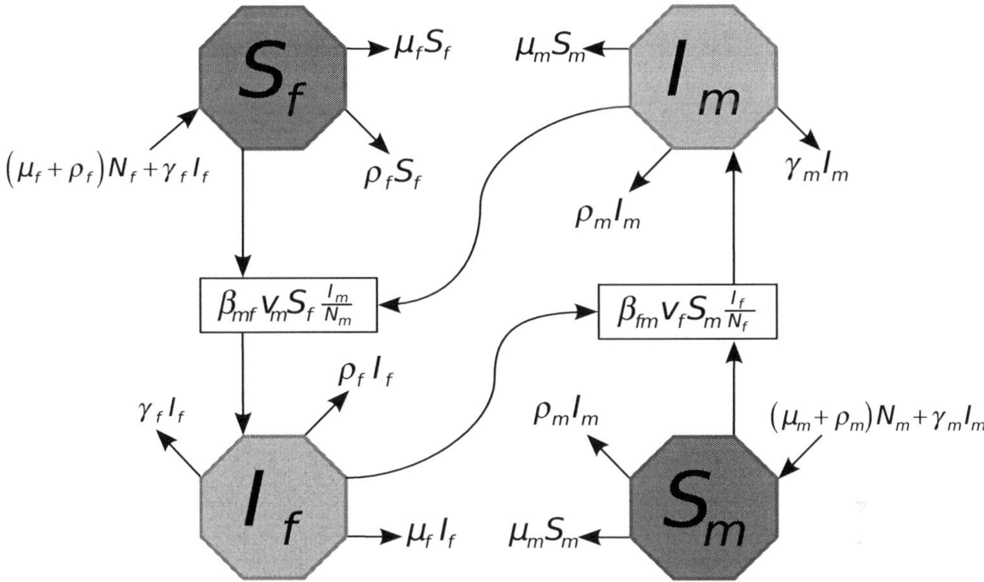

Figure 10.1. *A compartmental diagram for the system in* (10.37). *(This schematic diagram was modified from Figure* 1 *of* [63, p. 4].*)*

an infected female per contact and ξ_{mf} denotes the probability that a susceptible female contracts the disease from an infected male per contact, then the total number of effective contacts per unit of time is given by $\beta_{mf}\xi_{mf}^{-1}\nu_m N_f$ and $\beta_{fm}\xi_{fm}^{-1}\nu_f N_m$, respectively. Thus, we arrive at the following system shown in flowchart form in Figure 10.1:

$$\begin{aligned}
\dot{S}_f &= \left(\left(\mu_f+\rho_f\right)N_f+\gamma_f I_f\right)-\left(\mu_f+\rho_f\right)S_f-\beta_{mf}\nu_m\frac{I_m}{N_m}S_f,\\
\dot{S}_m &= (\mu_m+\rho_m)N_m+\gamma_m I_m-(\mu_m+\rho_m)S_m-\beta_{fm}\nu_f\frac{I_f}{N_f}S_m,\\
\dot{I}_f &= \beta_{mf}\nu_m\frac{I_m}{N_m}S_f-(\gamma_f+\mu_f+\rho_f)I_f,\\
\dot{I}_m &= \beta_{fm}\nu_f\frac{I_f}{N_f}S_m-(\gamma_m+\mu_m+\rho_m)I_m.
\end{aligned} \tag{10.37}$$

Here, the total population of truck drivers is $N_m = S_m + I_m$ and of sex workers is $N_f = S_f + I_f$. The assumption that the sizes of N_f and N_m are constant reduces (10.37) to

$$\begin{aligned}
\dot{I}_f &= \beta_{mf}\nu_m\frac{I_m}{N_m}\left(N_f-I_f\right)-(\gamma_f+\psi_f)I_f,\\
\dot{I}_m &= \beta_{fm}\nu_f\frac{I_f}{N_f}(N_m-I_m)-(\gamma_m+\psi_m)I_m.
\end{aligned} \tag{10.38}$$

Since the populations are constant or asymptotically constant, then we can reformulate (10.38) in terms of the proportions of the respective infected core groups. Let $X = \frac{I_f}{N_f}$

and $Y=\frac{I_m}{N_m}$. Substituting ψ for $\mu+\rho$ gives the system

$$\begin{aligned}\dot{X} &= \beta_{mf}\nu_m Y(1-X)-(\gamma_f+\psi_f)X,\\ \dot{Y} &= \beta_{fm}\nu_f X(1-Y)-(\gamma_m+\psi_m)Y,\end{aligned} \tag{10.39}$$

which is analyzed in the next section.

Remark. The mathematical model and results in this subsection appeared in [63].

10.5.2 Mathematical analysis

System (10.39) supports two equilibria: a disease-free equilibrium $E_0=(0,0)$ and an endemic equilibrium E_1. The basic reproductive number $\mathcal{R}_0$, using the next generation operator (see [36] or [42]) at the disease-free equilibrium E_0, is given by

$$\mathcal{R}_0=\sqrt{\frac{\beta_{mf}\beta_{fm}\nu_m\nu_f}{(\gamma_m+\psi_m)(\gamma_f+\psi_f)}}. \tag{10.40}$$

It can be shown that E_0 is globally asymptotically stable if $\mathcal{R}_0<1$ (see [64]). For the endemic equilibrium, we have that $E_1=(\tilde{X},\tilde{Y})$ is given by

$$\tilde{X}=\frac{\beta_{mf}\beta_{fm}\nu_m\nu_f-(\gamma_m+\psi_m)\left(\gamma_f+\psi_f\right)}{\beta_{fm}\nu_f\left(\beta_{mf}\nu_m+\gamma_f+\psi_f\right)}, \tag{10.41a}$$

$$\tilde{Y}=\frac{\beta_{mf}\beta_{fm}\nu_m\nu_f-(\gamma_m+\psi_m)\left(\gamma_f+\psi_f\right)}{\beta_{mf}\nu_m\left(\beta_{fm}\nu_f+\gamma_m+\psi_m\right)}, \tag{10.41b}$$

or, equivalently, we have that values of $\tilde{I}_f$, $\tilde{S}_f$ $\tilde{I}_m$, and $\tilde{S}_m$ are

$$\tilde{I}_f=\tilde{X}N_f,\ \tilde{S}_f=(1-\tilde{X})N_f,\ \tilde{I}_m=\tilde{Y}N_m,\ \tilde{S}_m=(1-\tilde{Y})N_m. \tag{10.42}$$

Hence, the linearized Jacobian of (10.39) at E_1 is given by

$$\mathbf{J}=\begin{bmatrix} -\frac{\beta_{fm}\nu_f(\beta_{mf}\nu_m+\gamma_f+\psi_f)}{\beta_{fm}\nu_f+\gamma_m+\psi_m} & \frac{\beta_{mf}\nu_m(\gamma_f+\mu_f)(\beta_{fm}\nu_f+\gamma_m+\psi_m)}{\beta_{fm}\nu_f(\beta_{mf}\nu_m+\gamma_f+\psi_f)} \\ \frac{\beta_{fm}\nu_f(\gamma_m+\psi_m)(\beta_{mf}\nu_m+\gamma_f+\psi_f)}{\beta_{mf}\nu_m(\beta_{fm}\nu_f+\gamma_m+\psi_m)} & -\frac{\beta_{mf}\nu_m(\beta_{fm}\nu_f+\gamma_m+\psi_m)}{\beta_{mf}\nu_m+\gamma_f+\psi_f} \end{bmatrix}.$$

Letting r_{mf} denote the number of female infections generated by an infected male truck driver in a disease-free population before the first infected female is removed from the sexually active population (e.g., by progression to AIDS, or death, etc.), and by r_{fm} the corresponding value for male infections caused by females, leads to the ratios

$$r_{mf}=\frac{\beta_{mf}\nu_m}{\gamma_f+\psi_f} \quad \text{and} \quad r_{fm}=\frac{\beta_{fm}\nu_f}{\gamma_m+\psi_m}. \tag{10.43}$$

The basic reproductive number is actually the geometric mean of the above values, namely, $\mathcal{R}_0=\sqrt{r_{mf}\cdot r_{fm}}$. Appropriate substitutions for $\beta_{mf}\nu_f$ and $\beta_{fm}\nu_m$ lead to the system

$$\dot{X} = (\gamma_f + \psi_f)\big(r_{mf}Y(1-X) - X\big), \quad \dot{Y} = (\gamma_m + \psi_m)\big(r_{fm}X(1-Y) - Y\big). \tag{10.44}$$

Rewriting the values $\tilde{X}$ and $\tilde{Y}$ in terms of r_{mf} and r_{fm} results in the following expressions:

$$\tilde{X} = \frac{r_{mf}r_{fm} - 1}{r_{fm}\left(r_{mf}+1\right)} \quad \text{and} \quad \tilde{Y} = \frac{r_{mf}r_{fm} - 1}{r_{mf}\left(r_{fm}+1\right)}. \tag{10.45}$$

Since

$$\operatorname{trace}(\mathbf{J}) = -\left(\beta_{fm}\nu_f\left(\frac{r_{mf}\left(r_{fm}+1\right)}{r_{fm}\left(r_{mf}+1\right)}\right) + \beta_{mf}\nu_m\left(\frac{r_{fm}\left(r_{mf}+1\right)}{r_{mf}\left(r_{fm}+1\right)}\right)\right) < 0,$$

and $\det(\mathbf{J}) = \beta_{mf}\beta_{fm}\nu_m\nu_f\frac{\mathcal{R}_0^2-1}{\mathcal{R}_0^2} > 0$ whenever $\mathcal{R}_0 > 1$, we thus have that E_1 is a locally stable node.

Next, we place the origin at the endemic equilibrium and use the proportions $U = 1 - X/\tilde{X}$ and $V = 1 - Y/\tilde{Y}$. Then if $r_{fm} > 1$, the substitution $r_{mf} = \mathcal{R}_0^2/r_{fm}$ in (10.44) and the Lyapunov function given by

$$L_{E_1} = \frac{\left(r_{fm}+1\right)}{(\gamma_f+\psi_f)}|U| + \frac{\left(\mathcal{R}_0^2 + r_{fm}\right)}{(\gamma_m+\psi_m)}|V|$$

allow us to establish the global stability of the endemic state. In fact, since

$$\dot{L}_{E_1} = -\left(\mathcal{R}_0^2 - \theta\right)\left(r_{fm}-1\right)(1-U)|V| - H,$$

where $H = 2\left(\mathcal{R}_0^2 + r_{fm}\right)(1-V)|U|$ if $UV < 0$ and $H = 0$ if $UV > 0$ with $\theta = \operatorname{sign}(UV)$, then $\mathcal{R}_0 > 1 \Rightarrow \dot{L}_{E_1} \leq 0$. In the case $r_{fm} < 1$ the substitution $r_{fm} = \mathcal{R}_0^2/r_{mf}$ in (10.44) and the use of the symmetry argument lead to $\dot{L}_{E_1} \leq 0$ whenever $\mathcal{R}_0 > 1$.

Remark. The mathematical model and results in this subsection appeared in [63].

10.5.3 Sensitivity analysis on $\mathcal{R}_0$

The results of the sensitivity analyses of $\mathcal{R}_0$ (10.40), with respect to each of the eight parameters β's, ν's, γ's, and ψ's, using $\mathcal{R}_0$'s normalized sensitivity index (elasticity) (see [39, Chapter 9] or [57]), are summarized below. First, we note that

$$\frac{z}{\mathcal{R}_0}\frac{\partial\mathcal{R}_0}{\partial z} = \frac{1}{2} \text{ for } z = \beta_{fm}, \beta_{mf}, \nu_m, \nu_f, \text{ while } \left|\frac{z}{\mathcal{R}_0}\frac{\partial\mathcal{R}_0}{\partial z}\right| < \frac{1}{2} \text{ for } z = \gamma_m, \gamma_f, \psi_m, \psi_f.$$

We have shown in [63] that $\mathcal{R}_0$ is less sensitive to changes in the rate of removal, due to AIDS progression, of HIV infected individuals as well as to the turnover rate than to the rates of HIV transmission (in both classes), the fraction of truck drivers, and the fraction of sex workers in the general population. Decreases in $\mathcal{R}_0$ may arise from changes in the values of β's and/or ν's.

Obviously, changing the fraction s of truck drivers using condoms with female sex workers would lead to decreases in HIV transmission rates (as s decreases) from reductions in the rates of female-to-male transmission, and vice versa. We explore reductions through the use of $\beta_i^{new} = k \cdot \beta_i^{old}$, where $k = 1 - s$ and $i = mf$ or fm (use the same k in both directions). The values of r_{fm} and r_{mf} are replaced by

$$r_{fm} \to k \cdot r_{fm} \quad \text{and} \quad r_{mf} \to k \cdot r_{mf}. \tag{10.46}$$

We now consider only the truck driver group. The use of the substitution of (10.45) in (10.42) using expression (10.46) leads to the following new value $\tilde{I}_m^{new}$ of the infected truck drivers at E_1 (assuming that a fraction k of them will not wear condoms):

$$\tilde{I}_m^{new} = \frac{k^2 r_{mf} r_{fm} - 1}{k r_{mf} \left(k r_{fm} + 1 \right)} N_m, \quad 0 < k \leq 1. \tag{10.47}$$

In order to determine the impact in the endemic population size that results from truck drivers wearing condoms, we consider the ratios

$$J_m(k) = \frac{\tilde{I}_m(k)}{\tilde{I}_m(1)} \quad \text{and} \quad J_f(k) = \frac{\tilde{I}_f(k)}{\tilde{I}_f(1)}, \tag{10.48}$$

where the latter is for sex workers. The percentage *decrease* in endemic HIV cases among truck drivers is calculated from $\mathcal{P}(s) = (1 - J(1-s)) \cdot 100\%$. The dependence of $\mathcal{P}$ on s for truck drivers ($\mathcal{P}_m$) and sex workers ($\mathcal{P}_f$) is collected in Figure 10.2. The graphs collect the

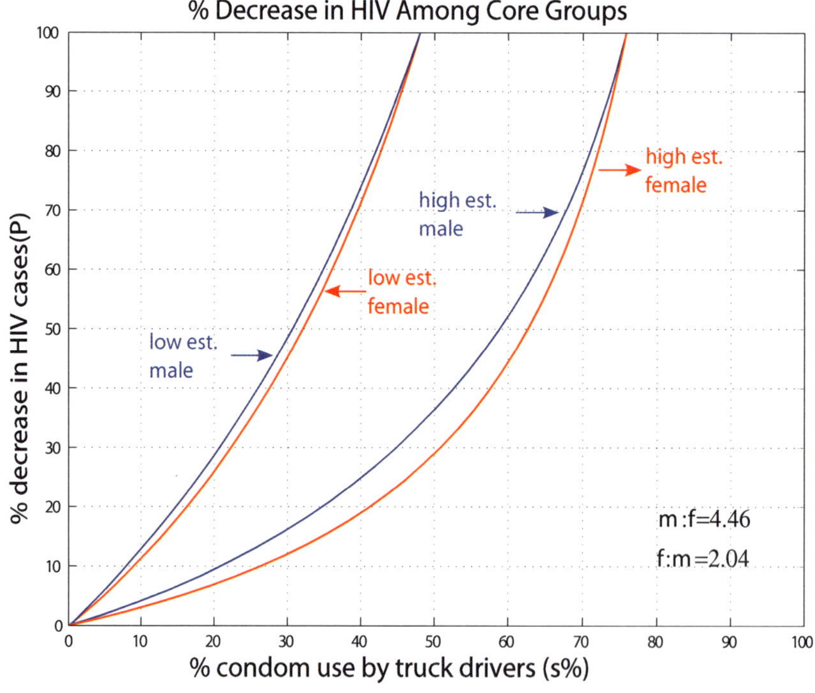

Figure 10.2. *The effect of condom use by truck drivers on the prevalence of HIV in the core populations; modified from the corresponding figure in* [63].

Table 10.2. *Effect of condom use by truck drivers on HIV cases as presented in* [63].

% of truck drivers wearing condoms	% decrease in HIV cases among truck drivers	% decrease in HIV cases among sex workers
10%	4–12%	3–11%
20%	10–27%	7–24%
30%	16–46%	12–42%
40%	25–70%	19–67%
50%	37–100%	29–100%
60%	53–100%	45–100%
70%	79–100%	74–100%
80%	100%	100%
90%	100%	100%

high and low HIV-prevalence estimates that emerge from variations in transmission rates. The selected values are listed in Table 10.2.

From Table 10.2 and Figure 10.2 we see that 50% condom use among truck drivers leads to within-group HIV-case reduction in the 37–100% range and in female sex workers in the 29–100% range.

10.6 Coupling of the Core and General Populations

The growth of HIV infections in the general population is tied to HIV prevalence in the core. A model that includes the coupling between the core and noncore groups is introduced (see Figure 10.3). The transmission rates for this two-sex multigroup model are defined in Table 10.3.

In our notation, β_{m2f2} and β_{f2m2} correspond to β_{mf} and β_{fm}, the equivalent parameters in the isolated core model in Section 10.5.1. The rate of progression to AIDS is assumed to be the same for males and females $(\gamma_f = \gamma_m = \gamma)$. We take the same value μ_f for core and noncore women and the same value μ_m for core and noncore men.

S_{m1} and S_{f1} denote the number of susceptible males and females in the general population, while I_{m1} and I_{f1} denote the number of infected males and females in the general population. S_{m2} and S_{f2} denote the number of susceptible truck drivers and female sex workers, while I_{m2} and I_{f2} denote the number of infected male truck drivers and female sex workers, respectively. Further, the parameters ρ_{f2} and ρ_{m2} denote the per-capita rates of retirement. The entire population is assumed to be well mixed, and N_m and N_f comprise the entire population of sexually active males and females.

The HIV dynamics in core and noncore (general) populations are naturally rather complex. We have built in [63] a manageable system that can address, in as simple a setting as possible, the following questions of interest: What is the role of the core in noncore HIV dynamics? Can we manage to express the general population dynamics as a function of the core group HIV-transmission dynamics? A large number of rough simplifications and crude assumptions have been made in [63] that lead to a highly simplified and crude system. The approach is driven by efforts to address some of the challenges posed by HIV dynamics in

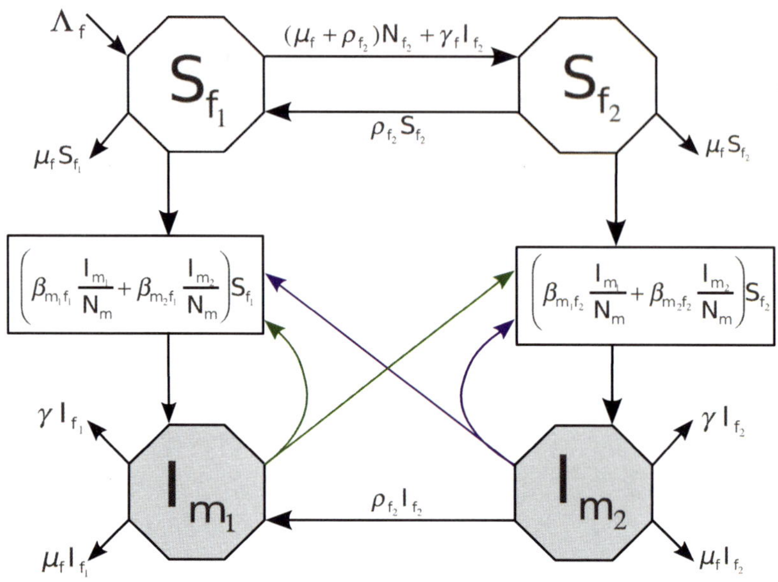

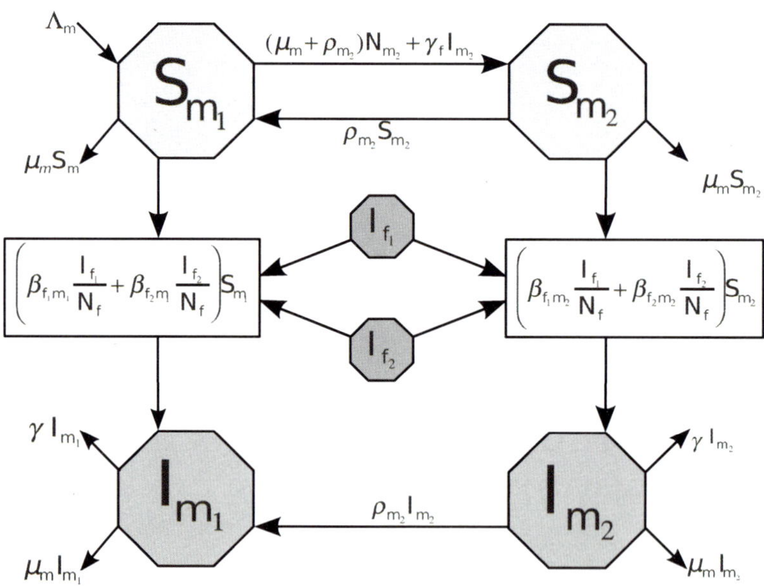

Figure 10.3. *A compartmental diagram for the system* (10.49). *(This figure was modified from Figure* 1 *of* [63, p. 10].*)*

Table 10.3. *Disease transmission rates between subpopulations. (Modified from* [63].*)*

from ↓ \ to ⟶	Females general pop.	Males general pop.	Females sex workers	Males truck drivers
Females, general pop.		β_{f1m1}		β_{f1m2}
Males, general pop.	β_{m1f1}		β_{m1f2}	
Females, sex workers		β_{f2m1}		β_{f2m2}
Males, truck drivers	β_{m2f1}		β_{m2f2}	

Nigeria. In other words, the situation of Nigeria is used as a prototypical underlying case study. Simulation based on Nigeria core group data is shown later (Figure 10.6) [96].

This philosophy (driven by a rather specific question) leads us to choose to model the core-group HIV-transmission dynamics with a slightly modified version of system (10.37). The slight modifications arise from the inclusion of an extra source of HIV infection, a source tied to the dynamics of sexual activity between members of the core and the general population. The HIV-transmission dynamics within the general population (noncore groups) is assumed to follow, with different parameter values, those within the core group, except that the losses in the core ("retirement") are moved into the noncore. In addition, uninfected noncore individuals are the only source of new drivers and sex workers; the overall rate of recruitment into the sexually active population is assumed to be given by the constant Λ, with all recruits joining the uninfected noncore. Further, in order to guarantee nonnegative subpopulation sizes, it is assumed that $\Lambda_f \geq (\mu_f + \rho_{f2} + \gamma) I_{f2}$ and $\Lambda_m \geq (\mu_m + \rho_{m2} + \gamma) I_{m2}$.

The use of simplifying assumptions and definitions leads to a "manageable" nonlinear system for coupled HIV-transmission dynamics that involves core and noncore subpopulations:

$$\begin{aligned}
\dot{S}_{f1} &= \Lambda_f - \left(\beta_{m1f1}\frac{I_{m1}}{N_m} + \beta_{m2f1}\frac{I_{m2}}{N_m}\right) S_{f1} + \rho_{f2} S_{f2} - ((\mu_f + \rho_{f2}) N_{f2} + \gamma I_{f2}) - \mu_f S_{f1},\\
\dot{I}_{f1} &= \left(\beta_{m1f1}\frac{I_{m1}}{N_m} + \beta_{m2f1}\frac{I_{m2}}{N_m}\right) S_{f1} + \rho_{f2} I_{f2} - (\mu_f + \gamma) I_{f1},\\
\dot{S}_{m1} &= \Lambda_m - \left(\beta_{f1m1}\frac{I_{f1}}{N_f} + \beta_{f2m1}\frac{I_{f2}}{N_f}\right) S_{m1} + \rho_{m2} S_{m2} - ((\mu_m + \rho_{m2}) N_{m2} + \gamma I_{m2}) - \mu_m S_{m1},\\
\dot{I}_{m1} &= \left(\beta_{f1m1}\frac{I_{f1}}{N_f} + \beta_{f2m1}\frac{I_{f2}}{N_f}\right) S_{m1} + \rho_{m2} I_{m2} - (\mu_m + \gamma) I_{m1},\\
\dot{S}_{f2} &= ((\mu_f + \rho_{f2}) N_{f2} + \gamma I_{f2}) - \left(\beta_{m1f2}\frac{I_{m1}}{N_m} + \beta_{m2f2}\frac{I_{m2}}{N_m}\right) S_{f2} - (\mu_f + \rho_{f2}) S_{f2},\\
\dot{I}_{f2} &= \left(\beta_{m1f2}\frac{I_{m1}}{N_m} + \beta_{m2f2}\frac{I_{m2}}{N_m}\right) S_{f2} - (\mu_f + \rho_{f2} + \gamma) I_{f2},\\
\dot{S}_{m2} &= ((\mu_m + \rho_{m2}) N_{m2} + \gamma I_{m2}) - \left(\beta_{f1m2}\frac{I_{f1}}{N_f} + \beta_{f2m2}\frac{I_{f2}}{N_f}\right) S_{m2} - (\mu_m + \rho_{m2}) S_{m2},\\
\dot{I}_{m2} &= \left(\beta_{f1m2}\frac{I_{f1}}{N_f} + \beta_{f2m2}\frac{I_{f2}}{N_f}\right) S_{m2} - (\mu_m + \rho_{m2} + \gamma) I_{m2}.
\end{aligned} \tag{10.49}$$

10.6.1 Pseudoformal and rough modeling approximations

The study of HIV dynamics in core and noncore populations is rather complex but our interest in the question "What is the role of the core group in noncore HIV dynamics in situations like Nigeria?" makes it possible to use a large number of approximations that, we hope, allow us to learn something from modeling. Hence, we proceed to find a way of expressing the dynamics of the noncore population as a function of HIV-transmission dynamics in the core within a model that keeps key features of the full model. Our approach is based on a slightly more sophisticated "back-of-the envelope" computation that manages to generate model simplifications in a nonrigorous way through the use of some of the underlying features observed in the HIV situation in Nigeria.

Here noncore and core subpopulations are $N_{f1}=S_{f1}+I_{f1}$, $N_{f2}=S_{f2}+I_{f2}$, $N_{m1}=S_{m1}+I_{m1}$, $N_{m2}=S_{m2}+I_{m2}$, $N_f=N_{f1}+N_{f2}$, $N_m=N_{m1}+N_{m2}$, respectively, and the rates of change in the noncore and core subpopulations are given by the system

$$\begin{aligned}
\dot{N}_{f1} &= \dot{S}_{f1}+\dot{I}_{f1}=\Lambda_f-\mu_f\left(N_{f1}+N_{f2}\right)-\gamma\left(I_{f1}+I_{f2}\right),\\
\dot{N}_{m1} &= \dot{S}_{f2}+\dot{I}_{f2}=\Lambda_m-\mu_m\left(N_{m1}+N_{m2}\right)-\gamma\left(I_{m2}+I_{m1}\right),\\
\dot{N}_{f2} &= \dot{S}_{f2}+\dot{I}_{f2}=0, \quad \dot{N}_{m2}=\dot{S}_{m2}+\dot{I}_{m2}=0.
\end{aligned}$$

The use of a constant recruitment rate (appropriate over some time horizon) means that equilibria will be supported by the model. In fact, at the disease free state, we have that

$$\mu_f\left(\tilde{N}_{f1}+\tilde{N}_{f2}\right)=\Lambda_f,\quad \mu_m\left(\tilde{N}_{m1}+\tilde{N}_{m2}\right)=\Lambda_m.$$

And once an endemic equilibrium is reached, we will have that

$$\mu_f\left(\tilde{N}_{f1}+\tilde{N}_{f2}\right)+\gamma\left(\tilde{I}_{f1}+\tilde{I}_{f2}\right)=\Lambda_f,\quad \mu_m\left(\tilde{N}_{m1}+\tilde{N}_{m2}\right)+\gamma\left(\tilde{I}_{m2}+\tilde{I}_{m1}\right)=\Lambda_m.$$

It is at this stage that we make additional *drastic* assumptions, namely, that the noncore population reaches equilibrium quickly (disease-free state) and that the noncore population size does not change much due to the disease, an appropriate assumption if the prevalence is low within the noncore but relatively large when compared the size of the core population. These additional simplifying assumptions lead to the following "quasi-steady state" relations:

$$\begin{aligned}
\dot{N}_{f1} &= \dot{S}_{f1}+\dot{I}_{f1}\approx 0, \qquad & \dot{N}_{f2} &= \dot{S}_{f2}+\dot{I}_{f2}=0,\\
\dot{N}_{m1} &= \dot{S}_{m1}+\dot{I}_{m1}\approx 0, \qquad & \dot{N}_{m2} &= \dot{S}_{m2}+\dot{I}_{m2}=0.
\end{aligned}$$

Under the assumption that the total subpopulations are constant, the above system turns out to be equivalent to the following nonlinear system:

$$\begin{aligned}
\dot{I}_{f1} &= \left(\beta_{m1f1}\frac{I_{m1}}{N_m}+\beta_{m2f1}\frac{I_{m2}}{N_m}\right)\left(N_{f1}-I_{f1}\right)-\left(\mu_f+\gamma\right)I_{f1}+\rho_{f2}I_{f2},\\
\dot{I}_{m1} &= \left(\beta_{f1m1}\frac{I_{f1}}{N_f}+\beta_{f2m1}\frac{I_{f2}}{N_f}\right)\left(N_{m1}-I_{m1}\right)-\left(\mu_m+\gamma\right)I_{m1}+\rho_{m2}I_{m2},\\
\dot{I}_{f2} &= \left(\beta_{m1f2}\frac{I_{m1}}{N_m}+\beta_{m2f2}\frac{I_{m2}}{N_m}\right)\left(N_{f2}-I_{f2}\right)-\left(\mu_f+\rho_{f2}+\gamma\right)I_{f2},\\
\dot{I}_{m2} &= \left(\beta_{f1m2}\frac{I_{f1}}{N_f}+\beta_{f2m2}\frac{I_{f2}}{N_f}\right)\left(N_{m2}-I_{m2}\right)-\left(\mu_m+\rho_{m2}+\gamma\right)I_{m2}.
\end{aligned} \tag{10.50}$$

Further, the use of subpopulation fractions leads to

$$X_1 = \frac{I_{f1}}{N_{f1}}, \quad X_2 = \frac{I_{f2}}{N_{f2}}, \quad Y_1 = \frac{I_{m1}}{N_{m1}}, \quad \text{and} \quad Y_2 = \frac{I_{m2}}{N_{m2}},$$

We now introduce the following subpopulation gender-specific ratios (ν's):

$$\nu_{f1} = \frac{N_{f1}}{N_f}, \quad \nu_{f2} = \frac{N_{f2}}{N_f}, \quad \nu_{m1} = \frac{N_{m1}}{N_m}, \quad \text{and} \quad \nu_{m2} = \frac{N_{m2}}{N_m},$$

The incorporation of these ratios leads to the the following useful simplification, a system for the dynamics of the proportions

$$\begin{aligned}
\dot{X}_1 &= \left(\beta_{m1f1}\nu_{m1}Y_1 + \beta_{m2f1}\nu_{m2}Y_2\right)(1-X_1) - \left(\mu_f + \gamma\right)X_1 + \rho_{f2}\frac{N_{f2}}{N_{f1}}X_2,\\
\dot{Y}_1 &= \left(\beta_{f1m1}\nu_{f1}X_1 + \beta_{f2m1}\nu_{f2}X_2\right)(1-Y_1) - (\mu_m + \gamma)Y_1 + \rho_{m2}\frac{N_{m2}}{N_{m1}}Y_{m2},\\
\dot{X}_2 &= \left(\beta_{m1f2}\nu_{m1}Y_1 + \beta_{m2f2}\nu_{m2}Y_2\right)(1-X_2) - \left(\mu_f + \rho_{f2} + \gamma\right)X_2,\\
\dot{Y}_2 &= \left(\beta_{f1m2}\nu_{f1}X_1 + \beta_{f2m2}\nu_{f2}X_2\right)(1-Y_2) - (\mu_m + \rho_{m2} + \gamma)Y_2.
\end{aligned} \tag{10.51}$$

Can we simplify further? Well, in the context of Nigeria, the terms $\rho_{f2}\frac{N_{f2}}{N_{f1}}X_2$ and $\rho_{m2}\frac{N_{m2}}{N_{m1}}Y_{m2}$ are tiny ($10^{-4} - 10^{-3}$, whereas the size of the next smallest terms are around 10^{-2}). Hence, the replacement of ψ_f by $\mu_f + \rho_{f2}$ and ψ_m for $\mu_m + \rho_{m2}$ leads to

$$\begin{aligned}
\dot{X}_1 &= \left(\beta_{m1f1}\nu_{m1}Y_1 + \beta_{m2f1}\nu_{m2}Y_2\right)(1-X_1) - \left(\mu_f + \gamma\right)X_1,\\
\dot{Y}_1 &= \left(\beta_{f1m1}\nu_{f1}X_1 + \beta_{f2m1}\nu_{f2}X_2\right)(1-Y_1) - (\mu_m + \gamma)Y_1,\\
\dot{X}_2 &= \left(\beta_{m1f2}\nu_{m1}Y_1 + \beta_{m2f2}\nu_{m2}Y_2\right)(1-X_2) - \left(\psi_f + \gamma\right)X_2,\\
\dot{Y}_2 &= \left(\beta_{f1m2}\nu_{f1}X_1 + \beta_{f2m2}\nu_{f2}X_2\right)(1-Y_2) - (\psi_m + \gamma)Y_2.
\end{aligned} \tag{10.52}$$

As was done in Section 10.4 we proceed to introduce the expressions

$$\begin{aligned}
r_{m1f1} &= \frac{\beta_{m1f1}N_{m1}}{\left(\mu_f + \gamma\right)N_m}, & r_{f1m1} &= \frac{\beta_{f1m1}N_{f1}}{(\mu_m + \gamma)N_f},\\
r_{m1f2} &= \frac{\beta_{m1f2}N_{m1}}{\left(\psi_f + \gamma\right)N_m}, & r_{f1m2} &= \frac{\beta_{f1m2}N_{f1}}{(\psi_m + \gamma)N_f},\\
r_{m2f1} &= \frac{\beta_{m2f1}N_{m2}}{\left(\mu_f + \gamma\right)N_m}, & r_{f2m1} &= \frac{\beta_{f2m1}N_{f2}}{(\mu_m + \gamma)N_f},\\
r_{m2f2} &= \frac{\beta_{m2f2}N_{m2}}{\left(\psi_f + \gamma\right)N_m}, & r_{f2m2} &= \frac{\beta_{f2m2}N_{f2}}{(\psi_m + \gamma)N_f}.
\end{aligned} \tag{10.53}$$

These parameters, again, denote the number of new cases within each subpopulation before the first case in that subpopulation recovers (given that the disease was introduced into a disease-free subpopulation) times the fraction of that sex-specific subpopulation.

Use of the second generation operator [36, 42] yields the basic reproductive number for this system:

$$\mathcal{R}_0 = \sqrt{\tfrac{1}{2}\left(r_{f1m1}r_{m1f1} + r_{m1f2}r_{f2m1} + r_{f1m2}r_{m2f1} + r_{m2f2}r_{f2m2}\right)} \times \sqrt{1 + \sqrt{1 + \frac{4(r_{m1f1}r_{m2f2} - r_{m1f2}r_{m2f1})(r_{f1m2}r_{f2m1} - r_{f2m2}r_{f1m1})}{(r_{f1m1}r_{m1f1} + r_{m1f2}r_{f2m1} + r_{f1m2}r_{m2f1} + r_{m2f2}r_{f2m2})^2}}}. \tag{10.54}$$

The endemic equilibrium is determined from the solution of the following nonlinear system:

$$\begin{aligned} \frac{\tilde{X}_1}{1-\tilde{X}_1} &= r_{m1f1}\tilde{Y}_1 + r_{m2f1}\tilde{Y}_2, & \frac{\tilde{Y}_1}{1-\tilde{Y}_1} &= r_{f1m1}\tilde{X}_1 + r_{f2m1}\tilde{X}_2, \\ \frac{\tilde{X}_2}{1-\tilde{X}_2} &= r_{m1f2}\tilde{Y}_1 + r_{m2f2}\tilde{Y}_2, & \frac{\tilde{Y}_2}{1-\tilde{Y}_2} &= r_{f1m2}\tilde{X}_1 + r_{f2m2}\tilde{X}_2. \end{aligned} \tag{10.55}$$

Specific assumptions that make use of the situation in Nigeria allow us to approximate the HIV dynamics in the general population as a function of the core group dynamics:

$$\begin{aligned} \dot{X}_1 &\approx (\mu_f + \gamma)\left(\left(r_{m1f1}\left(\frac{r_{f2m1}}{r_{f2m1}X_2 + 1}\right)X_2 + r_{m2f1}Y_2\right)(1 - X_1) - X_1\right), \\ \dot{Y}_1 &\approx (\mu_m + \gamma)\left(\left(r_{f1m1}\left(\frac{r_{m2f1}}{r_{m2f1}Y_2 + 1}\right)Y_2 + r_{f2m1}X_2\right)(1 - Y_1) - Y_1\right). \end{aligned} \tag{10.56}$$

The terms

$$\left(\frac{r_{f2m1}}{r_{f2m1}X_2 + 1}\right), \qquad \left(\frac{r_{m2f1}}{r_{m2f1}Y_2 + 1}\right)$$

can be interpreted as the "strength" of the coupling between gender-specific core groups with the noncore group of the *same* sex. At the endemic equilibrium we have approximately that

$$\tilde{X}_1 \approx \frac{r_{m2f1}\tilde{Y}_2\left(1 + r_{f2m1}\tilde{X}_2\right) + r_{m1f1}r_{f2m1}\tilde{X}_2}{\left(1 + r_{m2f1}\tilde{Y}_2\right)\left(1 + r_{f2m1}\tilde{X}_2\right) + r_{m1f1}r_{f2m1}\tilde{X}_2}, \tag{10.57a}$$

$$\tilde{Y}_1 \approx \frac{r_{f2m1}\tilde{X}_2\left(1 + r_{m2f1}\tilde{Y}_2\right) + r_{f1m1}r_{m2f1}\tilde{Y}_2}{\left(1 + r_{f2m1}\tilde{X}_2\right)\left(1 + r_{m2f1}\tilde{Y}_2\right) + r_{f1m1}r_{m2f1}\tilde{Y}_2}. \tag{10.57b}$$

We define the relative potential force of infection,

$$\phi_{mf} = \frac{r_{m1f1}}{r_{m2f1}} = \frac{\beta_{m1f1}N_{m1}}{\beta_{m2f1}N_{m2}} \quad \text{and} \quad \phi_{fm} = \frac{r_{f1m1}}{r_{f2m1}} = \frac{\beta_{f1m1}N_{f1}}{\beta_{f2m1}N_{f2}}. \tag{10.58}$$

Thus,

$$\tilde{X}_1 \approx \frac{r_{m2f1}\tilde{Y}_2\left(1+r_{f2m1}\tilde{X}_2\right)+\phi_{mf}r_{m2f1}r_{f2m1}\tilde{X}_2}{\left(1+r_{m2f1}\tilde{Y}_2\right)\left(1+r_{f2m1}\tilde{X}_2\right)+\phi_{mf}r_{m2f1}r_{f2m1}\tilde{X}_2}, \tag{10.59a}$$

$$\tilde{Y}_1 \approx \frac{r_{f2m1}\tilde{X}_2\left(1+r_{m2f1}\tilde{Y}_2\right)+\phi_{fm}r_{f2m1}r_{m2f1}\tilde{Y}_2}{\left(1+r_{f2m1}\tilde{X}_2\right)\left(1+r_{m2f1}\tilde{Y}_2\right)+\phi_{fm}r_{f2m1}r_{m2f1}\tilde{Y}_2}. \tag{10.59b}$$

Assuming that ϕ_{mf} and ϕ_{fm} are small (much less than 1) leads to

$$\tilde{X}_1 \approx \frac{r_{m2f1}\tilde{Y}_2}{1+r_{m2f1}\tilde{Y}_2}, \qquad \tilde{Y}_1 \approx \frac{r_{f2m1}\tilde{X}_2}{1+r_{f2m1}\tilde{X}_2}. \tag{10.60}$$

Further, in the case where the relative rates of infections are very small we have that

$$\tilde{X}_1 \approx r_{m2f1}\tilde{Y}_2, \qquad \tilde{Y}_1 \approx r_{f2m1}\tilde{X}_2. \tag{10.61}$$

(The parameters ϕ_{mf} and ϕ_{fm} may provide a useful index of the influence of the core group on the general population. The indices $\varkappa_m = \frac{(\mu_m+\gamma_m)\beta_{m2f1}N_{m2}}{(\psi_m+\gamma_m)\beta_{m1f1}N_{m1}}$ and $\varkappa_f = \frac{(\mu_f+\gamma_f)\beta_{f2m1}N_{f2}}{(\psi_f+\gamma_f)\beta_{f1m1}N_{f1}}$, relative reproductive numbers at the potential maximum number of infected for the respective subpopulations, resemble some of the measures generated in [74], like vectorial capacity, in the context of vector-borne diseases.)

10.6.2 Prevention exercise

In order to roughly assess the effects of condom use by truck drivers on decreasing HIV prevalence in the general population, all rates of infection involving truck drivers are multiplied by the factor k, leading to

$$\tilde{X}_1^{new}(k) \approx r_{m2f1}\frac{k^3 r_{m2f2}r_{f2m2}-1}{k r_{m2f2}\left(k r_{f2m2}+1\right)}. \tag{10.62}$$

As was done before in this lecture, the effect of condom use by truck drivers in the general population is assessed via the quotient

$$J_{f1}(k) = \frac{\tilde{X}_1^{new}(k)}{\tilde{X}_1^{new}(1)} = k J_{m2}(k), \tag{10.63}$$

with $J_{m2}(k)$ replacing the expression that used when we were studying a decoupled core group model (10.48). Hence, the left-hand side of the above expression gives the fraction of the initial endemic number of infected women in the general population. The percentage *decrease* of endemic HIV cases among truck drivers can be estimated from $\mathcal{P}_{f1}(s) = (1 - J_{f1}(1-s)) \cdot 100\%$.

We find a substantial decrease in the prevalence of HIV in the noncore population of women, a decrease that is way above the expected decrease in the prevalence of HIV among sex workers (compare Figure 10.4 with Figure 10.2).

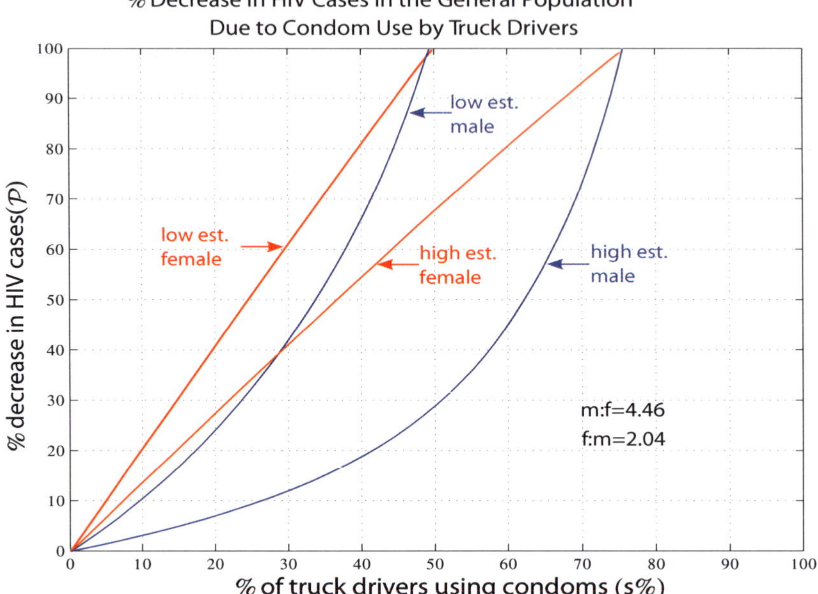

Figure 10.4. *The effect of condom use by truck drivers on prevalence of HIV in the general population (modified from* [63]*).*

The situation of males in the noncore population is assessed from

$$\tilde{Y}_1^{new}(k) \approx r_{f1m2} \frac{k^2 r_{m2f2} r_{f2m2} - 1}{k r_{f2m2} \left(k r_{m2f2} + 1\right)} \tag{10.64}$$

via the quotient

$$J_{m1}(k) = \frac{\tilde{Y}_1^{new}(k)}{\tilde{Y}_1^{new}(1)} = k J_{f2}(k), \tag{10.65}$$

where $J_{f2}(k)$ is as in the core group model (10.48). The impact of condom usage for males and females in the general population is as above, that is, a greater decrease is observed in the males and females than in the core. The case where men (from core and noncore) use condoms can be assessed with the quotient

$$J_{m1}(k) = \frac{\tilde{Y}_1^{new}(k)}{\tilde{Y}_1^{new}(1)} = k J_{f2}(k) \tag{10.66}$$

and leads to a dramatic reductions in HIV (as expected); see Figure 10.5.

The presence of an almost linear curve highlights the significance of the effects of condom use on the general population; that is, they are much greater than the effects of their use just within the core groups.

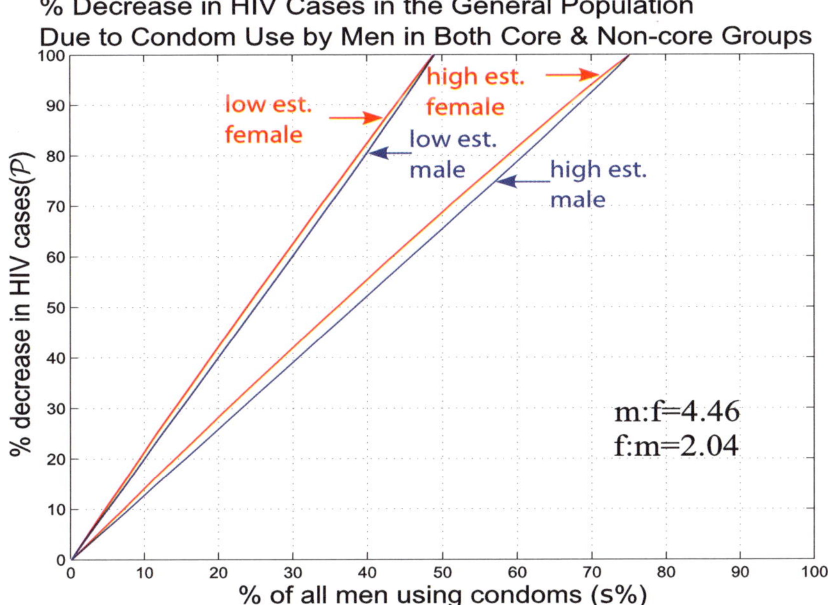

Figure 10.5. *The effect of condom use by all men on prevalence of HIV in the general population (modified from* [63]*).*

Table 10.4. *Effect of condom use on HIV cases (see* [63]*).*

% of all men wearing condoms	% decrease in HIV cases among general pop. men	% decrease in HIV cases among general pop. women
10%	13–20%	14–21%
20%	26–40%	28–42%
30%	38–60%	41–62%
40%	51–80%	55–82%
50%	65–100%	68–100%
60%	78–100%	81–100%
70%	92–100%	94–100%
80%	100%	100%
90%	100%	100%

From Figure 10.4, we conclude that if 50% of all truck drivers use condoms, then HIV cases will be reduced among men in the general population by 29–100%, and among women by 68–100%. From the simulations in Figure 10.5, we conclude that if 50% of all men use condoms, HIV cases will be reduced among men in the general population by 65–100%, and among women by 68–100%. Further, the percentage of truck drivers (assume all to be men) that should wear condoms in order to meet the goal of reducing the prevalence

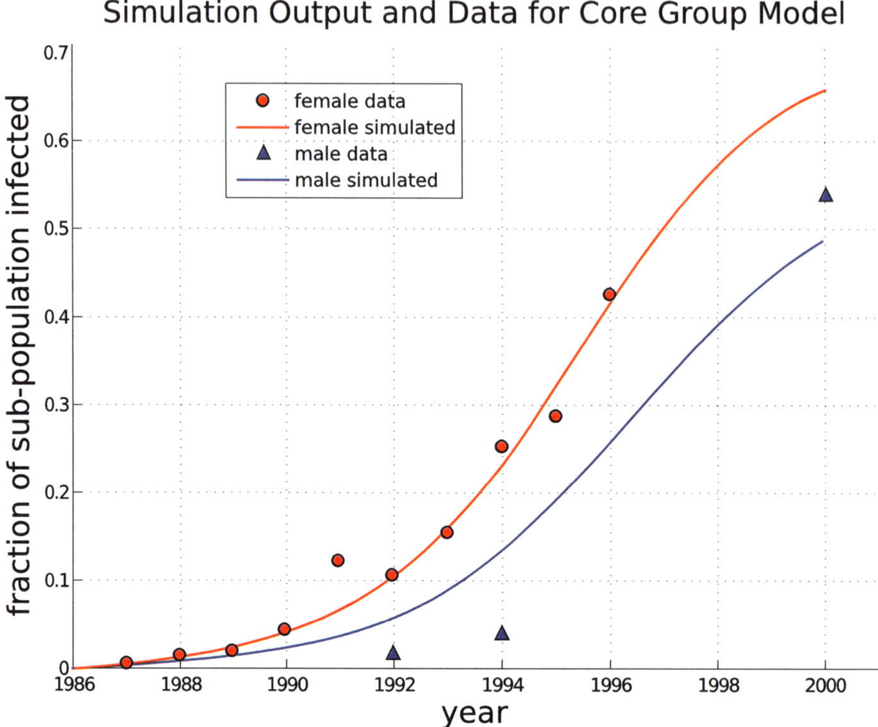

Figure 10.6. *Estimate of rates of infection from fitting system* (10.39) *parameters to data in Table* 10.3 *as reported in* [63].

by 50% turns out to be (from these simulations) to be 34–62%. Further, we observe that 25–39% condom usage by truck drivers would reduce HIV cases among men in the general population by roughly 50%. Similarly, 24–36% condom usage by truck drivers would also reduce HIV cases in women in the general population by half. In other words, as expected, the main source of infection in (all) women can be traced back to the proportion of infected truck drivers.

10.7 Conclusions and Final Thoughts

In this lecture, we have provided a rough overview of some of the challenges associated with the study of the transmission dynamics, control, and evolution of STDs. We reviewed some of our past work on STD multistrain competition using single-and two-sex models. Gonorrhea is the underlying motivating disease throughout the first part of this lecture. We have also highlighted the challenges faced by researchers working on specific applications, primarily by discussing modeling simplifications with an eye on the HIV situation in Nigeria. In the case of Nigeria, the need to incorporate the impact of core groups, within a two-sex model, on HIV dynamics was central. The challenges that emerged from the analysis of the highly complex nonlinear models led us to search for ways of constructing related simplified models that allowed us to assess the impact of control measures on HIV dynamics.

The limitations in the models and the crudeness of the approximations used have probably made most of the readers of these notes (if any are left) to question the value of these models in practical situations. Given the seriousness of the challenges and the lack of a full set of data, we argue that we have no option but to work with what we have.

The challenges that we faced in connecting models to data were buried in the background. In order to give you some idea of how the parameters used were chosen or estimated, we conclude this lecture with a typical example: contact rates. Statistical and numerical details, including to technical references, can be found in [63].

The parameters β_{fm} and β_{mf} are estimated from whatever we know about reciprocals of the average time to the HIV infectious state from the time a person entered the core group (his/her risk increased) under the assumption that all encounters are with infected individuals. The rates of infectious contact, β_{fm} and β_{mf}, depend on the total number of contacts per person per year, and the probability of transmission per contact (see [80] and [64]). The risks of STD infection are quantified from "partners studies" (see [15]). Under the assumption that most truck drivers are clients of sex workers, we consider the rate at which truckers are infecting the sex workers. (In a prospective cohort study of 1,948 initially HIV-uninfected female sex workers in Senegal [51] it was established that the rate of male to female transmission is 0.000311–0.000561 for HIV-1 and 0.0000733–000119 for HIV-2.)

Data from [90], [75], and [66] helped generate the per-contact probability of female to male transmission range of 0.003–0.010 and for the per-contact probability of male to female transmission of 0.006–0.080. The results in various studies and sources ([48] and [86, 87]) are used to justify the assumption that the average range of contacts for a truck driver with sex workers is 3–6 times per week and for a female sex worker with truck drivers it is 6–30 contacts per week. Calculating β as the probability of transmission per contact $\times$ number of contacts per person per time leads to

$$\begin{aligned}\beta_{fm} &= (0.003 \times 3 \text{ contacts/wk} \times 52 \text{ weeks/yr}, 0.01 \times 6 \text{ contacts/wk} \times 52 \text{ weeks/yr})\\ &= \left(0.468 \text{ years}^{-1}, 3.12 \text{ years}^{-1}\right),\end{aligned}$$

that is, roughly speaking, it would take truck drivers, on the average, between 4 and 24 months to become infected in a scenario where all sex workers were HIV positive.

$$\begin{aligned}\beta_{mf} &= (0.006 \times 6 \text{ contacts/wk} \times 52 \text{ weeks/yr}, 0.08 \times 30 \text{ contacts/wk} \times 52 \text{ weeks/yr})\\ &= \left(1.87 \text{ years}^{-1}, 124.8 \text{ years}^{-1}\right),\end{aligned}$$

or, roughly speaking, it would take sex workers between 3 and 180 days to become infected if all truck drivers were HIV positive (see Table 10.5 for some comparisons).

Model output (see (10.6)) from just the core groups (system (10.39)) generated estimates of $\beta_{fm} v_f = 0.382 \pm 0.125$ (95% confidence interval).

Similar approaches were used in [63] to estimate turnover rates, that is, the rates at which truck drivers retire, die, or are removed from the profession for all reasons except HIV); the natural turnover rate ψ_f of female sex workers, the reciprocal of the average time that a female sex worker spends in the profession following recruitment; and AIDS-related removal rates taken from a multitude of sources that include, for example, [61].

The study of STD models is full of the challenges and opportunities that are common to interdisciplinary and transdisciplinary research. The importance of creating working teams that involve social and behavioral scientists, epidemiologists, statisticians, modelers,

Table 10.5. *Percentage of prevalence in core groups (data from* [100], [85] *and* [48]*) as reported in* [63].

Year	Sex workers (rural)	Sex workers (urban)	Sex workers (avg.)	Truckers
1987	0.35%		0.35%	
1988	1.25%		1.25%	
1989		1.7%	1.7%	
1990	4.3%		4.3%	
1991		12.3%	12.3%	
1992	11.5%	9.9%	10.7%	1.6%
1993		15.4%	15.4%	
1994	21.4%	29.1%	25.2%	4%
1995	24%	33.3%	28.7%	
1996	54.7%	30.5%	42.6%	
2000				54%

and mathematicians should be obvious from this lecture and this volume. Building collaborative teams around the solution of problems involving health and economic disparities is central to the success of an enterprise that must assess its impact through the quality of its solutions to questions that are critical to the dynamics, control, and evolution of diseases, including STDs.

Bibliography

[1] Anderson, R.M. and R.M. May (1982) Coevolution of hosts and parasites. Parasitology, **85**, 411–426.

[2] Anderson, R. and R. May (1991) *Infectious Diseases of Humans: Dynamics And Control*, Oxford Science Publications, Oxford University Press.

[3] Avert.org (2011) *HIV/AIDS in South Africa*, http://www.avert.org/africa-hiv-aids-statistics.htm.

[4] Beck, K. (1984) *Coevolution: Mathematical analysis of host-parasite interactions*, J. Math. Biol. **19**: 63–77.

[5] Blythe, S.P. and C. Castillo-Chavez (1989) *Like-with-like preference and sexual mixing models*, Math. Biosc. **96**: 221–238.

[6] Blythe, S., C. Castillo-Chavez, J. Palmer, and M. Cheng (1991) *Toward a unified theory of sexual mixing and pair formation*, Math. Biosc. **107**: 379–405.

[7] Blythe, S.P., C. Castillo-Chavez, and G. Casella (1992) *Empirical methods for the estimation of the mixing probabilities for socially structured populations from a single survey sample*, Mathematical Population Studies **3**: 199–225.

[8] Blythe, S., F. Brauer, C. Castillo-Chavez, and J. Velasco-Hernandez (1993) *Sexually Transmitted Diseases with Recruitment*, Technical Report BU-1193-M, Cornell University, Ithaca, NY.

[9] Blythe, S., S. Busenberg, and C. Castillo-Chavez (1995) *Affinity in paired event probability*, Math. Biosc. **128**: 265–284.

[10] Brauer, F., S.P. Blythe, and C. Castillo-Chavez (1992) *Demographic Recruitment in Sexually Transmitted Disease Models*, Technical Report BU-1154-M, Cornell University, Ithaca, NY.

[11] Brauer, F., C. Castillo-Chávez, and J. Velasco-Hernandez (1996) *Recruitment effects in heterosexually transmitted disease models*, Advances in Mathematical Modeling of Biological Processes, International Journal of Applied Science and Computation **3**: 78–90.

[12] Brauer, F., C. Castillo-Chavez, and J. Velasco-Hernandez (1997) *Recruitment into a core group and its effect on the spread of a sexually transmitted disease*, in Advances in Mathematical Population Dynamics–Molecules, Cells, and Man: Proceedings of the 4th International Conference on Mathematical Population Dynamics, O. Arino, D.E. Axelrod, M. Kimmel, and V. Capasso, eds., World Scientific, Singapore: 477–486.

[13] Bremermann, H.J. and J. Pickering (1983) *A game-theoretical model of parasite virulence*, J. Theor. Biol. **100**: 411–426.

[14] Bremermann, H.J. and H.R. Thieme (1989) *A competitive exclusion principle for pathogen virulence*, J. Math. biol. **27**: 179–190.

[15] Brookmeyer, R. and M.H. Gail (1994) *AIDS Epidemiology: A quantitative Approach*, Vol. 22, Oxford University Press.

[16] Busenberg, S. and C. Castillo-Chavez (1989) *Interaction, pair formation and force of infection terms in sexually transmitted diseases*, in Mathematical and Statistical Approaches to AIDS Epidemiology, C. Castillo-Chavez, ed., Springer-Verlag, New York: 289–300.

[17] Busenberg, S. and C. Castillo-Chavez (1991) *A general solution of the problem of mixing of subpopulations and its application to risk- and age-structured epidemic models for the spread of AIDS*, Mathematical Medicine and Biology **8**: 1–29.

[18] Castillo-Chavez, C., H. Hethcote, V. Andreasen, S. Levin, and W. Liu (1988) *Cross-immunity in the dynamics of homogeneous and heterogeneous populations*, in Mathematical Ecology: Proceedings of the Autumn Course Research Seminars: International Centre for Theoretical Physics, T.G. Hallam, L.J. Gross, and S.A. Levin, eds., Miramare, Trieste, World Scientific, Teaneck, NJ: 303–316.

[19] Castillo-Chávez, C. (1989) *Mathematical and Statistical Approaches to AIDS Epidemiology*, Vol. 83, Springer-Verlag.

[20] Castillo-Chavez, C., H.W. Hethcote, V. Andreasen, S.A. Levin, and W.M. Liu (1989) *Epidemiological models with age structure, proportionate mixing, and cross-immunity*, J. Math. Biol. **27**: 233–258.

[21] Castillo-Chavez, C., K. Cooke, W. Huang, and S. Levin (1989) *Results on the dynamics for models for the sexual transmission of the human immunodeficiency virus*, Appl. Math. Lett. **2**: 327–331.

[22] Castillo-Chavez, C., K. Cooke, W. Huang, and S. Levin (1989) *The role of long periods of infectiousness in the dynamics of Acquired Immunodeficiency Syndrome* (AIDS), in Mathematical Approaches to Problems in Resource Management and Epidemiology: Proceedings of a Conference Held at Ithaca, NY, 1987, C. Castillo-Chavez, S.A. Levin, and C.A. Shoemaker, eds., Springer-Verlag, Berlin: 177–189.

[23] Castillo-Chavez, C. and S. Busenberg (1990) *On the solution of the two-sex mixing problem*, in Proceedings of the International Conference on Differential Equations and Applications to Biology and Population Dynamics, Lect. Notes in Biomath. **92**, Springer-Verlag, New York: 80–98.

[24] Castillo-Chavez, C., S. Busenberg, and K. Gerow (1991) *Pair formation in structured populations*, in Differential Equations with Applications in Biology, Physics, and Engineering, J.A. Goldstein, F. Kappel, and W. Schappacher, eds., *Lect. Notes in Pure and Appl. Math.* **133**, Marcel Dekker, New York: 47–65.

[25] Castillo-Chavez, C., S. Shyu, G. Rubin, and D. Umbauch (1992) *On the estimation problem of mixing/pair formation matrices with applications to models for sexually transmitted diseases*, AIDS Epidemiology: Methodology Issues **384**: 402.

[26] Castillo-Chevez, C. and H.R. Thieme (1993) *Asymptotically autonomous epidemic models*, in Mathematical Population Dynamics: Analysis of Heterogeneity. Volume One, Theory of Epidemics, Wuerz Publishing: 33–50.

[27] Castillo-Chávez, C., J. Velasco-Hernández, and S. Fridman (1994) *Modeling contact structures in biology*, in Frontiers in mathematical biology, S.A. Levin, ed., Lect. Notes in Biomath. **100**, Springer-Verlag, New York: 454–491.

[28] Castillo-Chavez, C. and W. Huang (1995) *The logistic equation revisited: The two-sex case*, Math. Biosc. **128**: 299–316.

[29] Castillo-Chavez, C., W. Huang, and J. Li (1996) *On the existence of stable pairing distributions*, J. Math. Biol. **34**: 413–441.

[30] Castillo-Chavez, C., W. Huang, and J. Li (1996) *Competitive exclusion in gonorrhea models and other sexually transmitted diseases*, SIAM J. Appl. Math. **56**: 494–508.

[31] Castillo-Chavez, C., W. Huang, and J. Li (1996) *Dynamics of multiple pathogen strains in heterosexual epidemiological models*, in Differential Equations and Applications to Biology and to Industry: Proceedings of the June 1–4, 1994 Claremont International Conference Dedicated to the Memory of Stavros Busenberg (1941–1993), S.N. Busenberg and M. Martelli, eds., World Scientific, Singapore.

[32] Castillo-Chavez, C., W. Huang, and J. Li (1997) *The effects of females' susceptibility on the coexistence of multiple pathogen strains of sexually transmitted diseases*, J. Math. Biol. **35**: 503–522.

[33] Castillo-Chavez, C. and S.-F. Hsu Schmitz (1997) *The evolution of age-structured marriage functions: It takes two to tango*, in Structured-Population Models in Marine, Terrestrial, and Freshwater Systems, Vol. 18, S. Tuljapurkar and H. Caswell, eds., Chapman and Hall: 533–553.

[34] Castillo-Chavez, C. and J. Velasco-Hernandez (1998) *On the relationship between tight coevolution and superinfection*, J. Theor. Biol. **192**: 437–444.

[35] Castillo-Chavez, C., W. Huang, and J. Li (1999) *Competitive exclusion and coexistence of multiple strains in an SIS STD model*, SIAM J. Appl. Math. **59**: 1790–1811.

[36] Castillo-Chavez, C., Z. Feng, and W. Huang (2002) *On the computation of ro and its role in global stability*, in Mathematical Approaches for Emerging and Reemerging Infectious Diseases: An Introduction, C. Castillo-Chavez, S. Blower, P. van den Driessche, D. Kirschner, and A.-A. Yakubu, eds., IMA Vol. Math. Appl. **125**, Springer-Verlag, New York: 229–250.

[37] Castillo-Chavez, C. and B.T. Li (2008) *Spatial spread of sexually transmitted diseases within susceptible populations at demographic steady state*, Math. Biosc. & Eng. **5**: 713–727.

[38] Castillo-Chavez, C. and G. Chowell (2011) *Special Issue on Mathematical Models, Challenges, and Lessons Learned from the 2009 A/H1N1 Influenza Pandemics PREFACE*, Math. Biosc. & Eng. **8**.

[39] Caswell, H. (2001) *Matrix Population Models: Construction, Analysis, and Interpretation*, 2nd ed., Sinauer Associates.

[40] Cooke, K.L. and J.A. Yorke (1973) *Some equations modelling growth processes and gonorrhea epidemics*, Math. Biosc. **16**: 75–101.

[41] Crawford, C., S. Schwager, and C. Castillo-Chávez (1990) *A Methodology for Asking Sensitive Questions among College Undergraduates*, Technical Report BU-1105-M, Cornell University, Ithaca, NY.

[42] Diekmann, O., J.A.P. Heesterbeek, and J.A.J. Metz (1990) *On the definition and the computation of the basic reproduction ratio R_0 in models for infectious diseases in heterogeneous populations*, J. Math. Biol. **28**: 365–382.

[43] Dietz, K. (1979) *Epidemiologic interference of virus populations*, J. Math. Biol. **8**: 291–300.

[44] Dushoff, J., W. Huang, and C. Castillo-Chavez (1998) *Backwards bifurcations and catastrophe in simple models of fatal diseases*, J. Math. Biol. **36**: 227–248.

[45] Dwyer, G., S.A. Levin, and L. Buttel (1990) *A simulation model of the population dynamics and evolution of myxomatosis*, Ecological Monographs **60**: 423–447.

[46] Ewald, P.W. (1993) *The evolution of virulence*, Scientific American **268**: 86–93.

[47] Ewald, P.W. (1994) *Evolution of Infectious Disease*, Oxford University Press.

[48] Family Health International (2000) HIV/AIDS *Behavioral Surveilance Survey, Nigeria* 2000, Report and Data Sheets, http://gametlibrary.worldbank.org/FILES/689_BSS%20Nigeria%202000.pdf.

[49] Fenner, F. and K. Myers (1978) *Myxoma virus and myxomatosis in retrospect: The first quarter century of a new disease*, in Viruses and Environment, J. Cooper and F. MacCallum, eds., Academic Press, London: 539–570.

[50] Fenner, F. and F.N. Ratcliffe (1965) *Myxomatosis*, Cambridge University Press.

[51] Gilbert, P.B., I.W. McKeague, G. Eisen, C. Mullins, A. Guéye-NDiaye, S. Mboup, and P.J. Kanki (2003) *Comparison of HIV-*1 *and HIV-*2 *infectivity from a prospective cohort study in Senegal*, Statistics in Medicine **22**: 573–593.

[52] Hadeler, K. and C. Castillo-Chavez (1995) *A core group model for disease transmission*, Math. Biosc. **128**: 41–55.

[53] Hadeler, K. (2012) *Pair formation*, J. Math. Biol. **64**: 613–645.

[54] Heiderich, K., W. Huang, and C. Castillo-Chavez (2002) *Nonlocal response in a simple epidemiological model*, in Mathematical Approaches for Emerging and Reemerging Infectious Diseases: An Introduction, C. Castillo-Chavez, S. Blower, P. van den Driessche, D. Kirschner, and A.-A. Yakubu, eds., IMA Vol. Math. Appl. **125**, Springer-Verlag, New York: 129–151.

[55] Hethcote, H.W. (2000) *The mathematics of infectious diseases*, SIAM Rev. **42**: 599–653.

[56] Hethcote, H.W. and J.A. Yorke (1984) *Gonorrhea Transmission Dynamics and Control*, Springer-Verlag, New York.

[57] Hicks, J. (1939) *Value and Capital. An Inquiry into Some Fundamental Principles of Economic Theory*, Oxford University Press.

[58] Hsieh, Y.H. and C. Hsun Chen (2004) *Modelling the social dynamics of a sex industry: Its implications for spread of HIV/AIDS*, Bull. Math. Biol. **66**: 143–166.

[59] Huang, W., K.L. Cooke, and C. Castillo-Chavez (1992) *Stability and bifurcation for a multiple-group model for the dynamics of HIV/AIDS transmission*, SIAM J. Appl. Math. **52**: 835–854.

[60] Huang, W. and C. Castillo-Chavez (2002) *Age-structured core groups and their impact on HIV dynamics*, in Mathematical Approaches for Emerging and Reemerging Infectious Diseases: Models, Methods and Theory, C. Castillo-Chavez, S. Blower, P. van den Driessche, D. Kirschner, and A. Yakubu, eds., IMA Vol. Math. Appl. **126**, Springer-Verlag, New York: 261–273.

[61] Hyman, J.M.J., J.J. Li, and E.A.E. Stanley (1999) *The differential infectivity and staged progression models for the transmission of HIV*, Math. Biosc. **155**: 77–109.

[62] Idoko, J. (2004) *The plague among us: Where is the cure?*, in Unijos Inaugural Lectures.

[63] Kasseem, G., S. Roudenko, S. Tennenbaum, and C. Castillo-Chavez (2006) *The role of transactional sex in spreading HIV/AIDS in Nigeria: A modeling perspective*, in Mathematical Studies on Human Disease Dynamics: Emerging Paradigms and Challenges, A. Gumel, C. Castillo-Chavez, D.P. Clemence, and R.E. Mickens, eds., American Mathematical Society, Providence, RI: 367–389.

[64] Kribs-Zaleta, C.M., M. Lee, C. Roman, S. Wiley, and C.M. Hernandez-Suarez (2005) *The effect of the HIV/AIDS epidemic on Africa's truck drivers*, Math. Biosc. Eng. **2**: 771–788.

[65] Lajmanovich, A. and J.A. Yorke (1976) *A deterministic model for gonorrhea in a nonhomogeneous population*, Math. Biosc. **28**: 221–236.

[66] Lazzarin, A., A. Saracco, M. Musicco, and A. Nicolosi (1991) *Man-to-woman sexual transmission of the human immunodeficiency virus. Risk factors related to sexual behavior, man's infectiousness, and woman's susceptibility. Italian study group on HIV heterosexual transmission*, Arch. Intern. Med. **151**: 2411–2416.

[67] Levin, S. and D. Pimentel (1981) *Selection of intermediate rates of increase in parasite-host systems*, The American Naturalist **117**: 308–315.

[68] Levin, S.A. (1983) *Co-evolution*, in Population Biology: Proceedings of the International Conference Held at the University of Alberta, Edmonton, Canada, June 22–30, 1982, H. Freedman and C. Strobeck, eds., Lect. Notes in Biomath. **52**, Springer-Verlag, New York.

[69] Levin, S.A. (1983) *Some approaches to the modeling of co-evolutionary interactions*, in Coevolution, M.H. Nitecki ed., University of Chicago Press.

[70] Levin, S.A., J. Dushoff, and J.B. Plotkin (2004) *Evolution and persistence of influenza A and other diseases*, Math. Biosc. **188**: 17–28.

[71] Lin, J., V. Andreasen, R. Casagrandi, and S.A. Levin (2003) *Traveling waves in a model of influenza A drift*, J. Theor. Biol. **222**: 437–445.

[72] Lotka, A. (1923) *Contribution to the analysis of malaria epidemiology*, American Journal of Hygiene **3** (Suppl.): 96–112.

[73] Luo, X. and C. Castillo-Chavez (1993) *Limit behavior of pair-formation for a large dissolution rate*, Journal of Mathematical Systems, Estimation, and Control **3**: 247–264.

[74] Macdonald, G. (1957) *The Epidemiology and Control of Malaria*, Oxford University Press.

[75] Mastro, T., G. Satten, T. Nopkesorn, S. Sangkharomya, and I. Longini (1994) *Probability of female-to-male transmission of HIV-*1 *in Thailand*, Lancet **343**: 204–207.

[76] May, R.M. and R.M. Anderson (1983) *Epidemiology and genetics in the co-evolution of parasites and hosts*, Proceedings of the Royal Society of London. Series B. Biological Sciences **219**: 281–313.

[77] May, R.M. and R.M. Anderson (1990) *Parasite—host coevolution, Parasitology* **100**: S89–S101.

[78] Mena-Lorca, J., J.X. Velasco-Hernandez, and C. Castillo-Chavez (1999) *Density-dependent dynamics and superinfection in an epidemic model*, IMA Journal of Mathematics Applied in Medicine and Biology **16**: 307–317.

[79] Morin, B.R., C. Castillo-Chavez, S.-F. Hsu Schmitz, A. Mubayi, and X. Wang (2010) *Notes from the heterogeneous: A few observations on the implications and necessity of affinity*, Journal of Biological Dynamics **4**: 456–477.

[80] Morison, L., H.A. Weiss, A. Buve, M. Carael, S.C. Abega, F. Kaona, L. Kanhonou, J. Chege, and R.J. Hayes (2001) *Commercial sex and the spread of HIV in four cities in sub-Saharan Africa*, AIDS **15** (Suppl 4): S61–S69.

[81] Nuño, M.A. (2005) *Mathematical Models for the Dynamics of Influenza at the Population and Host Level*, Ph.D. Thesis, Cornell University, Ithaca, NY.

[82] Nuño, M., Z. Feng, M. Martcheva, and C. Castillo-Chavez (2005) *Dynamics of two-strain influenza with isolation and partial cross-immunity*, SIAM J. Appl. Math. **65**: 964–982.

[83] Nuño, M., C. Castillo-Chavez, Z. Feng, and M. Martcheva (2008) *Mathematical models of influenza: The role of cross-immunity, quarantine and age-structure*, in Mathematical Epidemiology, F. Brauer, P. van den Driessche, and J. Wu, eds., Lect. Notes in Math. **1945**, Springer-Verlag, Berlin, Heidelberg: 349–364.

[84] Nuño, M., M. Martcheva, and C. Castillo-Chavez (2009) *Immune level approach for multiple strain pathogens*, Journal of Biological Systems **17**: 713–737.

[85] Ogboi, S.J., K. Sabitu, P.U. Agu, H.O. Ogboi, and O. Ayegbusi (2001), *Prevalence of HIV Transmission in Nigerian Transit Towns among Long Distance Drivers*, Laboratory Survey.

[86] Orubuloye, I.O., P. Caldwell, and J.C. Caldwell (1993) *The role of high-risk occupations in the spread of AIDS: Truck drivers and itinerant market women in Nigeria*, International Family Planning Perspectives **19**: 43–48.

[87] Orubuloye, I.O. and F. Oguntimehin (1999) *Intervention for the Control of STDs Including HIV among Commercial Sex Workers, Commercial Drivers and Students in Nigeria*, pp. 121–129.

[88] Panchaud, C., V. Woog, S. Singh, J.E. Darroch, and A. Bankole (2002) *Issues in measuring HIV prevalence: The case of Nigeria*, African Journal of Reproductive Health **6**: 11.

[89] Ross, R. (1911) *The Prevention of Malaria*, 2nd ed. (with Addendum), John Murray, London.

[90] Royce, R.A., A. Seña, W. Cates, and M.S. Cohen (1997) *Sexual transmission of HIV*, New England Journal of Medicine **336**: 1072–1078.

[91] Rubin, G., D. Umbach, S.-F. Shyu, and C. Castillo-Chavez (1992) *Using mark-recapture methodology to estimate the size of a population at risk for sexually transmitted diseases*, Stat. Med. **11**: 1533–1549.

[92] Schmitz, S. (1994) *Some Theories, Estimation Methods and Applications of Marriage Functions and Two-Sex Mixing Functions in Demography and Epidemiology*, Ph.D. Thesis, Cornell University, Ithaca, NY.

[93] Schmitz, S.-F.H. and C. Castilla-Chavez (1994) *Parameter estimation in nonclosed social networks related to the dynamics of sexually transmitted diseases*, in Modeling the AIDS Epidemic: Planning, Policy and Prediction, E.H. Kaplan and M.L. Brandeau, eds., Raven Press: 533–559.

[94] Schmitz, S.-F. and C. Castillo-Chavez (2000) *A note on pair-formation functions*, Mathematical and Computer Modelling **31**: 83–91.

[95] Smith, H.L. (1988) *Systems of ordinary differential equations which generate an order preserving flow. A survey of results*, SIAM Rev. **30**: 87–113.

[96] Sunmola, A.M. (2005) *Sexual practices, barriers to condom use and its consistent use among long distance truck drivers in Nigeria*, AIDS Care **17**: 208–221.

[97] Thieme, H. (1992) *Convergence results and a Poincaré-Bendixson trichotomy for asymptotically autonomous differential equations*, J. Math. Biol. **30**: 755–763.

[98] Thieme, H.R. and C. Castillo-Chavez (1993) *How may infection-age-dependent infectivity affect the dynamics of HIV/AIDS?*, SIAM J. Appl. Math. **53**: 1447–1479.

[99] Thieme, H.R. (1993) *Asymptotically autonomous differential equations in the plane*, Rocky Mountain Journal of Mathematics **24**: 351–380.

[100] UNAIDS (2004), *Epidemiological Fact Sheets on HIV/AIDS and STI: Nigeria*, 2004 update, http://data.unaids.org/Publications/Fact-Sheets01/nigeria_en.pdf.

[101] Velasco-Hernández, J.X., F. Brauer, and C. Castillo-Chavez (1996) *Effects of treatment and prevalence-dependent recruitment on the dynamics of a fatal disease*, Mathematical Medicine and Biology **13**: 175–192.

[102] Von Reyn, C. (1990) *Epidemiology of HIV infection in Africa*, AIDS and Society **3**.

Index